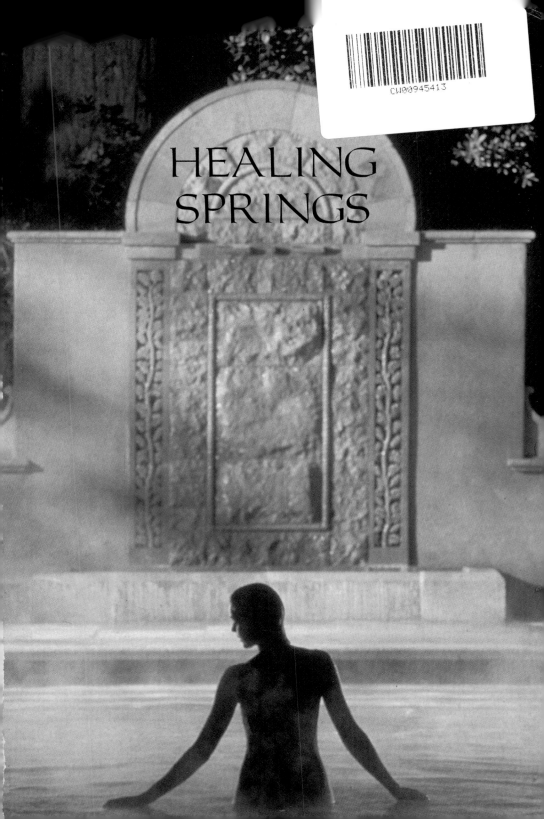

HEALING
SPRINGS

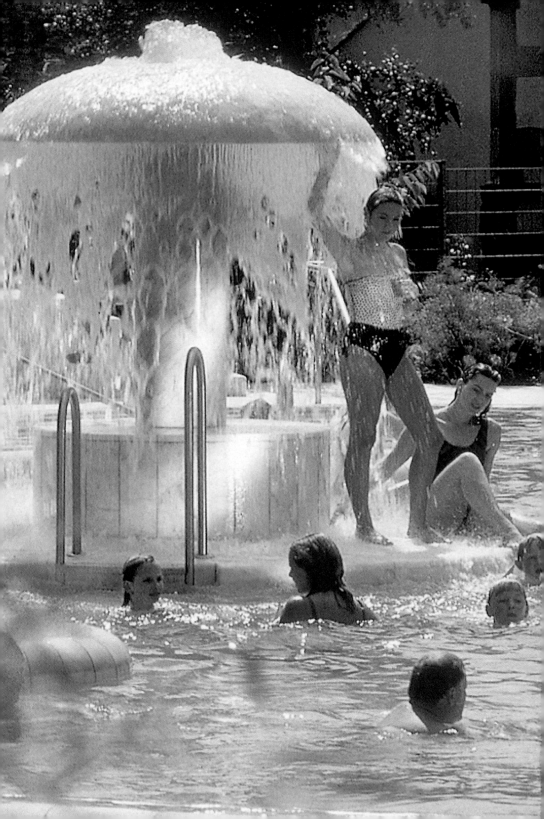

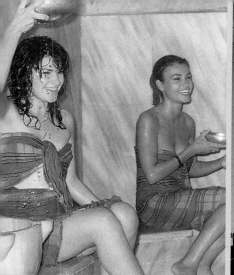

Overleaf: Sonoma Mission Inn & Spa,
California

Above: Bursa, Turkey

Right: Baden-Baden, Germany

Below: Yangmingshan, Taiwan

Opposite: Baden-Baden, Germany

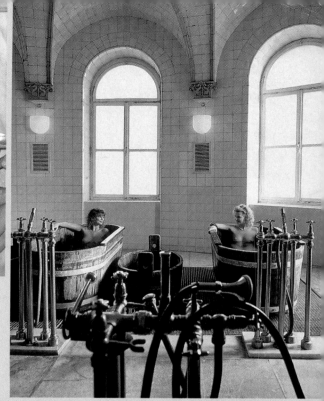

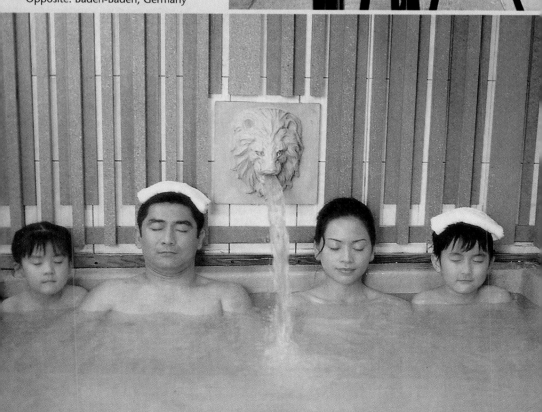

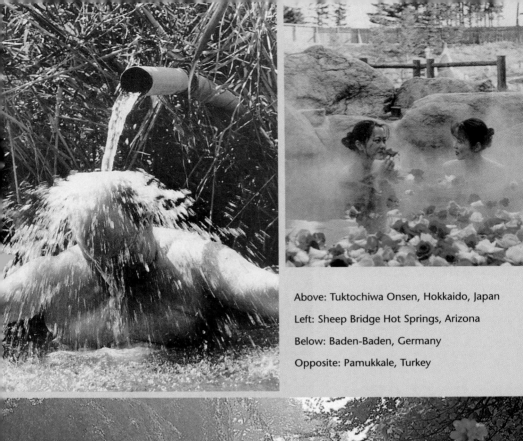

Above: Tuktochiwa Onsen, Hokkaido, Japan

Left: Sheep Bridge Hot Springs, Arizona

Below: Baden-Baden, Germany

Opposite: Pamukkale, Turkey

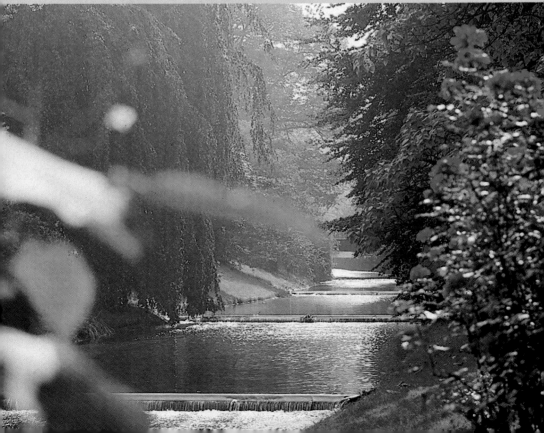

HEALING SPRINGS

THE ULTIMATE GUIDE
TO TAKING THE WATERS

From hidden springs
to the world's greatest spas

NATHANIEL ALTMAN

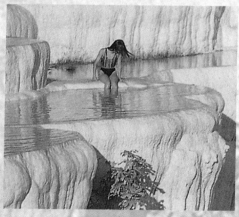

Healing Arts Press
Rochester, Vermont

Healing Arts Press
One Park Street
Rochester, Vermont 05767
www.InnerTraditions.com

Healing Arts Press is a division of Inner Traditions International

Library of Congress Cataloging-in-Publication Data

Altman, Nathaniel.
    Healing springs : the ultimate guide to taking the waters / Nathaniel Altman.
        p. cm.
    Includes index.
    ISBN 0-89281-836-0 (alk. paper)
    1. Health resorts. 2. Mineral waters. 3. Hot springs. I. Title.

    RA794 .A465 2000
    613'.122—dc21

00-056736

Printed and bound in Canada

10 9 8 7 6 5 4 3 2 1

Text design and layout by Priscilla Baker
This book was typeset in Berkeley and Stone Sans, with Carolus as a display
face.

Opposite and background: Sycamore Mineral Springs Resort, California

CONTENTS

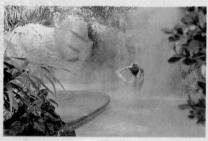

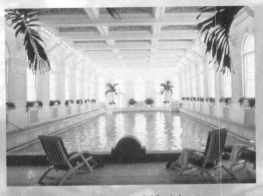

The Homestead, Virginia

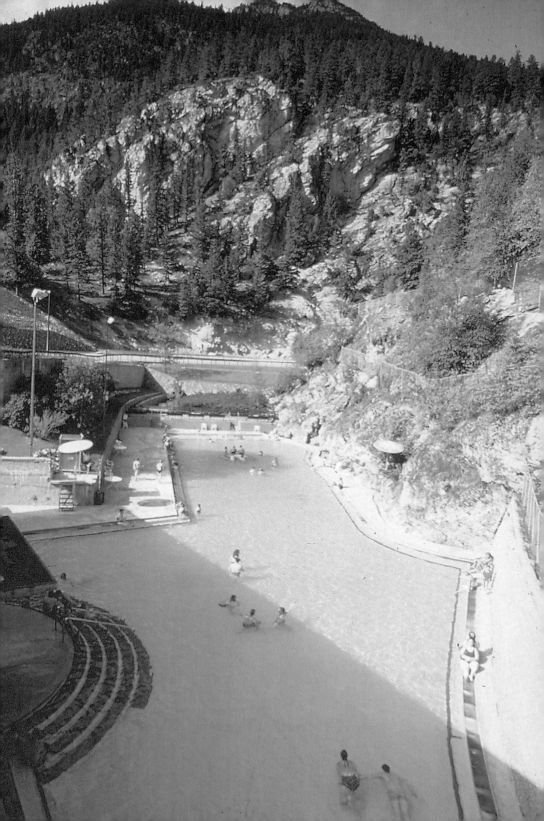

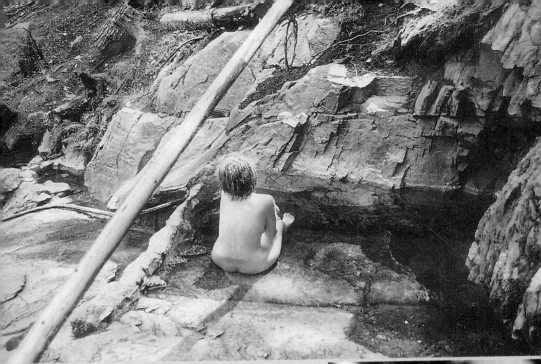

Opposite: Radium Hot Springs, British Columbia, Canada

Above: St. Leon Hot Springs, British Columbia, Canada

Right: Baden-Baden, Germany

Below right: Thermes de Vittel, France

Below left: Patch Adams and Wavy Gravy at Vichy Springs, California

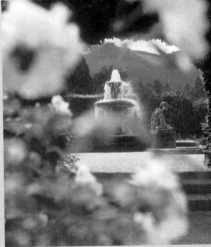

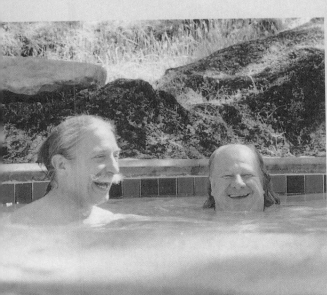

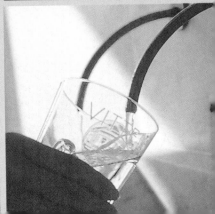

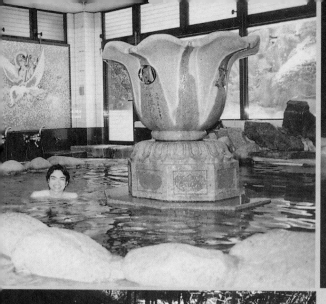

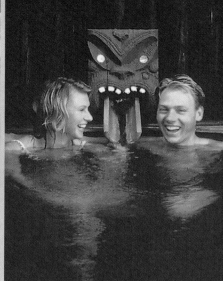

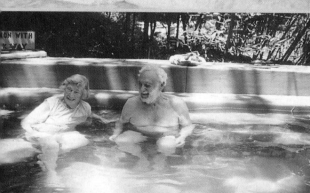

Above right: Polynesian Spa, Rotorua, New Zealand

Above left: Kobono-yu Onsen, Hakone, Japan

Left: Author's aunt and uncle at Gilroy Hot Springs, California

Below: Pott's Ranch Hot Spring, Nevada

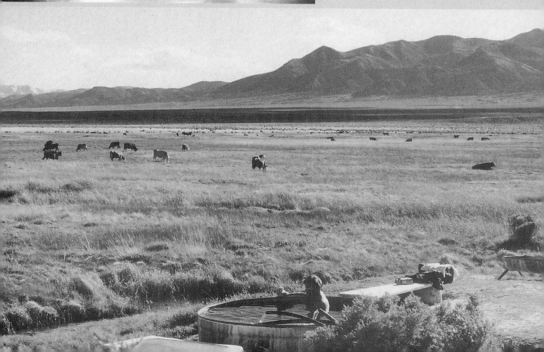

NOTE TO THE READER

The author of this book is not a physician. The following material is presented in the spirit of historical, philosophical, and scientific inquiry and is *not* offered as medical advice, diagnosis, or treatment of any kind.

Although studies have attested to the safety of balneology and hydrotherapy, it should be remembered that hot springs bathing is not for everyone, including those who are pregnant, or who are suffering from serious cardiovascular disease, high blood pressure, or cancer. The author and publisher advise against self-treatment with hot springs bathing. Any medical treatment should be done under the supervision of a qualified health practitioner.

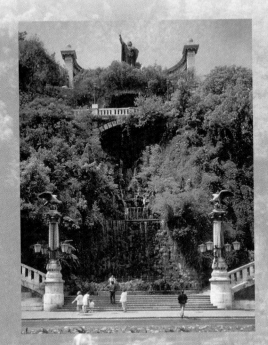

Budapest, Hungary

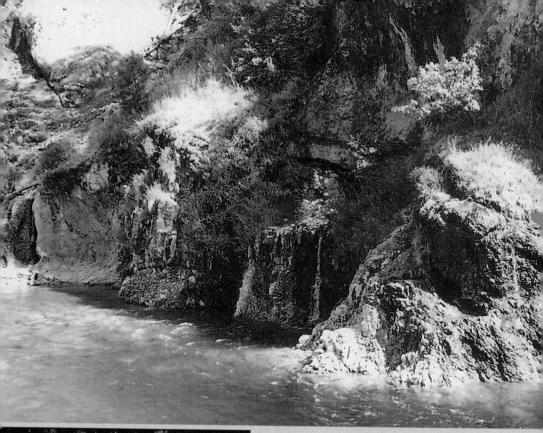

Above: Brown's Creek, Idaho

Left: Harrison Hot Springs Resort, British Columbia, Canada

Below: Atami Onsen, Japan

Opposite: Vichy Springs, California

Following Acknowledgments: Gold Strike Hot Springs, Nevada

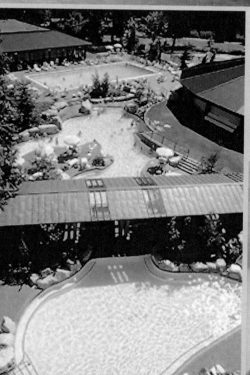

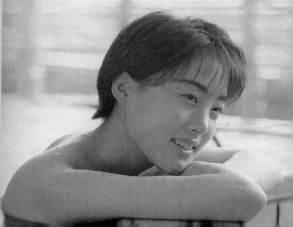

ACKNOWLEDGMENTS

I owe a tremendous debt of gratitude to many individuals who assisted me in the research and writing of this book, including Helmut G. Pratzel, M.D., President of the International Society of Medical Hydrology and Climatology (I.S.M.H.), for his suggestions and valuable reference materials; Marie-José Crussaire at the Syndicat National des Établissements Thermaux (S.N.E.T.) in Paris, for generously providing reference materials and guidebooks; Michel Boulangé, M.D., Director of the Department of Balneology and Climatology at the Medical School of the Université Henri Poincaré in Nancy, France, for his reference materials, advice, and permission to do research at the extensive library on medical balneology and climatology at the Medical School, and Chantal Faye for her gracious assistance at the library; Yuko Agishi, M.D., for providing numerous reference materials, as well as his wise advice and practical guidance during my research trip to Japan; Kazuo Kubota, M.D., for providing reference materials and generous assistance at Kusatsu Onsen; Lawrence Charles Parish, M.D., for providing his excellent bibliography on balneology and dermatology; Hijiri Harada for his astute guidance and patient assistance during my research trip to Japan; and Yi-Shan Shei for her drawings. Thanks are also due to Shi-Wei Shei, Edward Gasser, Den Rasplicka, Norman Goldstein, Thomas Laubscher, Bryan McAllister, Hiroshi Motoye, Michael Aissen, Mildred Aissen, and my literary agent, Stephany Evans, for their assistance, suggestions, and support. And thanks to my editor, Jeanie Levitan, whose skillful attention to detail, commonsense wisdom, and patient good humor make her the kind of editor most authors can only dream of having.

I would also like to thank the following organizations for permission to reproduce copyrighted illustrations in this book: *Hot Springs Gazette;* Foto Wolkersdorfer, Bad Hofgastein, Austria; Calistoga Spa, Harbin Hot Springs, the Sharpsteen Museum Association, Sonoma Mission Inn and Spa, Sycamore Mineral Springs Resort, and Vichy Springs, California; Canadian Rockies Hot Springs and Harrison Hot Springs Resort, Canada; Medicinal Spa Mariánské Lázně Corporation, Czech Republic; Thermes de La Bourboulle, La Roche-Posay, and Vittel, France; Baden-Baden Marketing GmbH, Bad Wildbad, and the German National Tourist Board, Germany; the Hungarian National Tourist Office; Icelandic Nature Health Society; the Italian Government Tourist Office; Chico Hot Springs, Montana; Polynesian Spa, New Zealand; *Spa Lady* magazine, Taiwan; the Turkish Tourism and Information Bureau; and the Homestead, Virginia.

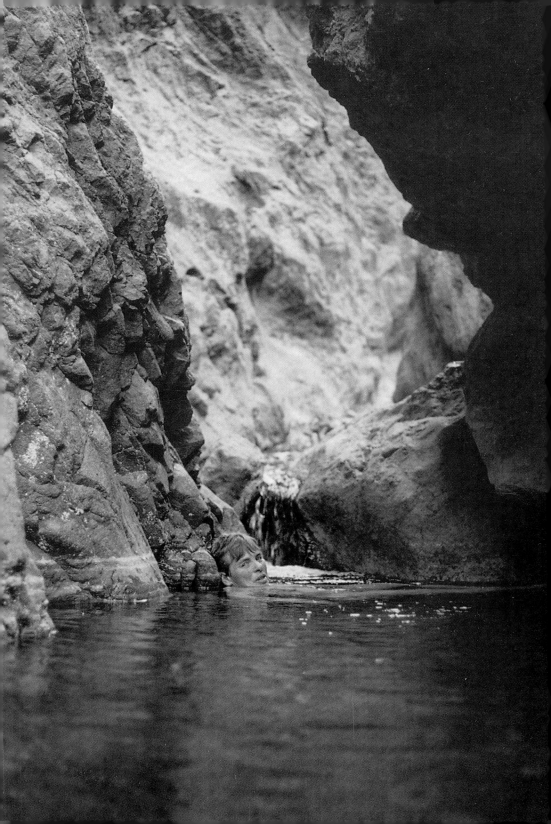

THE BEST-KEPT SECRET

I first visited a hot spring in Bolivia during the spring of 1973. While traveling around South America, I spent several days visiting friends in Cochabamba, a city in an Andean valley renowned for its year-round spring weather and excellent archaeological museum. One Saturday morning, about five of us piled into a battered Jeep and headed into the mountains. After an hour of speeding along a paved highway toward Santa Cruz, our driver suddenly turned onto a narrow dirt road that obviously hadn't been maintained in years. The next 30 minutes were a bone-crushing ordeal as we bounced around hairpin curves, forded rushing streams, and pounded over potholes that would have destroyed the suspension system of an ordinary car.

We reached the crest of a hill and suddenly came upon an old stone building with steam coming up from behind it. Battered and bruised, we piled out of the Jeep and were welcomed by the owner of the spa, a smiling man named Juan Antonio, who was busy chopping firewood. Putting down his hatchet, he showed us to a dressing room, where we changed into bathing suits and made our way to the hot spring itself, located behind the building.

The rustic pool was lined with cobblestones. A small waterfall fed the pool with steaming water, which smelled strongly of sulfur.* As I gingerly joined my friends, who were already lounging in the steaming water, I experienced a wonderful feeling of relaxation and warmth that was far more pleasant than any ordinary bath. All the muscle aches from the trip to the spring seemed to disappear as we swam, floated, and frolicked in the hot sulfur spring. I spent about 15 minutes swimming and soaking, and left the pool feeling pleasantly tired. After an hour's nap and a light lunch of salad and soup with my friends, I felt both rejuvenated and relaxed. On that crisp April afternoon in the Andes, I became hooked on hot springs.

---

*Editor's note: Throughout this book, we use the American spelling, sulfur, except when direct quotations or place-names use the alternative spelling, sulphur.

Since then I have visited thermal springs in many parts of the United States, Canada, Latin America, and Eastern and Western Europe as well as on the volcanic islands of Japan, New Zealand, Taiwan, Iceland, and the Azores. I've always been impressed at the amazing variety of springs, their often beautiful natural surroundings, and their ability to make both my body and soul feel rejuvenated and relaxed. After bathing in some springs, such as the mud-brown Terra Nostra thermal pool on São Miguel Island in the Azores, I noticed that some minor skin problems had completely disappeared, and I experienced almost instant relief from chronic muscle and joint pain. During a week as the only guest at the rustic Termas de Palguín in Chile, I took long walks on its mountain trails and grew to appreciate hot springs as "power spots" in nature that facilitate healing, increase our appreciation of the earth, and enable us to become more sensitive to our body and its natural rhythms.

People have used geothermal waters and mineral waters for bathing and improving their health for thousands of years. Balneology, the practice of using natural mineral spring water for the prevention and cure of disease, can be traced back about 5,000 years to the Bronze Age, although there is evidence that humans have been using hot springs for more than 600,000 years.

The healing value of spas has long been accepted by the medical community, especially in Europe and Japan, where they are used both for the prevention and the treatment of disease. The former Soviet Union has 3,500 spas, where "taking the waters" remains a normal part of Russian life. In the Czech Republic and Slovakia, there are 52 health spas and more than 1,900 mineral springs, including the famous triad of Bohemian spas at Karlovy Vary (Carlsbad), Mariánské Lázně (Marienbad), and Františkovy Lázně (Franzenbad). Every year, some 220,000 Czech and Slovak citizens are granted free spa treatment for 3 weeks, paid for by their countries' respective national health insurance programs. Japan boasts over 12,300 volcanic hot springs (known as *onsen*), which attract more than 100 million visitors every year. The first medical study of hot springs in Japan was undertaken in 1709, and no fewer than six universities have established medical research institutes at hot springs to evaluate their therapeutic benefits on an ongoing basis.

There are over 200 commercial hot springs and mineral springs in the United States and Canada, along with thousands of smaller noncommercial springs, many accessible only on foot or by horseback. Many of these springs enjoyed their heyday in the latter part of the nineteenth century, when thousands of city dwellers boarded steam trains and converged on spa towns every summer for several weeks of vacation. Many of these hot springs resorts were modeled after the famous European spas, and they attracted their own variety of royalty, including presidents, writers, musicians, and artists.

During this time, it was popular for spa owners to claim that their waters would cure an impressive list of ailments, including heart disease, diabetes, and cancer. Government regulations later prohibited such health claims, and interest in "taking the waters" began to decline in America. As people began to favor urban entertainment and theme parks and glitzy seaside resorts toward the middle of this century, many hot springs resorts began to close.

However, today's growing interest in natural lifestyles, physical fitness, and alternative healing has brought about a renewed interest in healing springs, both for bathing and for drinking. Spa towns that experienced a decline in popularity in the 1940s such as Calistoga in California, Hot Springs in Arkansas, and Saratoga Springs in New York are becoming popular tourist destinations once again. Government regulations concerning health claims have led people to appreciate hot springs primarily for their calming effects and recreational value, although many people feel that the hot mineralized water found in these spas has a marked therapeutic effect on the body. Few are aware that balneotherapy is an accepted form of mainstream medicine in Europe and Japan, where an abundance of medical evidence shows that in addition to relieving stress, certain mineral waters can help the body heal itself from heart, liver, and kidney problems; skin diseases; asthma; digestive disorders; arthritis; and a host of other health problems. Many of these findings are presented to the English-speaking public for the first time in this book.

In addition to the curative waters themselves, many of today's hot springs resorts have licensed health professionals on staff and provide natural and complementary health treatments such as acupuncture, homeopathy, massage, mud baths, herbal wraps, fasting programs, relaxation classes, and fitness training. However, hot springs and mineral springs also appeal to those who seek sensual pleasure and relaxation through delicious cuisine, comfortable accommodations, beautiful gardens, and congenial people, as the popularity of thermal resorts such as Desert Hot Springs and Palm Springs in California, Hot Springs in Arkansas, Glenwood Springs in Colorado, and Banff in Alberta would suggest.

As testimony to the growing interest in healthy lifestyles, mineral waters such as Calistoga, Arrowhead Spring, Poland Spring, and Saratoga, along with European imports such as Evian, Perrier, Spa, San Pellegrino, and Volvic are among the most popular beverages on the market, with sales surpassing $5 billion a year.

The success of guidebooks such as *Fodor's Spa Guide, Hot Springs and Hot Pools,* and *Great Hot Springs of the West* also attests to the renewed interest in spas and mineral springs to promote health and well-being in North America. Yet, despite the popularity of some of the springs mentioned above, most healing springs in the United States and Canada are woefully underutilized. Most Americans know little about the therapeutic value of hot springs and mineral springs and are unfamiliar with the abundance of scientific and medical literature from Europe and Japan that has documented the healing properties of mineral and thermal waters.

WHAT MAKES A HEALING SPRING A HEALING SPRING?

Healing waters vary tremendously. They may be enjoyed in an undeveloped natural pool in the countryside that can accommodate only one bather or in an Olympic-sized swimming pool at a luxury resort. They also can be piped into soaking pools, whirlpool baths, bathtubs, or drinking fountains. The water may be enjoyed naturally cold or hot, or may be artificially cooled or heated as necessary for swimming, showering, or bathing. In some spas described in this book, the water may be chemically treated to ensure purity, or it may flow through the pool at such a rate that it requires no additional treatment.

Generally speaking, a spring can be classified as "therapeutic" if it contains a minimum amount of one or more minerals per liter or kilogram of water: the type and amount of minerals is determined by individual government standards. In some countries, the water must flow from the earth at a minimum temperature as well. In Japan, for example, a spring is considered therapeutic if spring waters flow from the earth at a temperature of at least 25°C (77°F) and contain at least a minimum amount of one of the following components: total dissolved solids (1000 milligrams [mg]), free carbon dioxide (1000 mg), copper (1 mg), iron (20 mg), aluminum (100 mg), hydrogen (1 mg), arsenic (.7 mg), sulfur (2 mg), or radon (8.25 mache units). The Japanese also classify spring waters by temperature:

Cold: under 25°C (77°F)

Tepid: 25–34°C (77–93°F)

Warm: 34–42°C (93–108°F)

Hot: over 42°C (108°F)[1]

As we'll see later on, in addition to temperature, the presence of specific minerals and gases in the water helps determine the medicinal qualities of a spring. In some springs, minerals such as sulfur, calcium, or magnesium may predominate. Other springs may have trace amounts of lithium, arsenic, or silica. Some springs may include a gas such as carbon dioxide, while others may contain trace amounts of radon. Each of these elements provides specific therapeutic benefits to bathers as we will see in part 2, "Just What's in that Water?" While some springs may contain one primary element, such as sulfur, many healing springs contain a combination of up to several dozen different elements, often in unique proportions. For example, the unusual combination of free carbon dioxide with sodium chloride and bicarbonates of sodium, calcium, and magnesium helped make Saratoga Springs, New York, a popular center for treating heart disease, arthritis, and skin problems throughout much of the nineteenth and the first half of the twentieth centuries.

The book you are holding in your hands presents bathing in mineral springs and drinking their waters as part of a holistic approach to health and well-being, and it includes a review of the healing modalities that best complement both bathing in and drinking medicinal waters. Each discussion of a disease or disorder in part 3 is followed by a brief list of springs around the world where that disorder is treated. In addition, part 4 contains a directory of several hundred hot springs in the world, ranging from the best-known to the more obscure. This directory briefly describes each spring, the type of water(s) it contains, and what health conditions are best treated there. It also includes the names and addresses of government tourist bureaus to contact for more detailed information about healing springs and related accommodations. No matter where in the world you visit, the chances are good that you can find one or more thermal or mineral springs to enjoy.

ARE THE WATERS SAFE?

Many hot springs and mineral springs around the world were first discovered thousands of years ago and were often considered sacred healing sites. Over the centuries, these medicinal springs have "stood the test of time" not only for safety, but for their ability to help treat a wide variety of human ailments, including arthritis, skin problems, circulatory disorders, wound healing, and digestive complaints. Concurrent with the evolution of modern science, many springs around the world were analyzed for their chemical and medicinal properties, and physicians often made evaluations on why certain types of springs helped heal specific health problems. Springs that were determined by scientists and physicians to be unsafe (whether due to their chemical content or pollution) were often closed for bathing and drinking.

In the United States, Canada, and most other countries today, commercial hot springs operate under the jurisdiction of government health departments, which set standards for water clarity and purity, minimizing the risk of skin infections and other waterborne diseases. In California, for example, the cleanliness of all public pools and hot tubs are under the jurisdiction of the State Department of Health Services and are subject to regular inspection. In addition, many spas are required to meet county and municipal regulations and inspection standards as well.

Owners of hot springs are acutely aware of the importance of high sanitation standards and go to great lengths to maintain a high level of water purity and overall cleanliness of bathing and changing areas. In both the United States and abroad, most public pools are treated with chlorine, ozone, or other disinfectants. Other springs are able to meet government sanitation standards by operating their pools on a flow-through basis, water entering and draining from the pool continuously, or by emptying and cleaning individual soaking tubs after each use. Bathing in mineral springs—such as those containing sulfur and sulfates—have been found to strengthen the immune system and to kill bacteria and fungi, making them important centers for healing skin conditions and even venereal diseases,[2,3] without the risk of transmitting those conditions. Therapeutic spas in Europe and Japan are required to maintain the same levels of water purity and general sanitation as one would find in a hospital.

Unless they are providing actual balneotherapy for serious skin conditions (such as the medical spas of Europe and the hydrotherapy clinics in Japan), commercial hot springs will not allow persons suffering from poor health or skin conditions (including infections, boils, or pustules) from bathing with others.

Having said this, there is a small degree of risk from sharing a bath with strangers. However, these risks need to be viewed in context: your chances of getting infected from bathing in a hot spring (or any public pool) are far less than catching an airborne infection by commuting to work on the subway, taking a trip on a commercial airplane, working in an office building, or going to the hospital (whether as a patient or visitor), where staphylococcus, streptococcus, and other bacterial infections are common. Although some are afraid of contracting AIDS in a hot spring, several comprehensive studies have demonstrated that HIV cannot be transmitted through bathing with infected individuals.[4,5,6]

If you have concerns about the sanitary conditions of a hot spring or spa, call the establishment before you go, and address your questions to the manager. If you are uncomfortable about bathing with others, many hot spring establishments offer private pools for individuals that are emptied and cleaned after each use.

WHAT ABOUT PRICES?

The cost of hot springs therapy varies widely according to the facilities, services, and accommodations. A luxury spa in the United States such as the Homestead in Virginia or the Greenbrier in West Virginia, which offer their facilities primarily to overnight guests, normally costs up to $200 a day or more for accommodation and spa services, although package rates are often less. A 21-day stay at a luxury spa in Bad Gastein in Austria (with room, half board, nine balneological treatments, nine full body massages, and medical consultations) can cost 25,450 schillings, or roughly $2,000 (less than $100 a day). In Germany, a 7-night stay at a hotel in Bad Greisbach, including half-board and treatments, costs between 421 and 456 Euros, approximately $440–$480 (less than $70 a day). A 7-night stay at a three-star spa hotel at Montegrotto Terme in Italy, including full board and six treatments, costs just under 1.2 million lira, or approximately $635 (again, less than $100 a day). For many Europeans, a portion of the expenses is usually paid by social security or private health insurance if the person is being treated for a specific medical problem. At the time of this writing, spa stays in Eastern Europe are a bargain: a typical spa in the Czech Republic, Hungary, or Poland would charge the equivalent of only $30 to $50 a day for accommodation in a three-star hotel, including full board, medical examinations, daily use of the thermal pools, and a prescribed amount of treatments.

Day visits to hot springs are often reasonably priced. They can cost between $5 and $20 a day in the United States or Canada, depending on the resort. Taking the waters at one of the famous hot springs in Budapest costs between $2 and $4, and the use of the thermal indoor-outdoor swimming pool at Mondorf-les-Bains in Luxembourg is less than $10. A private bath at the famous spa of Baden-Baden in Germany costs DM 36 (approximately $19) and a bath followed by a massage is priced at a reasonable DM 48 (approximately $36). A private bath at Montegrotto Terme in Italy will set you back about $11, and an inhalation session with concentrated thermal water will cost approximately $7. Bathing in the hot springs in Japan can cost the equivalent of under $1 to $10 or more, depending on the level of luxury at the hotel or bathhouse, while a day visit to a *kuahausu* can run approximately $22 to $25. In some places such as Kusatsu Onsen, a beautiful spa town and ski resort about three hours from Tokyo, hot springs bathing in public bathhouses is available to the public free of charge.

WHAT THE SCIENTIFIC RESEARCH HAS TO SAY

One of my primary goals in this book is to present the evidence on the medical value of hot springs and mineral springs. Scientific research into the value of balneotherapy has taken various forms: the gathering and reporting of preliminary data and experiential data and, in a few cases, full-fledged research studies. But such research has often run up against several issues: financial obstacles, the integration of balneotherapy with other forms of treatment, and the requirements of double-blind studies.

Funding for medical research usually comes from governments and pharmaceutical companies. But these sources often do not grant financial support to studies in balneotherapy, except in countries such as Russia, Japan, and Hungary, where medical balneology has long been part of the medical mainstream.

In addition, it is often difficult to evaluate the effectiveness of bathing in and drinking mineral water because these waters are often used as part of a holistic approach. If you were being treated at a spa in Mariánské Lázně, for example, your therapy program would be very comprehensive. Besides soaking in a hot pool or drinking mineral water according to your physician's prescription, you would likely stay in a newly renovated century-old hotel, where you would enjoy a custom-designed spa diet and a special exercise regimen. To further enhance your treatment, you would be enjoying the town's beautiful surroundings, which provide a complete escape from the stresses of life at home or at work. Your days would be spent taking leisurely walks on forest trails, reading a book in one of the parks, listening to concerts, visiting art galleries, enjoying cappucino with friends at a sidewalk café, or admiring the many art nouveau buildings that make up most of the city. Although balneotherapy itself is the major component of healing at places such as Mariánské Lázně, it is certainly not the only one. Yet, most medical research these days bases its findings on objective criteria rather than on one's psychological and physical responses to nature, music, beauty, peace and quiet, or the company of friends. A scientific research study would isolate only one of these components—such as water—to measure its effect, and that is usually not practical.

Furthermore, the double-blind studies that have become the "gold standard" of scientific research, especially in the United States, are difficult to apply to the unique features of water-based treatments. In a double-blind study, neither the patient nor the investigator knows whether the patient is receiving the actual treatment or a placebo. The main advantage of this type of research is that complete objectivity is achieved, and measurable results can be obtained and evaluated. It also prevents the physician from giving preferential treatment to the patient. That, of course, is the primary drawback, because people in need of a valuable treatment may not be the ones to receive it.

In Europe, many physicians who have done research with medical balneology believe that double-blind studies are immoral. They maintain that water is not an experimental drug: bathing in hot springs and mineral springs has been used medically for hundreds of years. When used properly, water-related therapies have been shown to be safe and effective for millions of people. These European physicians believe that to deny a sick patient a treatment that is likely to relieve suffering or save life is a violation of the Hippocratic oath and an affront to the people who go to them for care.

Here in the United States the research director at the Saratoga Spa in New York, Oskar Baudisch, Ph.D., wrote about the significance of mineral water some 60 years ago.

> America possesses a rich treasure in its mineral springs, and it is possible to put this wealth to use. . . . Spas and watering places are important for the health and well-being of mankind. Mineral springs are a national asset, and any nation which fails to make wise use of these gifts of nature causes loss and damage to the economic strength of its people.[7]

Throughout this book you will find summaries of research into the medical benefits of balneology. References for all these studies and reports are given in the notes at the back. Having seen the evidence, readers may form their own conclusions, do additional research on their own, or study the findings in more detail.

Although Americans enjoy the most advanced medical care in the world, with the finest doctors, the most sophisticated diagnostic equipment, and the largest and most modern hospitals on Earth, our overall level of health is declining. Degenerative diseases such as cancer, diabetes, heart disease, and obesity continue to affect a large portion of the population. The use of prescription and over-the-counter medications increases each year, along with many of the adverse side effects these drugs can produce. Many billions of dollars are lost annually because of absenteeism from lower back pain, arthritis, and muscle aches alone.

As a result of their dissatisfaction with mainstream medicine, Americans are spending an estimated $12 billion a year on so-called alternative therapies such as chiropractic, acupuncture, herbal medicine, and homeopathy, which are often not covered by medical insurance. People are looking for safe, effective, inexpensive, and natural methods that enhance the body's innate healing processes for both the prevention and cure of disease.

As much of the material presented later in this book will show, using medicinal springs for wellness is a natural, effective, and enjoyable way to promote health and healing. Healing springs are a unique natural resource—a precious gift from the Earth Mother—that is unrecognized and unappreciated in this country. It is hoped that by understanding the medicinal value of healing springs, we will learn to appreciate their magical powers and strive to use them wisely for pleasure, personal reflection, and healing.

PART I

STEP INTO THE WATER

Over the past few years, bathing in healing springs has experienced a renaissance, especially in North America. Many hot springs resorts that were languishing as recently as twenty years ago are thriving as holistic health retreats and upscale spas, offering a wide variety of therapeutic and recreational services. Once the exclusive domain of Native Americans, hidden springs accessible only on foot or with an all-wheel-drive vehicle are becoming popular destinations for visitors throughout the American West. At the same time, the democratization of international travel has brought even the most exclusive European and Japanese spas within the reach of budget-minded tourists seeking healthy escapes in some of the world's most exotic—and often stunningly beautiful—locales.

Yet, many Americans are unfamiliar with the elements of bathing in hot springs. We know very little about what makes a healing spring a healing spring, and how therapeutic bathing can be one of the safest and most enjoyable ways to both prevent and heal a wide variety of common health problems.

This first section provides a grounding in the little-known science of therapeutic bathing, known scientifically as balneology. It shows how hot springs are formed and where they are found, as well as explaining what a typical spa treatment consists of, including examination, evaluation, and bathing protocols. In addition, we explore some of the natural therapies that are used to complement "taking the waters," such as mud therapy, massage, exercise, diet, and herbal wraps. We also compare bathing in, as opposed to drinking, therapeutic waters, including a comparison between the therapeutic action of water consumed at the source and that of commercial bottled mineral waters consumed weeks or months after their removal from the spring. And while healing springs are good for the vast majority of individuals, they are not for everyone. In addition to simple cautions concerning the risks of overheating and dehydration, we address the possible dangers of hot springs for individuals with cancer, immune system disorders, and advanced heart disease.

Many hot springs have fascinating histories, and a book about healing waters wouldn't be complete without a historical perspective of bathing in hot springs. Originally considered to be the abodes of gods and goddesses, their earthly pleasures attracted the likes of Japanese emperors, Roman legionnaires, and the cream of European royalty. Here in the United States, Presidents George Washington, Thomas Jefferson, and Franklin Roosevelt were frequent visitors to hot springs, along with a galaxy of famous writers, artists, military heroes, actors, and industrialists who spent their summers at American spas "taking the waters" and enjoying the wide range of recreational and social activities to be found there. Many of these historic springs remain popular tourist destinations today, to be enjoyed by a new generation of visitors seeking health, fun, and relaxation.

THE WATERS OF LIFE

Human beings have a natural affinity for water. In the beginning, life was created in a vast primal sea. Like the oceans of today, this vast sea was slightly saline, containing approximately 3 percent salt. While we develop in our mother's womb we live in a near-total aquatic environment (containing nearly 95 percent slightly saline water), protected from extreme heat, cold, noise, and injury. For many of us, relaxing in a warm bath—whether in a tub or a mineral spring—leads us to recall the primal feelings of security, comfort, and protection we first experienced in the womb.

Even though humans live and thrive on dry land, water is vital to our health and well-being. Our bodies are made up of more than 60 percent water by weight, thus making our bodies essentially an aquatic environment. Every single body cell is made up of water-rich intracellular fluid and is surrounded by a protective layer of extracellular fluid, also made primarily of water. Every one of our body's cells, tissues, and organs—as well as every one of the body's life-sustaining processes, such as thinking, nerve function, circulation, digestion, locomotion, and elimination—requires water in order to function properly.[1]

Though relatively stable, the water content in our body is constantly changing. Waste products are eliminated from the body in water by perspiration, breathing, urination, and bowel movements, with thirst being the body's way to tell us that we need to replace these lost fluids throughout the day. We normally consume approximately 2.5 liters of fluids daily in the form of pure water and fluids containing water, such as soup, juice, milk, beer, coffee and tea, although some physicians recommend that we consume at least eight to twelve 8-ounce glasses of water a day. We also consume water as food, primarily in the form of water-rich fruits and vegetables. Finally, we can absorb small amounts of water by soaking in a warm bathtub or in a natural source such as a lake, river, or spring.

Throughout human history, water has been considered essential for physical health and spiritual well-being, and it has long been part of ceremonial practices in many of the world's religions. The early Egyptians worshiped the Nile, and priests were required to bathe in the river twice daily before entering the sacred temples. In India, bathing in the Ganges has always been an important part of ritual purification. Hindus believe that the goddess Ganga transformed herself into the Ganges River, which flows from the big toe of the god Vishnu, "the preserver" in Hindu mythology. Among the Jews, the Talmud taught the importance of water in personal cleanliness, and Jewish women have long used the mikvah, a ritual cleansing bath, after menstruation. The first Christian baptisms took place in the sacred waters of the Jordan River, and Christians continue to be immersed in water during baptismal rites today. In many Christian religious services, water is combined with wine to represent the blood that flowed from Jesus' body when the soldier pierced him, and holy water is an essential aspect of ritual purification both in church and in the home. Muslims are required to wash the face, hands, and neck in a ritual manner five times a day before each of their daily prayers.[2]

WHAT ARE HEALING SPRINGS?

Healing springs are usually defined as springs of varying temperature containing minerals, gases, and vapors that are likely to bring about specific therapeutic effects on the human body, such as changes in body temperature and in the functioning of the glands, the heart, the circulatory system, the immune system, the muscles, and the skin.

The classification of mineral springs varies according to country. For example, French mineral springs may be classified as cold (under 20°C or 68°F), warm (20–35°C or 68–95°F), hot (35–50°C or 95–122°F) or very hot (over 50°C or 122°F).[3] In Japan, a hot spring is legally defined as "hot water, mineral water, water vapor, or other gases (except natural gas containing hydrocarbons at the main element) that issue from the ground with a temperature in excess of 25°C (77°F) or that contain more than a prescribed amount of designated substances" such as carbon dioxide, magnesium, fluoride, sulfur, or sodium bicarbonate.[4]

Springs are often classified as alkaline, neutral, or acidic, as expressed by the symbol pH (potential of hydrogen). A water that is neither acid nor alkaline is expressed as pH 7, an alkaline spring has a pH of over 8.5, and an acid spring has a pH value of less than 3. The pH value is determined primarily by the amount of calcium and magnesium salts the water contains: the greater the amount, the lower the pH. The pH of water has therapeutic significance. For instance, low-pH waters can be drunk therapeutically to improve digestion among those with low stomach acid, while drinking the high pH waters of Montecatini and other spas can help reduce stomach acid. Low-pH waters such as those found at Kusatsu in Japan are especially indicated for treating skin conditions such as dermatitis. Springs are also classified according to the predominant minerals they contain, such as sulfur, fluorides, calcium, magnesium, bicarbonate, sodium, and potassium.

WHAT IS A SPA?

The word *spa* traces its origin to a mountain town of that name near Liège in southeastern Belgium. Here, an iron-rich spring was used by an ironmaster in the fourteenth century to cure his rheumatism. He founded a health resort at the spring called Espa (meaning "fountain" in the Walloon language). Espa became so popular that the word known in English as *spa* became the common designation for health resorts around the world. Spa remains one of Europe's leading centers for "taking the waters" to this day.

In Europe, one would ordinarily take a vacation from daily life and travel to a spa for a prolonged time, usually 14 to 21 days. In countries such as

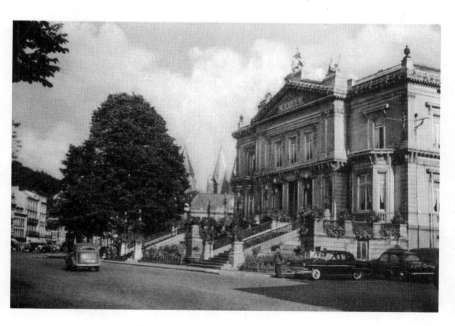

The baths in Spa during the 1950s.

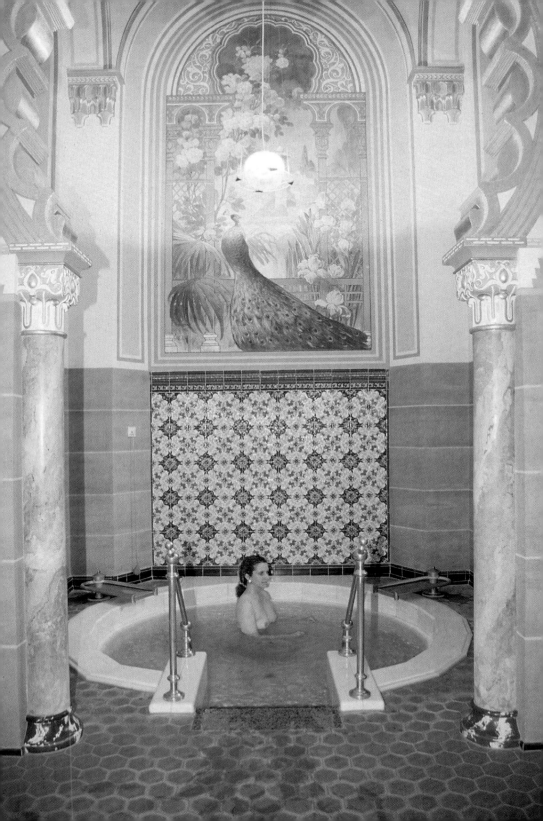

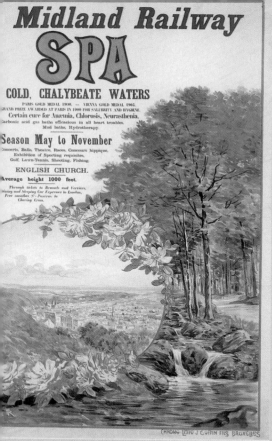

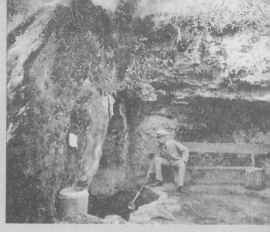

Overleaf: Palais Thermal, Bad Wildbad,
Germany

Above: Mark Twain at Vichy Springs,
California

Left: Publicity poster for Spa, Belgium

Below: Winter bathing at Kaikake Onsen,
Japan

Opposite above: Polynesian Spa, Rotorua,
New Zealand

Opposite below: Terme di Saturnia, Tuscany,
Italy

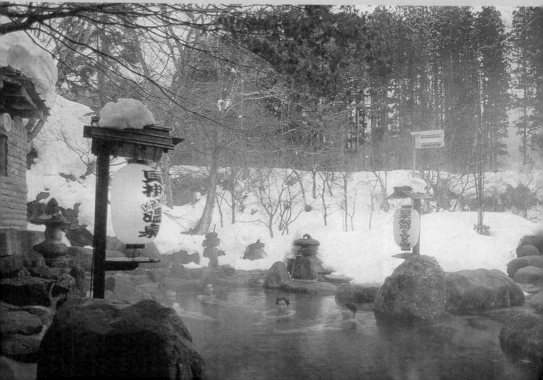

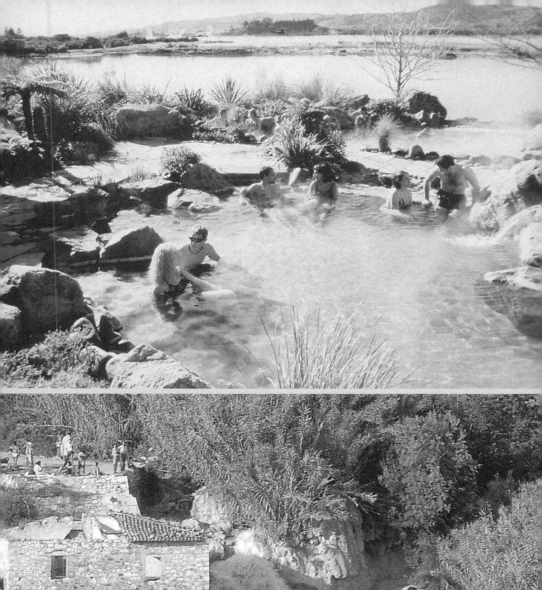
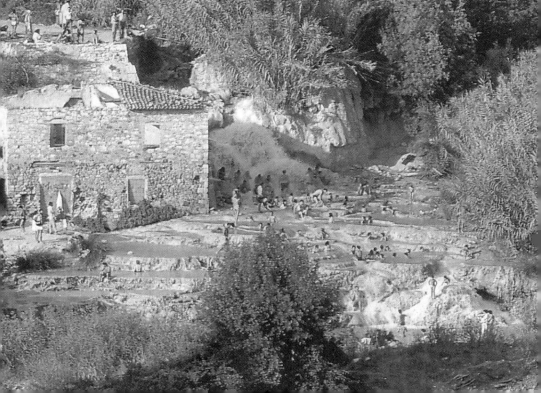

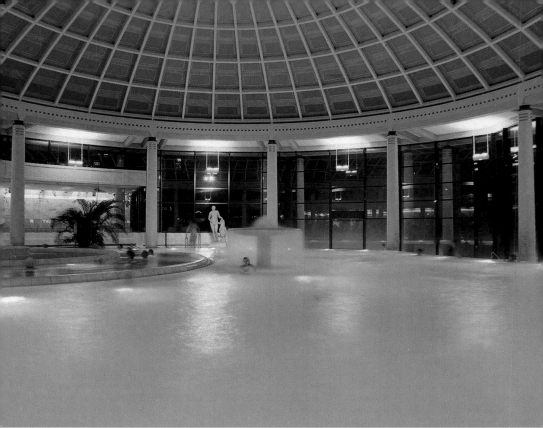

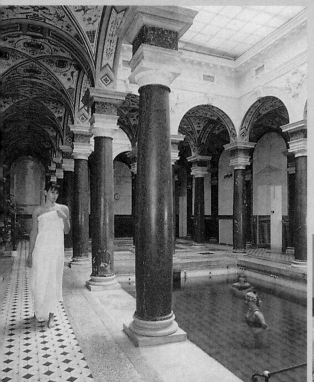

Above: Caracalla Terme, Baden-
    Baden, Germany

Left: Nové Lázně (New Bath),
    Mariánské Lázně, Czech Republic

Below: Mud bath at Calistoga Spa,
    California

Oppsite: Rác Medicinal Baths,
    Budapest

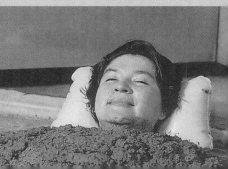

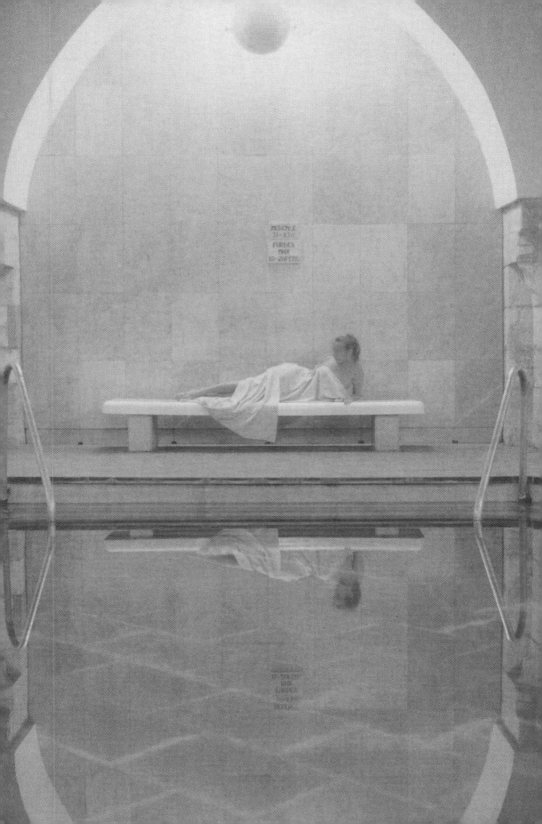

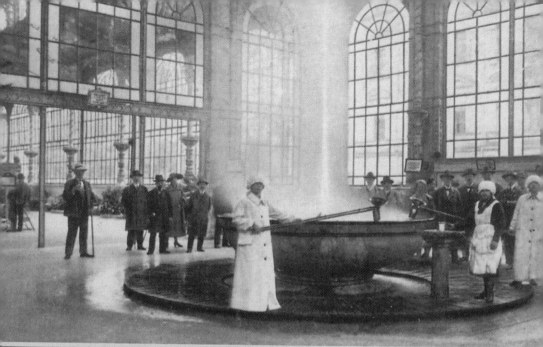

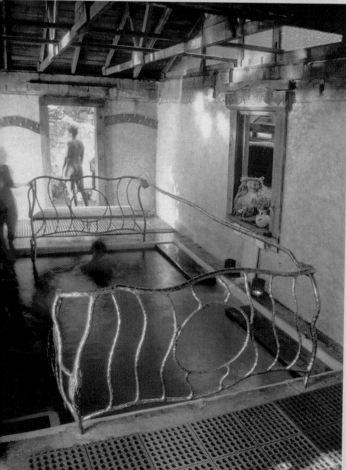

Above: Hot Spring Colonnade and Sprudel circa 1918, Karlovy Vary, Czech Republic

Left: The Hot Pool at Harbin Hot Springs, California

Below: Historic poster of Spa, Belgium

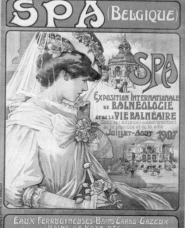

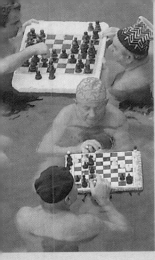

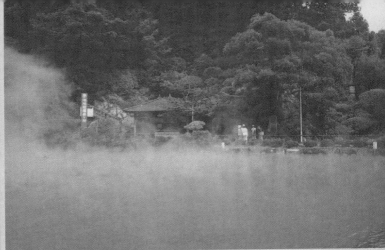

Above left: Playing chess at the Lido Pool of Széchenyi Medicinal Baths, Budapest, Hungary

Above right: Bloody Hell Pond, Beppu, Japan

Right: Yufuin Onsen, Japan

Below: Meadow Hot Springs, Utah

Overleaf: Caracalla Terme, Baden-Baden, Germany

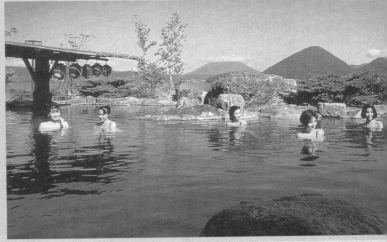

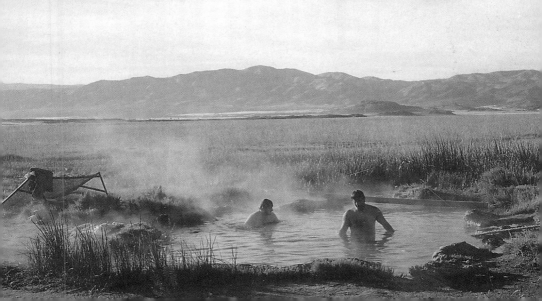

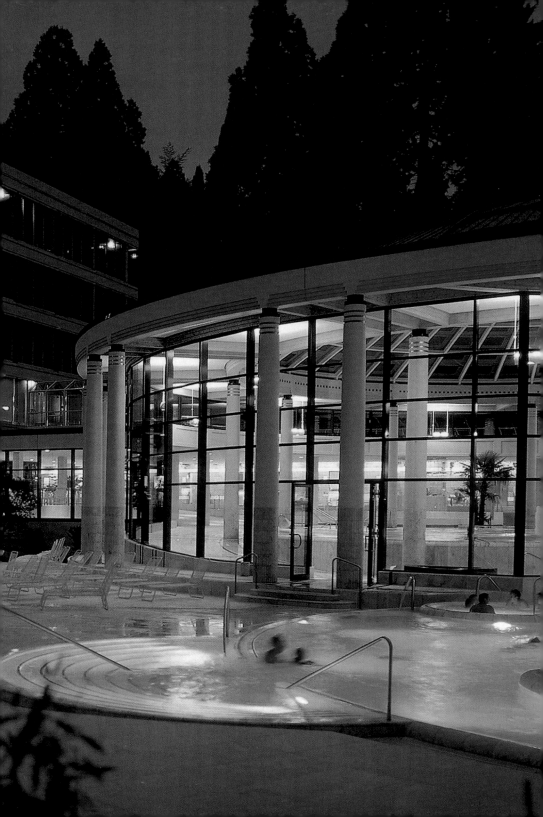

France, Italy, Spain, Germany, Hungary, Poland, Russia, or the Czech Republic, a 2- or 3-week course of spa therapy is prescribed by a physician and is paid for by social security. But for most Americans, a spa vacation costing several thousand dollars is beyond their budget, let alone taking 2 or 3 weeks off from work. Because of budgetary constraints and the fast pace of modern life, many people visit hot springs for much shorter periods of time, with stays of several hours to 2 or 3 days the norm.

Many have an image that a spa is mainly for older wealthy people who spend much of their time resting in bed or being given mud packs for their arthritis. While "taking the waters" is very popular with older people, especially in Japan and Europe, today's hot springs and mineral springs attract a diverse clientele of all ages. An elder is just as likely to take a 3-hour hike before enjoying a whirlpool bath as she would be to receive physical therapy for her arthritis. And it would be just as normal to see a teenager rush headfirst down a water slide in a thermal swimming pool as it would be to find his grandfather participating in a remedial exercise class. During a visit to the thermal spa at Bad Wildbad in the heart of the Black Forest in Germany, I was gratified (and, I must admit, somewhat surprised) to see three generations of family members enjoying the warm pools together, adhering to the "bathing suits optional" policy of the spa.

To attract short-term visitors, numerous spas have developed short 2- to 3-day programs to facilitate weight loss, reduce stress, and promote beauty enhancement. The vast majority of the world's mineral springs also offer innovative and healthy "spa cuisine," along with specialized exercise and recreation programs for all age groups. Many spas are located in beautiful natural environments and are surrounded by gardens, forests, lakes, and hiking trails. Some of the larger spa resorts in Europe and the United States offer a diverse range of recreational and cultural activities, such as water sports, cycling, boating, horseback riding, casino gambling, skiing, film screenings, concerts, and theater.

In Japan, some traditional hot springs are being developed into day spas known as *kuahausu* (derived from the old German term *kurhaus*). In addition to providing separate bathing areas for men and women containing a variety of mineral pools at different temperatures, a modern Japanese kuahausu might contain an enormous cold pool area (complete with fountains and water slides) for family swimming, a bowling alley, a well-equipped gym, spacious sauna and steam rooms, therapeutic massage services, relaxation rooms, a music room, several restaurants and bars, and a room filled with the latest video games for children and teens.

BALNEOTHERAPY: HEALING WITH WATER

One of the most improtant activities that takes place at a traditional spa is balneotherapy, a natural approach to health and healing that uses hot spring water, gases, mud, and climatic factors (such as heat) as therapeutic elements. In addition to bathing, modalities such as hydrotherapy, mud therapy, physical therapy, massage, steam baths, physical exercises, inhalation of water vapor, and drinking mineral water are often used as part of a complex therapy for both health preservation and treating disease.

Over the past four centuries, the science of balneology has evolved into a medical specialty in Europe and Japan, where special courses in balneotherapy are offered to both physicians and nurses by major medical schools. Doctors believe that thermal springs facilitate healing in a number of important ways:

- Bathing in hot springs gradually increases the temperature of the body, thus killing harmful germs and viruses.

- Thermal bathing increases hydrostatic pressure on the body, thus increasing blood circulation and cell oxygenation. The increase in blood flow also helps dissolve and eliminate toxins from the body.

- Hot springs bathing increases the flow of oxygen-rich blood throughout the body, bringing improved nourishment to vital organs and tissues.

- Bathing in thermal water increases body metabolism, including stimulating the secretions of the intestinal tract and the liver, aiding digestion.

- Repeated hot springs bathing (especially over a 3- or 4-week period) can help normalize the functions of the endocrine glands as well as the functioning of the body's autonomic nervous system.

- Trace amounts of minerals such as carbon dioxide, sulfur, calcium, magnesium, and lithium are absorbed by the body and provide healing effects to various body organs and systems. These healing effects can include stimulation of the immune system, leading to enhanced immunity; physical and mental relaxation; the production of endorphins; and normalized gland function.

- Mineral springs contain high amounts of negative ions, which can help promote feelings of physical and psychological well-being.

- The direct application of mineralized thermal waters (especially those containing sulfur) can have a therapeutic effect on diseases of the skin, including psoriasis, dermatitis, and fungal infections. Some mineral waters are also used to help the healing of wounds and other skin injuries.[5-9]

Indications for Balneotherapy

Over the several hundred years during which the science of medical balneology has developed, physicians have been able to identify the health conditions that can best be treated by healing springs. At the same time, they have developed specific protocols for safe and effective treatment. The following list of indications for balneotherapy is based on the research of Yuko Agishi, M.D., Professor Emeritus at the Hokkaido University School of Medicine and Director of the Arima Onsen Hospital near Kobe, Japan.

Chronic diseases

Chronic rheumatic diseases
Functional recovery of central and peripheral neuroparalysis
Metabolic diseases, especially diabetes, obesity, and gout
Chronic gastrointestinal diseases
Chronic mild respiratory diseases
Circulatory diseases, especially moderate or mild hypertension
Peripheral circulatory diseases (affecting the hands and feet)
Chronic skin diseases
Psychosomatic and stress-related diseases
Autonomic nervous system dysfunction
Vibration disorder (a middle ear disorder affecting balance)
Sequelae of (conditions resulting from) trauma
Chronic gynecological diseases

Rehabilitation

Sequelae of cerebrovascular disorders
Chronic rheumatic diseases
Sequelae of traffic accidents and sports-related injuries
Spinal paralysis
Treatment paralysis
Treatment after cerebral surgery or orthopedic surgery

Before and after surgical procedures

Hip replacements
Knee surgery

Preventive medicine

Prevention of adult diseases
Prevention of occupational diseases
Building up physical strength and general immunity[10]

Contraindications

Although bathing in thermal and mineral springs is both healthful and relaxing for the vast majority of individuals, Dr. Agishi and other medical balneologists point out it is not for everyone. People who have the following conditions should avoid bathing in hot springs unless they are under the direct supervision of a physician who is well versed in medical balneology:

Any disease involving high fever with progressing or exacerbating symptoms
Severe hypertension, uncompensated congestive heart failure
Malignant tumor (and cancer in general)
Serious liver, kidney, or circulatory disease
Serious heart arrhythmia (irregular heartbeat)
Recent heart attack or stroke
Any disease involving hemorrhage and severe anemia
Early and late stages of pregnancy
Severe mental illness[11]

In addition to the possible contraindications, several other words of caution are needed:

Avoid soaking in a hot spring alone.
If you are with children or elderly adults, be especially mindful of possible exhaustion or overheating.
If you are pregnant, avoid prolonged hot spring bathing; consult with a qualified health practitioner for guidance.
Do not enter a hot pool if you are under the influence of alcohol or drugs, especially heart medications.
Many people wrongly believe that if spending 10 minutes in a hot spring is good, 30 minutes is better. Avoid overheating, and do not remain in the water if you feel tired or uncomfortable. If you feel faint or dizzy, leave the pool immediately.
Drink plenty of cool water (not from the hot spring itself) to avoid dehydration.
Use private pools if you have a skin disease.

Certain types of infectious bacteria often thrive in hot springs. Commercial springs are carefully monitored for such bacteria, and are often filtered and treated with chemicals to maintain purity. If you decide to enjoy a noncommercial hot spring, keep your head above the water level because these bacteria can enter your body through the nose.

Finally, some springs contain heavy metals and other elements that may be good for your skin and sore muscles, but harmful if taken internally. For this reason, do not drink water from a medicinal spring unless you know that it is safe.[12]

THE HEALING TRIAD

Mineral springs can be used for health in three major ways.

Bathing

Immersing oneself in mineral water is the most popular form of balneotherapy. Therapeutic bathing may involve immersion into water at neck level, as we would do in an ordinary swimming pool, for approximately 15 to 20 minutes two or three times a day.

The time one can safely remain in a thermal pool varies according to both the temperature of the water and our own physical condition. For example, bathers can enjoy lounging in the outdoor pool at Harbin Hot Springs in California, which is slightly warmer than normal body temperature, for an hour or more at a time. However, few people can endure a 3-minute "time bath" at the famous Kusatsu hot spring in Japan, whose temperature remains a near-constant 52°C (125°F). Here, the bath master (known as a *yucho*) interviews each bather and determines if his or her condition merits taking the bath. The yucho also counts the minutes while the bather endures the scalding acidic waters. In a country known for its politeness and decorum, Kusatsu is probably the only place in Japan where yelling and swearing in public are acceptable.

In some cases, bathing in water at waist level or midchest level is recommended to relieve pressure on the body and avoid overheating during a bath in warm water. In addition to actual bathing, adjuncts such as physical therapy, aerobic exercise, stretching, and swimming are often recommended to help the bather achieve maximum benefit from the therapeutic waters. Some spas offer the unique Watsu massage method (derived from the words *water* and *shiatsu*), which was originally developed at Harbin Hot Springs. Watsu involves a specialized technique of massage and guided movement while the bather is in a mineralized thermal pool.

Mineral water is also applied as a shower, as a concentrated jet, as a douche, or in the form of hot or cold applications to the skin as water packs. In some European spas, a needle shower saturates the body with highly concentrated jets of water that stimulate the skin and massage the muscles and joints.

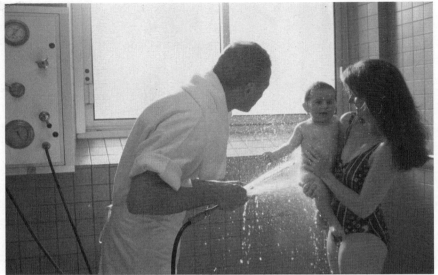

Mineral water applied as a concentrated jet.
Photo courtesy of Thermes de La Roche-Posay.

Drinking

The drinking cure is especially popular in Europe, where many types of mineral water are bottled for commercial use. After an examination by a spa physician, the patient goes to the source of the spring (often a beautiful pavilion), and drinks a prescribed amount of mineral water several times a day.

Minerals from spring water are absorbed into the bloodstream through the mucosa of the digestive tract. Not only do they affect the gastrointestinal, kidney, and other body functions (for example, drinking water rich in bicarbonates and sulfates before meals has been found to increase blood insulin levels), but also they provide vital nutrients such as calcium, magnesium, and iron. As we shall see later, there are many kinds of mineral waters with very different tastes as well as differing nutritional and medicinal properties. Some waters have been found, for example, to be very effective for treating liver problems; others are used to relieve urinary tract infections or intestinal complaints.

According to Dr. V. Digiesi of the Institute of Internal Medicine and Immunoallergiology at the University of Florence Medical School in Italy, drinking mineral water has several important nutritional benefits, especially when it is done under the guidance of a qualified nutritionist or health care professional:

• In addition to providing our normal daily requirement for water, mineral

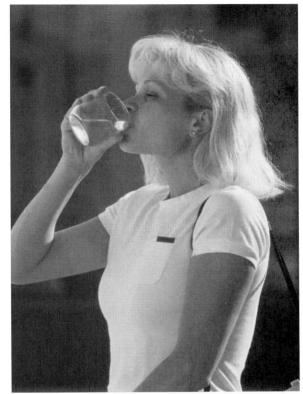

Drinking mineral water.
Photo courtesy of Thermes
de La Roche-Posay.

water contributes to our daily dietary allowance of both macroelements (such as iron) and trace elements (such as copper).

- Drinking mineral water helps treat certain gastrointestinal, kidney, metabolic, and cardiovascular diseases.

- The nutritional components of certain mineral waters can help prevent several kidney, bone, metabolic, and cardiovascular diseases. For example, water that is rich in calcium can help reduce the risks of osteoporosis, and water rich in magnesium may help prevent hypertension.[13]

Not all mineral waters are recommended for drinking. Some, such as those containing arsenic (which has been shown to be very good for treating fungal infections of the skin but can be poisonous when swallowed) should only be used externally. Other mineral waters, such as those containing large amounts of sulfur or iron, have such a disagreeable taste that no one wants to drink them!

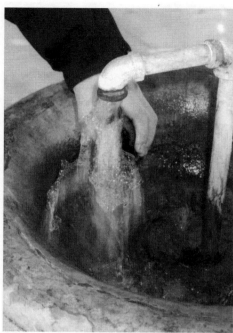

Hathorne Spring.
Saratoga Springs, New York.

In addition, mineral water consumed directly at the source of the spring is not the same as commercially bottled water taken from the same spring and processed at a bottling plant. Some minerals and gases tend to oxidize within hours after leaving the earth and may no longer have the therapeutic effects for which they are known. (This may also hold true for waters that are used for bathing.)[14]

For example, drinking a particular mineral water rich in calcium and magnesium at the source of the spring may aid digestion and promote regularity. Like a herbal remedy or a drug, doctors may recommend that we consume only half a glass (250 milliliters) of this water two or three times a day. By contrast, commercially bottled mineral water from the same spring can be consumed in unlimited amounts as a beverage and thirst-quencher. I learned about this important difference while doing research for this book in France. During a two-hour drive to Strasbourg I happily consumed a liter bottle of Contrexéville mineral water I had filled at the spring. Several emergency bathroom visits en route told me that I had not been drinking the familiar Contrexéville water I bought at the supermarket but had ingested a very efficient laxative that should have been taken in much smaller amounts over a longer period of time!

Inhalation

Inhaling mineral water as water vapor has been effective in helping people with asthma, sinus problems, allergies, and other respiratory problems. The water vapor takes the form of an extremely fine spray that can be released from a fountain not unlike a drinking fountain. By standing over the fountain and pushing a button, the person releases a fine mist from the fountain, which can be inhaled. In some European spa clinics, the mineral water mist is administered through an oxygen mask or through the kind of inhalers asthma patients use when taking medication. Other spas use eucalyptus oil or other herbal essences to help decongest the respiratory system.

A nontraditional but highly efficient method of inhaling mineral water can be found at the Rancho Río Caliente spa near Guadalajara, Mexico. At Río Caliente, the steam room is connected to one of the spa's hot mineral springs, which contains trace amounts of lithium. After one or two sessions of breathing in the therapeutic steam, even the most nervous or stressed-out guest becomes relaxed and very mellow. Therapeutic steam rooms are also found in many European spas.

In Europe, as well as in some of the most exclusive American spas, patients may be examined by a physician before undertaking any of the three basic forms of water cure. In this way, the doctor can formulate the most effective protocol of water therapy (along with selected adjunct therapies) to help the patient regain health and, at the same time, determine the safe limits for exposing the patient to thermal water, especially in cases of high blood pressure or other cardiovascular conditions.

In the Czech Republic and Slovakia, the spa regimen may be one of two types:

The *toughening regimen* utilizes a whole range of complex therapies designed to improve the patient's general health condition and raise his or her resistance to environmental factors, such as stress. In addition to the three types of balneotherapy mentioned above, this program includes fresh air, physical exercise, and active sports.

By contrast, the *conserving regimen* is designed to help the patient relax. It places less emphasis on exercise and focuses primarily on helping the patient benefit from rest and relaxation. For people experiencing stress or cardiovascular problems, or those recovering from acute illness, balneotherapy may be accompanied by massage and instruction in relaxation techniques. Depending on the patient's individual needs, moderate exercise may be included in this program as well.[15]

Music holds a special place in the treatment in many European spas. One of my most impressive memories of visiting Mariánské Lázně in the Czech Republic was listening to music from a Mozart concert wafting through the town as I visited various spas. According to the text *Spa Treatment in Czechoslovakia,* "As well as the regular music programs at the spa, which have a positive psychological effect and are mentally relaxing, it includes the direct therapeutic use of music, utilizing its possibilities for evoking tonic or relaxing conditioned reflex processes."[16] Ballroom dancing, disco, and other types of dance are also used as part of the therapeutic regimen in many Czech and Slovak spas for both their emotional and their physical benefits.

ADJUNCT THERAPIES

We mentioned that many spas offer a wide variety of adjunct therapies that complement the use of balneotherapy. While the effectiveness of some of these therapies has been scientifically documented (we'll explore them in the clinically oriented chapters later in this book), others have become popular with spa-goers because they are pleasurable, promote relaxation, or lead to feelings of overall well-being.

Acupressure is a form of Oriental finger massage that is designed to both relieve tension and stimulate the energy centers of the body. It is often used as part of *shiatsu* and traditional Chinese massage.

Acupuncture, an ancient form of healing developed in China, involves the use of needles to relieve tension and stimulate certain energy centers of the body. It is generally more precise than acupressure and should be done only by a qualified health care specialist.

Aromatherapy uses scented oils made from the essence of different flowers, often in massage. It is based on the ancient art of using perfumes for healing; certain odors are believed to promote relaxation, reduce anxiety, and relieve depression.

Body scrubs call for rubbing the body with a mixture of crushed apricot pits, mineral salts, seaweed, or other abrasive material combined with lotion or mineral oil. The goal is to cleanse the body by removing the outer layer of dead skin, leaving the body smooth and clean.

Colonic irrigation is a specialized type of enema that cleanses high into the colon. Some holistic spas utilize thermal spring water for this cleansing treatment.

Fangotherapy (also known as *pelotherapy*) calls for using a mud pack or coating parts of the body with mud. It is believed that mud helps remove toxins from the body, relieves arthritic and muscle pain, and helps heal the skin. In some spas, such as those in Calistoga and Palm Springs, California, fangotherapy involves total immersion in a tub of warm mud made with water from the mineral springs.

Fasting is the use of a supervised diet of water, juice, and possibly fruit to improve health and lose weight.

Herbal wraps are a popular adjunct to bathing. The body is wrapped in warm sheets and blankets infused with herbal essences, which penetrate the skin, promoting cleansing, healing, and relaxation.

Hydrotherapy is often an aspect of balneotherapy and encompasses several types of water therapies, including underwater massage with jets of water (hydromassage), alternating hot and cold showers or baths, hot and/or cold compresses, steam baths, colonic irrigations, or applying jets of water under pressure to various parts of the body.

The *Kneipp kur* is a specialized program of hydrotherapy that also includes a natural foods diet, exercise, and herbs. Developed by German cleric Sebastian Kneipp during the mid-1800s, it is still widely used in European spas today.

Massage involves manipulation, methodical pressure, friction, and kneading of different parts of the body. It is designed to relax the muscles, reduce stress, and improve body flexibility. Massage is a popular adjunct to different forms of balneotherapy (see *shiatsu* and *Swedish massage*).

Oxygen therapy is a general term used to describe the administration of supplemental oxygen to increase oxygenation of body tissues; however, it is often used to describe *ozone therapy* or the administration of small amounts of medical-grade hydrogen peroxide as an intravenous drip or added to bathwater.

Ozone therapy involves the use of mixing a small amount of therapeutic ozone and oxygen with the patient's blood, which is then reinfused into the patient. It has been used to treat a wide variety of diseases, including cancer, high blood pressure, HIV infection, and diabetes.

A *sauna* is usually a cedar-lined room where dry heat, from 70–98°C (160–210°F), is administered. Like the steam bath, a sauna increases body temperature, leading to increased circulation and elimination of toxins.

Shiatsu, a type of massage developed in Japan, uses finger pressure on meridians, or channels, that transport energy to different parts of the body.

A *Sitz bath* is the immersion of the lower part of the body in a warm bath, followed by cold water. It is intended to stimulate the immune system.

Spa cuisine is a rather vague term used to describe healthy natural foods with an emphasis on fresh fruits and vegetables, low-fat animal products, and a minimum of salt, artificial flavorings, and colorings.

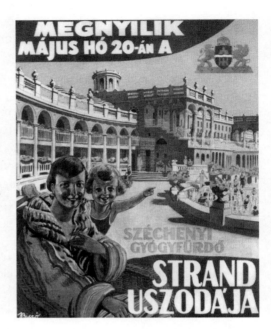

Poster advertising the Lido Pool at Széchenyi Medicinal Baths. Reprinted courtesy of the Hungarian National Tourist Office.

Steam baths take place in a room lined with ceramic tiles and heated with steam at temperatures of 43–70°C (110–160°F). The steam may or may not contain mineral water vapors, and is often better tolerated than a sauna. Like thermal bathing, steam baths increase blood circulation, raise body temperature, and aid in body cleansing.

Swedish massage, the most common type of massage in the West, involves kneading, stroking, and tapping different parts of the body to promote relaxation and relieve muscle and joint pain.

Thalassotherapy uses sea water, as well as seaweed wraps and breathing sea air. Some hot springs resorts located near the ocean or the Mediterranean Sea offer thalassotherapy along with traditional hot springs bathing regimens.

OTHER DIVERSIONS

A wide range of recreational and cultural activities have long been connected to hot springs. We mentioned earlier that in years past, many spa towns were exclusive vacation resorts, attracting royalty, military leaders, writers, artists, and philosophers. Some attracted a more diverse clientele. Hot Springs, Arkansas, was once viewed as a notorious center for illegal gambling and other forms of vice, and horse racing—and bootleg whisky smuggled in from nearby

Canada—made Saratoga Springs, New York, a preferred destination for organized crime figures from all over the East Coast during Prohibition. Throughout World Wars I and II, many of the spa towns in central Europe were active centers of spying and political intrigue; in France, Vichy served as the headquarters of the pro-Nazi government during the German occupation. By the beginning of World War II, the Peitou hot springs in Taiwan contained 72 bathhouses, many of them staffed with geishas and prostitutes. The best-known guests were kamikaze pilots (Japan occupied Taiwan from 1895 until 1945), who often spent their first—and last—night of pleasure at the bathhouses of Peitou, which nowadays promotes itself as a wholesome family resort.[17]

Although gambling and related entertainments can be found in numerous spa resorts today, many European spas feature more respectable pleasures, including museum exhibits, concerts, plays and film festivals, convention centers, golf courses, and facilities for tennis, volleyball, basketball, and horseback riding. The physical, thermal, and chemical effects of hot springs therapy combine with supportive natural therapies such as massage and aromatherapy designed to invigorate and relax; healthier diets available at the spas; the environmental climatic effects of beautiful natural surroundings; healthful activities such as walking, hiking, swimming, and other forms of outdoor exercise; the physical and emotional benefits of indoor exercises such as aerobics and strength-enhancing exercise; the social effects of interacting with others in a low-stress environment; cultural activities such as concerts and lectures; and increased opportunities for sleep and relaxation. With so many benefits available in one setting, balneologists are exploring the value of hot springs as a powerful form of preventive medicine that merits further study.[18]

2

DOWN FROM THE MOUNTAINS, UP FROM THE DEPTHS

Our planet is blessed with tens of thousands of hot springs and mineral springs. In the United States alone, there are over 115 major geothermal spas and many smaller ones, as well as over 1,800 bathing mineral springs throughout the country, primarily in the West. Other countries that are especially rich in hot springs and mineral springs include Russia (the former Soviet Union boasted 3,500 spas), Japan (1,500 spas with an estimated annual attendance of 100 million), and the Czech Republic and Slovakia (52 spas and more than 1,900 mineral springs),[1] as well as Romania, Bulgaria, Hungary, Poland, France, Germany, Italy, Spain, and Portugal. There are also numerous hot springs in Latin America, especially in Chile and Argentina, as well as in Brazil, Colombia, Ecuador, Peru, Venezuela, and Mexico. The directory listings in part 4 highlight many of these springs.

In times past, mineral and thermal springs inspired both fear and fascination. Because they seemed to originate from deep within the earth, they were viewed as passages to the underworld and were considered the homes of various divine beings who possessed the forces of life and death. In Japan, Shinto shrines can still be found next to many hot springs to acknowledge the presence of the *kami,* or spirit being, that is believed to inhabit the spring and guide its evolution.

Only during the past few hundred years have scientists determined that mineral and thermal springs are a natural part of the hydrological cycle of water, involving the natural processes of successive evaporation, condensation, and precipitation at levels deep within the earth. Although nearly every mineral spring is unique in temperature, mineral content, and mineral combination, there are essentially two basic types: filtration springs and primary springs.

FILTRATION SPRINGS

Filtration springs are common in the northeastern United States, France, Germany, Great Britain, Eastern Europe, and Korea. They originate at higher elevations and are nourished by normal rainfall, which percolates under pressure deep into the earth through fractures in various types of rock formations such as granite, iron, or gneiss. The water follows fractures and faults down into the earth and is heated (temperatures increase at about 37°C [100°F] for each kilometer beneath the earth's surface). The water then slowly travels back to the surface along fault lines in rock formations until it reaches the earth's surface—a process that can take thousands of years. Many of these springs contain oxygen and carbon dioxide as well as trace minerals such as calcium, iron, and magnesium that are leached from the rock formations.

Some filtration springs have an extraordinary geological history. The mineral waters of Saratoga, for example, owe their origin to the vast glaciers of the Pleistocene Age, when vast amounts of geological material and decaying plants were deposited in the area. The mineral-rich waters of the springs are actually part of a vast prehistoric sea found in deposits of limestone and dolomite; the surface of one of the faults is composed of an impervious layer of shale. The

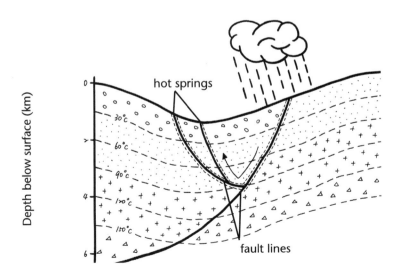

A simplified diagram of a filtration spring. Illustration by Yi-Shan Shei.

shale prevents the waters from reaching the surface except along fault lines where the surface is broken. At the same time, the shale keeps rainwater from reaching (and mixing with) the mineral waters.

Approximately eighteen springs discharge naturally carbonated mineral water at an average temperature of 13°C (55°F); most of the springs were drilled where carbon dioxide was found bubbling from the ground by Native Americans and early European settlers.[2] The Saratoga Springs area also contains the only geyser east of the Mississippi River. At present, ten springs are flowing freely at Saratoga Springs State Park and in the city of Saratoga Springs, where five different varieties of mineral water can be enjoyed by thirsty visitors. Bottled commercially since the 1820s, Saratoga waters have long been highly regarded and are said to rival those found in famous European spas such as Vichy, Aix-les-Bains, and Baden-Baden. At one time, waters similar to those of Saratoga were enjoyed at any of the four springs within the city limits of nearby Ballston Spa, which, sadly, are now closed.

The city of Hot Springs, Arkansas, contains 47 springs resulting from rainwater that percolated into deep rock formations containing Bigfork chert and Arkansas novaculite. The water is then heated at a depth of 6,040 feet (1,840 meters) and travels up along fault lines in the rock until it finally surfaces near what is now known as Hot Springs Mountain.[3] The area was described by J. J. Moorman, M.D., in *Mineral Springs of North America*, published in 1873:

> On the summit of the mountain are heavy pine and oak timber, abounding with clusters of grape-vines, huge masses of quartz rock apparently upheaved by some convulsion of nature; immediately below the summit, sharp-cornered honey-comb rocks, with sparkling surfaces; still lower, a

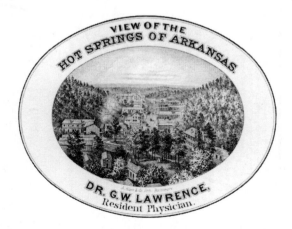

A view of Hot Springs, Arkansas (1873).

heavy undergrowth of pines and other trees, and from thence, where the Hot Springs flow to the base, calcareous tufa.[4]

Unlike the cooler water at Saratoga, water from Hot Springs, Arkansas, flowing at a rate of approximately 940,000 gallons a day, averages 62°C (143°F), which means that it must be allowed to cool before people can safely bathe in it. The water from these springs contains bicarbonate, calcium, silica, sulfate, and sodium; carbon 14 dating has shown that this water is over 4,000 years old.[5]

The most important spas in the Czech Republic—Karlovy Vary (Carlsbad) and Mariánské Lázně (Marienbad)—share similar geologic characteristics. Located in the western part of the country, they are part of a large system of carbonated waters that extends from France to Germany and through Bohemia to Silesia. The area contains rich marine sediments along with abundant minerals from the sedimentary rocks through which the waters circulate. The waters from the springs also result from unique combinations of various subterranean waters flowing under the Carpathian Mountains. Rainwater flows through fissures in the granite-rich rock formations down to a depth of more than

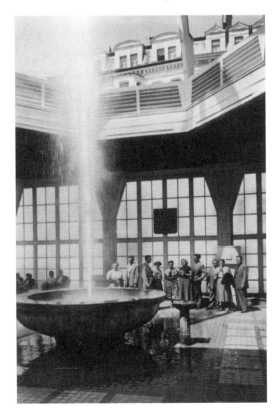

The Sprudel at Karlovy Vary, Czech Republic, circa 1955.

1,000 meters; it is then heated and flows toward the surface along fault lines.

Karlovy Vary, the more famous of the two, is a beautiful town framed by steep forested hills; the area where most of the spas are found is on a river and is often only one to two blocks wide. Over 130 springs can be found in Karlovy Vary, 12 of which are popular for drinking, including the famous Sprudel spring, which is not unlike a small geyser. Millions of cubic feet of carbon dioxide, as well as approximately 180 tons of mineral salts, are extracted from the springs at Karlovy Vary and exported for commercial and medicinal use each year.

Although smaller than its neighbor, the spa district of Mariánské Lázně boasts 40 filtration springs in an area of beautifully landscaped parks about a kilometer from the town center. In addition to its elegant healing centers and opulent colonnade, Mariánské Lázně gained renown in the nineteenth century as a romantic destination where one could pursue extramarital affairs. In *Taking the Waters,* a fascinating history of spas and bathing traditions, Alev Lytle Croutier mentioned that the ailing writer J. W. von Goethe first enjoyed the healing waters at Mariánské Lázně at the age of 74, but that the real cure probably came from courting a 19-year-old girl while he was vacationing there.[6]

PRIMARY SPRINGS

Primary springs occur mostly in the western United States and Canada, Italy, Taiwan, Japan, and New Zealand. They are more directly related to volcanic activity and contain minerals and other elements produced by volcanoes, such as sulfur, radon, and bromides. Unlike springs created primarily by filtration, the supply of water to volcanic springs is many miles beneath the earth, not only making the water hotter, but making the flow more constant and reliable. However, some of the mineral water also comes from rainfall.

When the Coast Range of California was formed nearly two million years ago, molten rock began to escape from deep within the earth. Volcanoes rose from weak areas of the earth's crust, and the extreme heat caused water to evaporate from the sea, returning as rain. Some seawater flowed into the earth through cracks in the earth's surface, where it was heated near the earth's core.

Hot springs occur when a magma chamber is located near the earth's surface. Within the vicinity of Harbin and Calistoga, for example, there is a large magma chamber about 13 miles in diameter located about 4 miles underground. Hot springs such as those in Harbin and Calistoga consist of heated circulating water augmented by steam rising from the molten magma. Some of this water is essentially heated groundwater that is the result of rain or snow. This water

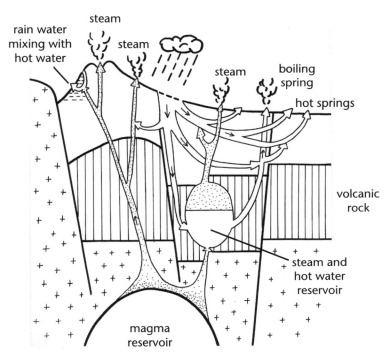

A diagram of the primary springs in Beppu, Japan.
Illustration by Yi-Shan Shei.

is heated and rises toward the surface as steam; as it cools it turns back into water and exits the earth through small fissures in the earth's crust.

Another type of water, juvenile water, has been trapped beneath the earth and never before reached the surface. Juvenile water, found in both primary and filtration springs, is often the remains of a vast, underground sea. Despite its name, juvenile water can be tens of millions of years old. These waters are stored in aquifers at various depths beneath the earth's surface at different temperatures before they finally flow toward the surface. This is one reason why mineral waters at a hot springs establishment can be found at various temperatures; in some places, a hot spring even can be found within a few meters of a cold spring. In some spas, springs are drilled and piped to a central bathing area, giving the appearance that the actual source of the springs is nearby, when in fact it may be hundreds of feet away.[7]

Among primary springs, perhaps the most extraordinary are found in and around the city of Beppu on Kyushu Island in southern Japan. Containing

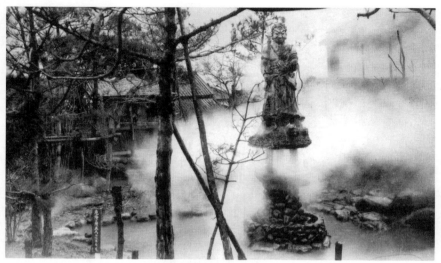

A scene of a Beppu jigoku.

over 3,800 hot springs and wells discharging an estimated 50,000 tons of thermal water per day (flowing at a rate of 9,200 gallons per minute), Beppu is one of the most thermally active places in the world. Though mostly hot (most Beppu waters must be cooled or diluted to make them safe for bathing), the thermal waters of Beppu reach the earth's surface at different temperatures. Beppu is considered a paradise for hot springs enthusiasts, who can have their choice of bathing in dozens of *onsen,* usually at hotels and public baths, as well as in traditional Japanese guest houses, known as *ryokan.*

Located near several volcanoes, the waters of Beppu are heated at great depth and bubble to the surface throughout the area. Passing through the Beppu region by train, one cannot help but notice the numerous steam vents that dot the landscape; many buildings in Beppu (including the biggest hotel in town, the Suginoi) generate their own electricity through small geothermal power plants.

Some of the most interesting attractions in Beppu are the *jigokus,* or "hell" ponds. They are steaming open springs that often contain a vast assortment of minerals, causing the waters (and often the bubbling mud) to appear in different colors. One famous hot spring, appropriately known as Bloody Hell Pond (*Chinoike jigoku*), contains a unique composition of ferrous oxide, magnesium oxide, and aluminum oxide that makes the waters bright red, while the *Umi jigoku* (Sea Hell) contains white mineral particles that reflect the color of the sky. Some of the Beppu waters are so hot (a few actually exceed the boiling point) that they are used to cook eggs and other foods.

OTHER SPRING CLASSIFICATIONS

Like any natural form, each hot spring or mineral spring is unique in form, size, temperature, and mineral content. Some springs may be classified as sulfate springs because they contain at least 1,000 milligrams of sodium, calcium, or magnesium sulfate per kilogram of water, while other springs are made up of a combination of many different minerals. For example, in Japan any spring that is 25°C (77°F) or hotter is classified as a simple thermal spring. Likewise a spring can be classified also as a mineral spring if it is composed of hot water containing at least 1,000 milligrams of minerals of various kinds per kilogram of water.[8]

The major types of springs include thermal, bicarbonate, sulfate (including sodium sulfate, calcium sulfate, and magnesium sulfate), sulfite (including sodium sulfite, calcium sulfite, and magnesium sulfite), chloride (including calcium chloride, magnesium chloride, and sodium chloride), sulfur, iron, or lithium. Springs also can contain gases such as carbon dioxide as well as radioactive elements such as radon. These springs, and the many different kinds of mud that can be derived from them, are described in detail in chapters 4 through 9.

3

A LONG-STANDING TRADITION

Soaking in a stream, lake, or tub has always ranked among the most pleasurable of human experiences, and people have enjoyed bathing in mineral springs since time immemorial. Traces of *Homo erectus* dating back 600,000 years have been found in the vicinity of some hot springs. Many mineral springs are distinguished by their warm or hot temperatures, and those rich in minerals such as sulfur, iron, and chloride often are distinguished by a distinctive color or odor that sets them apart from ordinary springs. In earlier times, many springs gained notoriety for their apparent ability to heal wounds and relieve the symptoms of arthritis and other diseases in those who bathed in them.

ANCIENT SPRINGS

The early Greeks enjoyed bathing in both private and public baths, and Homer, Hippocrates, and Asclepiades stressed the importance of both drinking water and bathing in water for health. A famous spring in the ancient city of Thermae—today's Loutraki—was held to be beloved of the gods and was the first health resort to be recorded in the annals of world history. The name Thermae comes from Artemis Thermia, the protectress of hot mineral springs. Both Apollo, the god of the sun and of spiritual peace, and Hera, the mother of the gods, were worshiped at temples there. The first written mention of the baths at Thermae is by Xenophon in his *Hellenica*. The early Romans were tremendously fond of bathing for both health and pleasure, and Roman baths, often large and luxurious establishments, served as centers of entertainment, gymnastics, debating, and art. As they conquered new territories, the Romans developed a network of thermal and mineral springs that had been discovered throughout the empire. Roman baths extended from Bath and Epsom in England to France (including Aix-les-Bains), Italy (including Titus and

38

Caracalla), Turkey, Romania, Hungary, and Bulgaria. During the Roman era, the military leader Sulla was cured by the springs of Loutraki, as were those who sought therapy at the Roman baths at Thermae. In addition to Loutraki, many other Roman springs are in use today throughout Europe.[1]

The Romans were believed to have discovered the abundance of medicinal waters in Budapest, which is unparalleled among traditional spa towns: over 70 million liters of water flow daily from 123 thermal and 400 mineral springs from 14 sources on the Buda side of the river along a geologic fault. The city contains seven thermal spas and eight swimming pools, some of which were built during the city's occupation by the Turks over 400 years ago. The Celts, who occupied the area after the Romans, named the city Aquincum, a name probably derived from the Latin *aqua quinque,* meaning "five waters." A record dating from 1178 notes that a hospital was established at the foot of Gellért Hill, the site of an important medicinal spring that is now the location of the Gellért Hotel and Spa.[2] Most of the waters flowing into the spas in Budapest are rich in calcium chloride, sodium bicarbonate, and calcium bicarbonate, although sulfur-rich waters flow from a deep well on Margaret Island, just up the river from the Parliament building.

Bathing in mineral springs has also long been popular in Japan, where over 2,000 cold, warm, and hot springs can be found. Tradition says that people

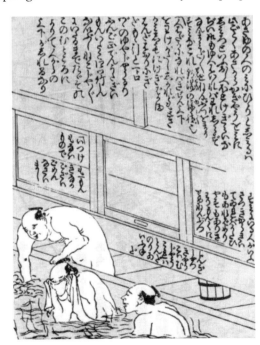

An old bathing scene, Japan.

have been acquainted with them since 700 B.C.E., with springs at Atami, Shuzenji, Suwa, and Dogo among the most ancient. Like those in Europe, many of the early Japanese medicinal springs were believed to be the abode of spiritual beings (known in Japan as *kami*), and their discovery, often by priests and other holy people, is often linked with spiritual vision and divine guidance. These discoveries were sometimes made with the help of animals regarded as messengers of the gods. For example, the discovery of the healing waters at Takeo on Kyushu Island was attributed to the empress Jingu, who came upon a white heron taking a bath in the warm waters.[3]

Many of the early Japanese springs were sponsored by rulers known as Daimyos. One Daimyo improved the bathing facilities at Domyo spa, building one room for the samurai (including the military noblemen and the priests), one room for women, and one for the general public. The popularity of hot springs in Japan was documented by early regional chronicles: the *Isumo Fudoki* reported that the Tamatsukuri Hot Spring, in Shimane Prefecture (known for its sodium bicarbonate and calcium sulfate waters), was extremely popular and that by "bathing once, the visitor was made fair of face and figure; bathing twice, all diseases were healed; its effectiveness has been obvious since the days of old."[4]

Native Americans have always considered mineral springs to be sacred healing grounds. Anthropological evidence uncovered at Lake Amatitlán near Guatemala City revealed that the Maya may have used thermal springs as early as 500 B.C.E. The Aztecs considered lakes, rivers, and springs to be the abodes of gods and goddesses. Because water was so highly regarded as essential to life in an area subject to frequent droughts, the mother of a newborn baby would often pray to these divinities for her child's protection and healing.[5] The hot springs in Central Mexico were important places of pilgrimage for Aztec priests and nobility; the warm healing waters at Agua Hedionda ("stinking water") near Cuautla in Morelos State were frequented by Montezuma and other Aztec leaders for both physical and spiritual renewal.

Farther north, the area now known as Hot Springs in Arkansas was originally called Valley of the Vapours, and was a sacred site of peace and healing for the Tunicas people. In 1541, the Spanish explorer Hernando DeSoto was the first European to visit these springs. He found it a place where members of warring tribes bathed, traded, and feasted in harmony.[6]

Many of the early North American hot springs were regarded sacred by native peoples who considered them gifts of the Great Spirit, who warmed them with his breath. As some tribes believed that the springs were the home of magical beings who could both heal and destroy, entering a hot spring was shrouded in ceremonial practice, and decorum and respect were observed by all who entered the healing waters. The springs at Saratoga were called Medicine Springs of the Great Manitou by the Mohawks, who considered them a gift of the Great Spirit. The Iroquois, Shawnee, and Tuscarora peoples often bathed together at Medicine Springs in what is now Bedford, Pennsylvania. In what is now Lake County, California, the Lake and Coast Miwok peoples used the present Harbin Hot Springs as a seasonal camp and sacred ground, with the hot springs both a place of healing and a path to the spiritual realms. According to Ellen Klages, writing in *Harbin Hot Springs: Healing Waters, Sacred Land:*

> To a shaman, the waters of a hot springs were an entrance way to the underworld. In a trance state, induced by meditating on such a point of entrance—a natural tunnel, rock crevasse or spring—a shaman could travel from the material world to the spirit realm. There he could talk to spirits and do healing work which, when returning to a non-trance state, be brought back to the people of his tribe. Since these natural openings to the spirit world are rare, the springs were considered to be a very special and sacred point in the already sacred material world.[7]

THE DECLINE AND REVIVAL OF TAKING THE WATERS

After the decline and fall of the Roman Empire, interest in bathing (especially communal bathing) declined. This was due in part to the Christian backlash against the widespread and notorious revelry that often took place at Roman springs, which included abundant wine, food, and occasional sexual activity.

Yet, toward the Middle Ages, bathing in medicinal springs made a comeback, with many of the present-day European spas tracing their early development from the fourteenth to the sixteenth centuries. We mentioned earlier that the word *spa* traces its origin to a mountain town near Liège in southern Belgium. Here a spring was used by an ironmaster in the fourteenth century to cure his rheumatism. He founded a health resort at the spring called Espa, meaning "fountain" in the Walloon language. Espa grew so popular that the word known in English as *spa* became the common designation for similar health resorts around the world.

In the present-day Czech Republic, popular legend relates that the famous Karlovy Vary springs were discovered by Charles IV, the king of Bohemia,

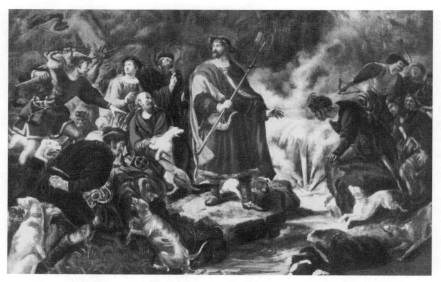

The discovery of the hot springs at Karlovy Vary by King Charles IV.

during a deer hunt in 1350. However, the founding of the town is probably the logical result of people arriving to the springs in search of a cure. From the Middle Ages until the first third of the sixteenth century, the cure at Karlovy Vary consisted of only one procedure: bathing. The popular drinking cure was introduced only after the physician Vaclav Payer published the first book about medical treatment at Karlovy Vary under the title *Tractatus de Thermis Caroll Quart Imperatoris* in 1522.

In Italy, an area rich in mineral springs, Ugolino wrote the famous treatise *De Balneis* in 1417, recommending the fabled mineral waters of Montecatini for the treatment of skin diseases, arthritis, and worms. France saw the development of numerous mineral springs, including those at Vichy and Bourbon-Lancy, and the English began to discover the famous mineral baths at Bath, Epsom, and Tunbridge Wells. The waters of Spa were not appreciated by scientists until 1737, the year *Demonstrations on the Usefulness of the Mineral Waters of Spa* was published.

During this time, the Japanese developed a growing appreciation for bathing in mineral springs, which were given names such as Meniyo (eye bath), Hiji-ori (elbow broken), and Tano-yu (ringworm bath) to identify their specific curative properties. By the seventeenth century, physicians from China and Japan began to evaluate and classify several medicinal springs, including those at Obama, Kinosaki, and Kusatsu. Goto Konzan, a doctor from Edo (now

Tokyo) initiated the first Japanese medical study of hot springs in 1709. Mineral water from Kusatsu was piped over 100 miles to Edo for the emperor's personal bath. After the founding of the Balneotherapy Institute in Beppu by Kyushu University in 1931, the Japanese began a more scientific and systematic research program in many parts of the country, and university research facilities were established at numerous hot springs throughout the country, including Beppu, Noboribetsu, Kirishima, and Kusatsu. By 1995, there were about 90 hospitals in spa stations in Japan, including 5 branch hospitals belonging to National Universities. In addition to pleasure and relaxation, hot springs in Japan are used therapeutically for the treatment of rheumatism; neuralgia; chronic diseases of the stomach, intestines, liver, and gallbladder; hypertension; skin diseases; and gout. People also go to hot springs after having undergone surgery or been through an accident.[8]

THE LEGENDARY EUROPEAN SPAS

By the seventeenth century, spas could be found throughout much of the European continent. Some of the most famous spas hosted many of Europe's "rich and famous," including a long and varied list of European royalty. Louis XIII, Anne of Austria, Cardinal Richelieu, and Louis XIV (and their numerous relatives and friends) enjoyed the waters of Bourbon-l'Archambault, Bourbon-Lancy, and Vichy in France, where they often spent the summer months. Napoleon

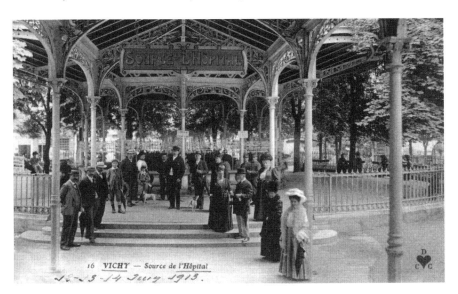

Enjoying the waters at Source de l'Hôpital, Vichy, circa 1913.

was said to have ridden his favorite horse into the healing waters at Piešťany Spa in Slovakia (Bulgarian Czar Ferdinand I used the Thermia Palace at Piešťany during the First World War as his headquarters), and Kaiser Wilhelm II was said to have plotted military strategy while staying at the springs of Baden-Baden. Among the variety of personalities who enjoyed the waters of Karlovy Vary were royalty such as Czar Peter the Great of Russia and King Edward VII of England, as well as the composers Wolfgang Amadeus Mozart and Ludwig von Beethoven.

This was also a time of increased interest in the medicinal value of mineral springs among scientists and physicians. During the eighteenth and nineteenth centuries, the waters of many European spas were meticulously studied and evaluated by chemists, and physicians developed specific protocols for patients with a variety of health disorders. During the nineteenth and early twentieth centuries, several important books about medical balneology were published. One such work was *The Principles and Practice of Medical Hydrology* (1913) by F. Fortescue Fox, M.D., the celebrated English balneologist who organized the International Society of Medical Hydrology in 1921, now the International Society of Medical Hydrology and Climatology (I.S.M.H.), with over 800 physician-members around the world.

During World War I, spas often became centers of hospitalization and convalescence for wounded servicemen. After the war, scientific interest in the medicinal value of spas increased, and chairs of hydrolgy and balneology were established at many medical schools. Over the years, an impressive amount of scientific and clinical evidence has been accumulated that testifies to the healing value of medicinal waters and related treatments, some of which is presented later in in this book. In Europe today, balneotherapy is considered an important part of mainstream medical practice in many countries, including France, Spain, Portugal, Luxembourg, Belgium, Germany, Austria, Italy, Greece, Turkey, the Czech Republic, Hungary, Poland, Romania, Slovenia, Slovakia, Russia, and other former Soviet republics. European physicians routinely refer their patients to spas for specialized treatments, which are often covered by national or private health insurance. European spas, some of which are affiliated with national universities and medical schools, are staffed by trained medical specialists under the careful supervision of the respective ministries of health.

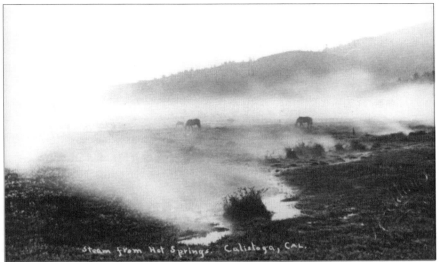

Early photograph showing steam from hot springs in Calistoga, California.
Reprinted courtesy of the Sharpsteen Museum Association, Calistoga, California.

SPRINGS AND SPAS IN NORTH AMERICA

We mentioned earlier that over 200 commercial hot springs and mineral springs can be found in the United States and Canada, along with thousands of smaller noncommercial springs. Interest in mineral springs developed soon after European colonists arrived in North America and learned about the many springs held sacred by the Native Americans in what are now Virginia, Pennsylvania, and New York. In addition to possessing a keen interest in trees and other plants, George Washington was fascinated by mineral springs. He first visited Berkeley Springs, West Virginia, in 1761, when he was 16 years old; later he returned to the healing springs when he was suffering from rheumatic fever at the age of 29. Berkeley Springs became a popular destination for others with this disorder. Washington first visited Saratoga Springs in 1783 and became so enamored with the waters and the land that he tried to purchase High Rock Springs from its owners.

Thomas Jefferson also was fascinated with hot springs and even designed the men's pool at Hot Springs, Virginia, in 1761. He devoted ten paragraphs to spas in his *Notes on the State of Virginia,* written in 1781 and 1782. He was a frequent guest at White Sulphur Springs, West Virgina (at that time, part of Virginia), and recommended that the Commonwealth of Virginia purchase the spring for public use.

Other early Americans who bathed in White Sulphur Springs included Daniel Webster, Davy Crockett, Francis Scott Key, John C. Calhoun, Henry Clay, and Presidents Martin Van Buren, John Tyler, Franklin Pierce, Millard Fillmore, and James Buchanan.[9, 10]

Many of the commercial springs enjoyed their heyday during the middle and latter parts of the nineteenth century, when thousands of city dwellers boarded steam trains and stage coaches and converged on spa towns every summer for several weeks of healing, entertainment, and relaxation. Many of the larger mineral springs resorts were modeled after the famous European spas, and they attracted their own variety of royalty, including presidents, writers, musicians, and artists. Some provided lavish entertainment, including theater, concerts, and costume parties; others offered more natural pleasures such as fishing, hunting, and boating.

Innovation was a major attraction at many spas. In addition to the latest healing modalities (the grape cure, first developed in Germany, was especially popular at the spas of Calistoga), new and novel forms of recreation were developed. The first golf course in the United States, for example, was built at White Sulphur Springs, West Virginia, in 1884.

Perhaps the most famous spa destination was Saratoga Springs in New York. In addition to political leaders such as the Marquis de Lafayette, Millard Fillmore, and James Buchanan, it attracted literary figures such as Robert Louis Stevenson, Edgar Allen Poe, and James Fenimore Cooper, who presumably found time to write while enjoying the myriad social and recreational activities offered at Saratoga Springs.

Several early North American hot springs were purchased by the federal government, the most famous being Hot Springs, Arkansas. As early as 1832, Congress set aside four sections of land there as a federal reservation. By 1878, over 3,500 people resided in the city of Hot Springs, which was attracting more than 50,000 visitors a year. Most of them had to endure a 12- to 14-hour trip by stagecoach from Little Rock, approximately 52 miles away. Featuring over a dozen bathhouses, each claiming to cure a specific disease, the springs were both inspected and regulated by the federal government. Though the springs attracted a wealthy clientele, bathing facilities were provided at no charge for the indigent; in 1911, over 220,000 persons bathed in the Free Bath House alone.

Some of the waters gained notoriety for healing venereal diseases, such as syphilis and gonorrhea. In 1918, the Division of Venereal Disease of the U.S. Public Health Service established a clinic and bathhouse hospital at Hot Springs, and treated people with mineral water, mercury, and the arsenical compound arsphenamine. With the development of penicillin in the early 1940s, the use of the waters at Hot Springs for treating venereal disease was abandoned.[11]

In 1896, the federal government signed a treaty with representatives of the Shoshone and Arapaho peoples in what is now Wyoming, allowing the Big Horn Spring at Thermopolis to be used by the general public. Rich in bicarbonate, sulfate, chloride, and sodium, this spring is now part of Hot Springs State Park, believed to be one of the largest hot spring complexes in the world. In times past, its waters attracted the likes of Buffalo Bill Cody, Butch Cassidy, and members of the notorious Hole in the Wall Gang.[12]

In addition to these large springs, literally hundreds of smaller spas opened in many parts of North America, including Virginia, West Virginia, Tennessee, North and South Carolina, Pennsylvania, and New England. As the Gold Rush and other economic opportunities attracted settlers to the West, additional hot springs in Colorado, Idaho, Oregon, New Mexico, and California were developed in the United States. Several Canadian springs were discovered and developed in Alberta and British Columbia, the most famous being the mineral springs in Banff, Alberta. With improved transportation after the conclusion of the Civil War, visits to spas increased tremendously, and even those in remote areas became accessible to city dwellers.

Physicians first began investigating the medicinal properties of North American mineral springs toward the end of the eighteenth century. The surgeon Samuel Tenney is believed to have been the first scientist to write about Saratoga Springs in 1783, and Samuel Latham Mitchell, destined to become one of the country's foremost early chemists, analyzed the Saratoga water in 1787, establishing its medicinal value scientifically. At the same time, Dr. Benjamin Rush, considered one of the most outstanding physicians of his time, dedicated a long paper to mineral springs in Pennsylvania, which created strong interest in the medicinal value of spring waters among fellow physicians.[13]

During the nineteenth century, chemists, physicians, and other researchers analyzed and classified the waters of hundreds of North American mineral and thermal springs. *On Baths and Mineral Waters,* written by the Philadelphia physician John Bell, stimulated scientific interest in mineral springs. During this time, numerous types of bathing were either developed or introduced from Europe: cold, warm, and hot showers; douches; sitz and vapor baths. By this time, doctors understood the therapeutic value of a natural environment, and adjunct therapies were often part of the bathing experience, including diet, relaxation, and exercise. In addition to boasting a variety of mineral springs

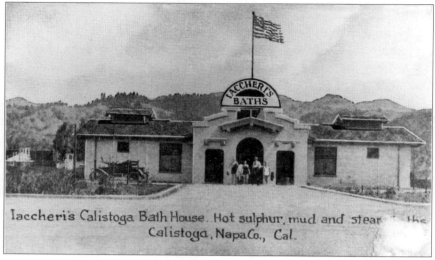

Iaccheri's Calistoga Bath House. Hot sulphur, mud and stear ' the Calistoga, Napa Co., Cal.

Iaccheri's bath house at Calistoga, California, featuring "hot sulphur, mud, and steam baths," circa 1925. Reprinted courtesy of the Sharpsteen Museum Association, Calistoga, California.

with "medicinal virtues applicable to every ill that flesh is heir to" along with an experienced physician in residence, the *Hand-Book of Calistoga Springs*, published in 1871, highlights a variety of other natural attractions, including "a spacious ornamental aviary, built on the lawn in front of the hotel, where will be gathered every species of the native wild birds of California . . . a large, well-appointed skating-rink, a natural steam-cooking spring, hunting grounds, an endless growth of roses and all garden flowers, and avenue drives of some seven miles on the premesis."[14]

Aside from the mineral and thermal springs themselves, interest in hydrotherapy increased tremendously in the United States during the nineteenth century, and by 1850, several hundred "water-cure" establishments had been set up throughout the eastern United States, including Lebanon Springs, New York; Brattleboro, Vermont; Lynn, Massachusetts; and Waterford, Maine. One of the largest overlooked Union Square in New York City. Under the direction of two hydrotherapists, one of whom had trained in Berlin, it contained 60 rooms and included a large plunge pool, a 25-foot-high cascading shower, two small plunge baths, and four small douches.

Hydrotherapy also attracted the interest of many physicians of the day, and facilities offering hydrotherapy were set up in numerous private, state, and federal hospitals to treat a wide range of diseases, including mental diseases and epilepsy. One of the most famous of these physicians was Dr. Simon Baruch, Professor of Balneology at the College of Physicians at Columbia University and an outstanding cardiologist. His *Use of Water in Modern Medicine,* published in 1893, became a classic. The Simon Baruch Research Institute, established at Saratoga Spa in 1933 and named in his honor, was the first institute for balneological research in the United States. Hydrotherapy became an established part of the medical mainstream by the 1900s, especially in the treatment of orthopedic problems. Facilities offering hydrotherapy were established at many well-known medical centers, including the Orthopedic Hospital in Los Angeles and Walter Reed Hospital in Washington, D.C. However, the most famous was the facility at Warm Springs, Georgia, which specialized in the treatment of polio. Franklin Delano Roosevelt was a frequent visitor to Warm Springs, where he found the exercise program known as hydrogymnastics highly beneficial.[15]

But by the end of the nineteenth century, many American spas had begun their decline, for various reasons. Fashion changed as vacationers, especially the rich and famous, shifted their interest to the newly established seaside resorts such as Atlantic City, New Jersey, and Newport, Rhode Island. In addition, the growth of scientific medicine made balneotherapy seem old-fashioned. Modern medications held out the promise for rapid cures of many chronic diseases, which seemed more attractive than several weeks of bathing and other water-related treatments. Because scientific proof of the curative value of spring waters was often scarce, few physicians remained convinced of their therapeutic value. In addition, unscrupulous charlatans made all sorts of unsubstantiated claims for hot springs bathing, and gradually the medical community and the general public lost interest in the curative value of spa therapy.

Nevertheless, Saratoga Springs attracted over 750,000 patients a year during the 1930s and 1940s. The construction of a magnificent new spa (advocated by Franklin Delano Roosevelt, the governor of New York before he was elected president in 1932) was completed in 1935, making Saratoga Spa the most complete government health facility in the country and one of the largest and best-equipped spas in the world, with the ability to treat over 4,500 patients a day. Under the direction of Walter S. McClellan, M.D., Associate Professor of Medicine at Albany Medical College, Saratoga Spa became a major center for balneology in the United States and educated many physicians in the benefits of this natural healing method.

The establishment in 1933 of the Baruch Institute at Saratoga Spa in the

United States held great promise. Unfortunately, the research center was dependent on funds from the state government from the time it opened. Although medical research was undertaken over the years, especially in cardiology and rheumatology, the center eventually closed its doors because of inadequate funding. The spa itself also suffered from major cuts in government funding (it has never been able to survive as a for-profit instutution), and attendance gradually declined.[16, 17] Today, many of its magnificent buildings stand abandoned, while others are used only partially. The beautiful Washington bathhouse was converted to a school, and a large portion of the Lincoln bathhouse, although still offering mineral baths to visitors, is rented to Saratoga County for courtrooms and offices.

While "taking the waters" remained popular in much of Europe and Japan, by the middle of the twentieth century both the American and the British public had lost interest in the medicinal value of mineral water and thermal springs, and many of the most important American spas closed: Manitou, Colorado; West Baden Springs, Indiana; Poland Spring, Maine; Siloam Springs, Missouri; Sharon Springs and Ballston Spa, New York; Panacea Mineral Springs, North Carolina; Bedford Springs, Pennsylvania; Buffalo Mineral Springs and Wyrick Springs, Virginia; and Capon Springs and Pence Springs, West Virginia. In Great Britain, once fashionable spa resorts such as Bath, Leamington Spa, Harrogate, Buxton, and Epsom lost their luster, and many former bathers either migrated to seaside resorts such as Blackpool and Brighton or "took the waters" in the spas of France, Germany, and Italy.

A major barrier to greater acceptance of the value of medicinal springs in the United States and Britain was the lack of objective scientific proof. The problem of proving scientifically that mineral and thermal waters produce specific healing effects was addressed by the British physician George Kersley, M.D. In an article about British spas in the *Journal of the Royal Society of Health,* he described a situation similar to the attitudes toward balneology in America:

> In England, however, especially in the 1930s, our super scientific outlook was suggesting that anything unproven did not exist and it was difficult to prove the efficacy of Spa treatment. To prove any specific effect, it would be necessary to treat thousands of patients in either spa or tap water, without their knowledge and would be therefore barely ethical.[18]

It has been said that the popularity of spas in the United States and Canada goes in cycles. After many years of popularity followed by many years of decline, a resurgence of interest in spas is now taking place, as seen by the popularity of spas such as the Greenbrier in West Virginia, the Homestead in Virginia, Calistoga in California, Hot Springs in Arkansas, and others. In addition to the healing waters themselves, modern spas offer services such as massage, aromatherapy, recreation, and extensive programs for beauty care and personal fitness. As more and more people pursue healthy lifestyles and choose natural forms of health care for themselves and their families, the popularity of hot springs and mineral springs for the prevention and treatment of disease will undoubtedly increase.

Nevertheless, North American and British spas have a distinct disadvantage when compared with European and Japanese spas: the absence of medical supervision caused by an almost complete lack of interest in balneotherapy among members of the medical community. While many European spas offer an extensive range of safe, effective, medically supervised therapies that can treat a wide range of health problems, the vast majority of spas in the United States and Canada are used only for relaxation and recreation. And although the mineral waters of many North American spas rank with the best of those in Europe, medical claims cannot be made for them.

This issue was addressed by Dr. Henry Sigerist in a talk presented at the Johns Hopkins University medical history club. Noting that thousands of Americans take health treatments at European spas every year, he outlined several priorities that could bring the use of North American spas in line with European standards:

- Insistence on the necessity of research.

- Provision of teaching facilities at major medical schools, including the creation of a chair for balneotherapy.

- Creation of a literature. Very few scientific books or research papers concerning balneotherapy have been written in the United States. (The vast majority of information presented in this book has been drawn from European and Japanese medical literature.)

- Organization of an American Society for the Science of Health Resorts (or whatever it may be called) to develop research in health resort medicine (now a function of the International Society of Medical Hydrology and Climatology).

- Organization of an American Association of Health Resorts that can be a central source of information about spas for both physicians and the public.

- A broadly conceived social program that would make American health resorts accessible to a larger percentage of the public. (Unlike many countries in Europe, health insurance and social security in the United States do not provide for spa treatments, placing balneotherapy out of the reach of most people.)

In his address, Dr. Sigerist concluded, "America is blessed with all curative forces nature can provide. It is up to us to use them intelligently for the benefit of the people."[19]

Sigerist offered these modest proposals in November 1941. In our own day, at a time of an aging population, along with an increase in degenerative disease and stress-related health problems, the needs he addressed are more important than ever before.

PART II

JUST WHAT'S
IN THAT WATER?

Nature has blessed humanity with a tremendous variety of healing springs, many of them located in some of the most beautiful natural settings on earth. Although our ancestors enjoyed bathing in and drinking medicinal waters since the dawn of human history, researchers did not begin to scientifically analyze their properties until four to five hundred years ago.

The following section examines the different types of waters (such as sulfur springs, radioactive springs, and iron springs) and their documented therapeutic effects on different organs of the body, such as the heart, liver, and skin. We also highlight specific therapies that often complement the use of each type (or types) of water, such as physical therapy and mud baths. At the end of each chapter, we offer a representative list of springs you can visit, which are described in detail in part 4.

BICARBONATE

Bicarbonate is a salt resulting from the incomplete neutralization of carbonic acid or the passing of excess carbon dioxide into a solution with a base. Many of these waters contain carbon dioxide, nitrogen, and oxygen and are often bubbly. There are two kinds of bicarbonate: sodium bicarbonate and calcium bicarbonate. Bicarbonate is a natural component of blood and is essential for proper digestion, metabolism, and overall functioning. The amount present is an indicator of the body's alkaline reserve, which keeps the body's acids in check.

Many bicarbonated mineral waters are rich in carbonic gas. In Spain, water is considered carbonic if it contains 250 milligrams per liter of free carbon gas. These waters are distinguished by their slightly acidic taste and their bubbly essence. Some of the world's favorite mineral waters, including Apollinaris, Badoit, Mattoni, Vichy San Yorré, Vichy Celestins, and Ferrarelli, naturally contain large amounts of both bicarbonate and carbonic gas. Other famous waters, such as Calistoga, Poland Spring, and Perrier, are artificially carbonated with carbon dioxide for drinking.

DRINKING

Water rich in bicarbonate stimulates the appetite and increases the secretion of the gastric juices necessary for proper digestion. Physicians recommend drinking small amounts (perhaps half a glass) of carbonated water an hour before mealtimes, and suggest drinking these waters during meals instead of ordinary table water.

At many European spas, such as Bad Ems in Germany, Mariánské Lázně in the Czech Republic, and Châtel-Guyon in France, drinking water rich in bicarbonate is one of the primary methods for treating patients with gastric disorders such as chronic dyspepsia, gastric ulcer, problems following stomach and duodenal operations, intestinal conditions (especially constipation and spastic colon), chronic ulcerative colitis, and irritable colon. These waters also have a positive

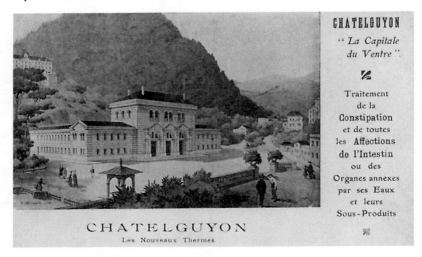

Early publicity card featuring the new thermal establishment at Châtel-Guyon,
"The Intestinal Capital," circa 1910.

effect on patients with diabetes, chronic recurring pancreatitis, and bile duct
conditions caused by hepatitis and other diseases.

The recommended amount of mineral water varies according to the spa
and the patient. At the famous Institute of Rheumatology and Physiotherapy
in Budapest, a 1,400-bed medical facility serving especially patients with muscle
and joint pain, a typical protocol recommends the consumption of 200 milliliters of medicinal water per day.

The numerous therapeutic effects of the drinking cure are based primarily
on the action of the dissolved salts in the water that finds its way into the
alimentary system. These salts influence the rate of absorption, secretion, and
excretion of the stomach, liver, gallbladder, pancreas, and intestines. Bicarbonate and other salts have anti-inflammatory and antispasmodic effects on the
gastrointestinal tract and relieve gastric and intestinal dyspepsia, normalize
bowel function, and promote restoration of kidney and liver function (including
bile synthesis and evacuation of the gallbladder). Drinking bicarbonate-rich
water has been clinically found to bring about these following benefits:

- It helps regulate the antiseptic activity of bile acids, which facilitate the
  digestion of fats.

- It also gently stimulates the pancreas, which activates the secretion of
  pancreatic juice—vital for proper digestion of proteins—into the small
  intestine.

- It helps regulate peristalsis, a wavelike movement in the alimentary tract. This enables the food to move more easily through the alimentary canal toward the stomach.

- It improves carbohydrate and fat metabolism.
- It assists the utilization of blood sugar by the body, resulting in lowered blood sugar levels in persons with diabetes.[1-4]

BATHING

Bathing in bicarbonate-rich water is especially popular in France and Germany, where the medically recommended protocol is a bath of 10 to 20 minutes at a temperature of 30–35°C (86–95°F). As a vasodilator, this water helps open the peripheral blood vessels of the body and improves circulation, especially to the extremities. It is also recommended for people with hypertension and moderate atherosclerosis; however, those with chronic cardiac insufficiency, hypertensive nephritis, and other forms of severe heart and circulatory disease should take warm bicarbonate baths only under the direction of a licensed health professional.

According to the noted balneologist Dr. Sigmund Forster, Professor Emeritus of Rehabilitative Medicine at the State University of New York College of Medicine in Brooklyn, carbon dioxide baths are especially recommended for the treatment of cardiovascular diseases, nervous exhaustion, and autonomic nervous system imbalance. He recommends a protocol involving three to five baths a week in water heated to 35–38°C (95–100°F) for 5 to 15 minutes, depending on the patient's needs and condition, for a total of ten to fifteen treatments per cure.[5]

Although water rich in bicarbonate can do much to help alleviate these health problems, physicians recommend that this type of water therapy should be considered as only one part of a holistic approach to health. Many diseases of the alimentary tract, such as constipation, peptic ulcer, and spasmodic colon, can be traced to emotional and physical stress. Similarly, stress, insufficient exercise, and diets high in fat and carbohydrates contribute to many gallbladder problems. Doctors have found a strong correlation between obesity and diabetes. For these reasons, proper diet, stress reduction, and exercise are often used as major complements to water therapy and have been clinically proven to promote long-term benefits.

Some Springs Rich in Bicarbonates

Argentina: Cachueta, Los Molles, Pismanta, Río Hondo, Rosario de la Frontera
Australia: Hepburn Springs, Moree

Austria: Bad-Deutch-Altenburg, Bad Gastein, Bad Goisern, Bad Hofgastein, Bad Shellerbach, Bad Tatzmannsdorf, Warmbad-Villach

Belgium: Chaudfontaine, Spa

Brazil: Caxambú, Poços de Caldas, São Lourenço, São Pedro

Bulgaria: Albena, Banya, Blagoevgrad, Hissarya, Kyustendil, Pavel Banya

Canada: Banff, Radium Hot Springs, Miette Hot Springs

Chile: Termas de Chillán

Colombia: Paipa

Cuba: San Miguel de los Baños, Santa Fe

Czech Republic: Františkovy Lázně, Jáchymov, Karlovy Vary, Lázně Poděbrady, Mariánské Lázně

Ecuador: El Tingo, Guapán, Guitig

Finland: Poorvo

France: Aix-les-Bains, Amélie-les-Bains, Barbotan, Bourbon-Lancy, Evian, Vichy, Vals, Royat-Chamalières, Châtel-Guyon, La Bourboulle, Ax-les-Thermes, La Roche-Posay

Germany: Bad Ems, Bad Homburg, Bad Kissingen, Bad Nauheim, Bad Wildbad

Hungary: Balatonfüred, Bükfürdo, Budapest, Hajdúszoboszló, Harkány, Héviz

Italy: Agnano Terme, Castrocaro Terme, Chianciano Terme, Montecatini Terme

Japan: Hakone, Narugo, Nikko Yumoto, Shiobara, Shirahama, Yugawara

Mexico: Ixtapán de la Sal, San José de Porúa, Tehuacán

New Zealand: Hamner Springs

Peru: Chancos, Monterrey, Yura

Poland: Cieplice Slaskie-Zdrój, Krynica, Kudowa, Polanica-Zarój

Portugal: Caldas do Geres, Furnas, Pedras Salgadas, Chaves

Romania: Băile Felix, Băile Herculane, Călimăneşti, Geoagiu Bai, Sovata

Russia: Essentuki, Kislovodsk, Pyatigorsk, Repino, Zheleznododsk

Slovakia: Čiz, Sliač

Slovenia: Moravske Toplice, Rogaška

Spain: Alhama de Aragón, Caldes de Malavalla, Jaraba

Taiwan: Peitou, Chipen, Wulai

Turkey: Bursa, Izmir-Balcova, Izmir-Çesme, Pamukkale

United States: Desert Hot Springs and Palm Springs, California; Saratoga Springs, New York; Hot Springs, Arkansas; Truth or Consequences, New Mexico; Hot Springs, South Dakota; Berkeley Springs, West Virginia; Thermopolis, Wyoming

Venezuela: Las Trincheras

SULFUR AND SULFATES

SULFUR

Sulfur springs abound wherever there is volcanic activity, although they can also be found in areas that are not highly volcanic. Sulfur springs contain free hydrogen sulfide, sulfurated alkaline metals, and their secondary products. They are easily identified by the strong aroma of the hydrogen sulfide gas emanating from the springs.

Sulfur springs assist in healing in several important ways. The gas itself is strongly antibacterial and also stimulates the mucous membranes, thus promoting expectoration. Breathing the vapors of waters rich in sulfur can help relieve problems of the nasal passages and the respiratory passages, including chronic bronchial catarrh. Such inhalations are known as phlegm baths in Japan and are often accomplished by bathing in the warm sulfur springs and breathing in the vapors for a prescribed amount of time.

People have long bathed in sulfur-rich waters to relieve a wide variety of health problems, including liver, digestive, and urinary conditions; chronic metallic poisoning; chronic skin diseases; scrofula; and even venereal diseases such as syphilis. It is also believed that the warmer the water, the greater the therapeutic benefits. In France, such waters are prescribed for treating gynecological problems, skin diseases, disorders of the respiratory passages, and rheumatism.[1-4]

After sulfur-rich waters reach the surface of the earth, they assist the formation of a variety of microorganisms, algae, and bacteria that are cultured and used therapeutically in the form of mud applications. In a full-body mud bath, a person's body is submerged, except the head, in a bathtub filled with warm mud for 15 or 20 minutes. Therapeutic mud may also be applied only to affected parts of the body. Mud made with sulfur-rich water is popular for treating both skin diseases and rheumatism, especially in France, Italy, and Japan.

Some Springs with Sulfurous Water

Argentina: Copahué, Los Molles

Austria: Baden bei Wien

Brazil: Araxá, Poços de Caldas, São Pedro

France: Aix-les-Bains, Ax-les-Thermes, Amélie-les-Bains, Luchon,
    Eugénie-les-Bains, Enghien-les-Bains

Germany: Bad Eilsen, Bad Herzburg, Bad Nenndorf

Great Britain: Harrogate

Israel: Ein Bokek, Ein Gedi, Tiberias

Italy: Acqui Terme, Castrocaro Terme, Sirmione Terme

Japan: Beppu, Katsuura, Tamagawa, Uizen, Yunomine

Mexico: Agua Hedionda

Portugal: Caldas da Rainha, Monte Real, São Padro do Sul

Romania: Băile Felix, Băile Herculane, Călimăneşti, Sovata

Spain: Archena

Switzerland: Bad Schinznach

Taiwan: Peitou, Yangmingshan

United States: Calistoga, Desert Hot Springs, and Palm Springs, California;
    Hot Springs, Virginia

SULFATES

Sulfates owe their chemical composition to sulfur, but in a form that renders it barely useful. The value of sulfates depends on their presence in one or more of the following chemical compounds:

Calcium sulfate is very soothing to the body overall; when ingested, it stimulates the secretion of bile and aids digestion. It has been used clinically in treating kidney disorders and certain metabolic diseases.

Sodium sulfate also stimulates bile secretion when ingested; it has a positive effect on problems relating to the liver and the bile ducts.

Magnesium sulfate has similar actions when ingested orally; when we bathe in waters rich in this compound, it soothes and tightens the skin while allowing the skin to retain moisture.

Sulfated waters result from the dissolution of underground salt deposits and other deposits containing calcium sulfate, sodium sulfate, and magnesium sulfate. For this reason, sulfated waters may contain a combination of these compounds in varying amounts, which will influence their medicinal value.

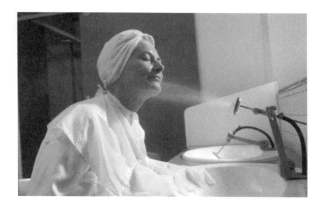

Inhaling mineral water as mist. Photo courtesy of Thermes de La Roche-Posay.

Because these waters change their chemical composition when exposed to air, they are most beneficial when used at or near the spring.

The diseases that are treated with sulfated waters include chronic infections of the respiratory tract, such as laryngitis, rhinopharyngitis, bronchial catarrh, and bronchial asthma; skin diseases, such as chronic eczema; rheumatism and other problems of the locomotor system; postoperative conditions relating to the locomotor system; and gynecological troubles.

Drinking sulfated waters to treat liver and gastrointestinal conditions is very popular in European spas, especially those whose waters also contain sodium bicarbonate. A typical prescription involves ingesting 50–200 milliliters of water (depending on the mineral content of the water and the patient's condition) two or three times on an empty stomach, usually before breakfast. If tolerated, this can be supplemented by another glass of water 1 or 2 hours before lunch and dinner.

Inhaling these waters in the form of a fine mist is often accomplished by breathing mineral water mist produced by a special misting device or with the aid of a nebulizer similar to the kind used by asthmatic persons. In European spas, this is done under the supervision of a qualified health professional. Depending on the needs of the patient, sulfated waters are also administered as douches or enemas to treat gynecological problems or gastrointestinal complaints, respectively.

Some Springs with Waters Rich in Sulfates

Argentina: Copahué, Los Molles, Pismanta, Reyes, Río Hondo, Rosario de la Frontera
Australia: Hepburn Springs

Austria: Bad-Deutch-Altenburg, Baden bei Wien, Bad Gastein, Bad
  Gosern, Bad Hofgastein
Belgium: Chaudfontaine
Brazil: Araxá, Poços de Caldas, Serra Negra
Bulgaria: Banya, Blagoevgrad, Kyustendil, Sophia
Canada: Harrison Hot Springs, Banff, Radium Hot Springs
Chile: Panimávida, Palguín
Colombia: Paipa, Tabio
Cuba: Ciego Montero, El Cedrón, Elguea, San Diego de los Baños
Czech Republic: Františkovy Lázně, Karlovy Vary, Mariánské Lázně
Ecuador: Papallacta
France: Aix-les-Bains, Amélie-les-Bains, Bagnères-de-Bigorre, Dax,
  Enghien-les-Bains, Eugénie-les-Bains, Vittel
Germany: Bad Bertrich, Bad Eilsen, Bad Harzburg, Bad Nenndorf,
  Hindelang
Great Britain: Bath, Cheltenham
Hungary: Budapest
Israel: Ein Gedi, Hamme Zohar, Tiberias
Italy: Bagni di Lucca, Chianciano Terme, Ischia Terme, Montecatini
  Terme, San Pellegrino Terme
Japan: Atami, Hakone, Katsuura, Kusatsu, Narugo, Nikko Yumoto,
  Noboribetsu, Tamagawa
Luxembourg: Mondorf
Mexico: Agua Hedionda, Ixtapán de la Sal, Tehuacán
Netherlands: Nieueschans
New Zealand; Hamner Springs, Rotorua
Peru: Baños del Inca
Poland: Ciechocinek
Portugal: Caldas da Rainha, Caldas do Geres, Termas da Curia, Monte Real
Romania: Baile Herculane
Russia: Kislovodsk, Zheleznovodsk
Slovakia: Pieštany, Sliač, Trenčianské Teplice
Spain: Ledesma, Peralta, Carabana, Santa Fé, Cofrentes, Cestoma
Switzerland: Bad Scoul-Tarasp-Vulpera, Baden, Leukerbad, Rheinfelden
Taiwan: Peitou, Chipen, Wulai, Yangminshan
Turkey: Bursa, Izmir-Çesme, Yalova
United States: Berkeley Springs and White Sulphur Springs, West Virginia;
  Hot Springs, South Dakota; Thermopolis, Wyoming
Venezuela: Aguas Calientes

6

CHLORIDE

Waters rich in chlorides are found throughout the world. Also popularly known as salt waters or muriated waters, they are primarily rich in sodium chloride (although they may contain other chlorides as well as other chemical compounds) and contain a high salt content, often derived from subterranean deposits of rock salt or sandstone containing sodium chloride. In years past, salt was often extracted from these waters to provide table salt.

Sodium is often considered to be the least popular of minerals, because many cardiologists recommend low-sodium diets for their patients. Nevertheless, sodium is an essential component in many body fluids, such as blood, tears, and perspiration. Chloride helps regulate fluids both in and out of the body cells, it facilitates the digestion of food and the body's absorption of nutrients, and it helps transmit nerve impulses to and from the brain.[1]

However, many of us consume excessive amounts of salt in our food. In addition to condiments such as table salt and soy sauce, small amounts of sodium are contained in a variety of foods, including cheese, eggs, celery, green leafy vegetables, apples, berries, and nuts.

Sodium chloride is a major component of many mineral springs, known as saline springs. It either is derived from a former sea (such as the water at Saratoga Springs) or is the result of water filtering through rock formations that contain sodium.

While drinking mineral water rich in sodium chloride is not recommended for those on low-sodium diets, salt waters are often recommended for bathing because they possess a variety of medicinal properties. According to Dr. Sigmund Forster, saline waters (ideally containing 0.5 percent to 3 percent sodium) at a temperature of 34–40°C (93–104°F) are indicated for treating rheumatic disorders, arthritis, central nervous system and peripheral nerve diseases, and posttraumatic, orthopedic, and postoperative disorders as well as gynecological diseases. Normally, three to five 10- to 25-minute baths a week are recommended, for a total of 15 to 20 treatments per cure.[2]

The chemical composition of many chloride springs is similar to that of seawater because some of these waters are derived from former oceans and prehistoric inland seas. In years past, the Great Salt Lake in Utah was renowned for its therapeutic saline waters (by the early 1900s, over a hundred bath-houses could be found along its shoreline), and it gained special mention in *Mineral Springs of North America* (it was described as a "wonderful saline reser-voir") by J. J. Moorman, M.D.[3]

One of the most famous salt water areas is the Dead Sea (Yam HaMelah) in Israel, an inland sea containing more than 30 percent salt (the Atlantic Ocean contains approximately 3 or 4 percent salt). Containing high concentrations of chlorides of sodium, calcium, sodium, and potassium, the Dead Sea has been renowned for its healing properties since Biblical times, when King Herod the Great used these thermal waters for relaxation and healing. Today, several famous Dead Sea resorts, including those at Ein Bokek, Hamme Zohar, and Ein Gedi, provide a wide variety of spa treatments and are considered the finest spas in the Mediterranean. These spas are extremely popular for the treatment of skin diseases, asthma and other respiratory problems, and joint disorders. The therapeutic mud there is widely used for beauty and cosmetic applications.

Waters with especially high concentrations of sodium chloride are also known as brine waters, and numerous spas in Europe offer brine bathing in naturally cold water. These include Rheinfelden and Bex in Switzerland, Ischl in Austria, Salsomaggiore in Italy, and Droitwich and Woodhall in England. Several European spas also offer thermal bathing in brine water: Wiesbaden and Baden-Baden in Germany, Montecatini in Italy, and Salins-les-Bains and Bourbonne-les-Bains in France. Saratoga Spa in New York and Glenwood Hot Springs in Colorado are perhaps the best-known chloride-rich springs in the United States.

Bathing in and drinking these waters is believed to help heal certain children's diseases, including hypotrophy (the progressive wasting away of cells and tissues), respiratory infections, and enuresis (involuntary urination). In adults, these waters are used to help heal diseases of the central and peripheral nervous systems, skin problems, and gynecological disorders. Bathing in these waters is also popular among those who have recently been in accidents or who have undergone surgery on the joints. These waters are considered valu-able when used with physical therapy, as well as in inhalation therapy, show-ers, and irrigations. Mild chloride waters are popular for drinking and are believed to increase the appetite, improve digestion, and relieve constipation.[4–7]

Some Spas Rich in Chlorides

Argentina: Cachueta, Los Molles, Río Hondo

Austria: Bad Aussi, Baden bei Wien, Bad Gleichenburg, Bad Hall, Bad Ischl, Salzburg

Belgium: Oostend

Bulgaria: Albena

Canada: Harrison Hot Springs

Chile: Panimávida, Huife, Palguín, Puyehue

Colombia: Paipa

Croatia: Lipik

Cuba: Amaro, Ciego Montero, Elguea

Czech Republic: Františkovy Lázně, Karlovy Vary

Ecuador: Baños (Azuay), El Tingo, Guapán, Guitig, Santa Elena, Tumbaco

France: Balaruc-les-Bains, Bourbon-Lancy, Bourbonne-les-Bains, Bourbonne-l'Archambault, La Bourboulle, Châtel-Guyon, Luchon, St. Honoré, Royat, Salins-les-Bains

Germany: Bad Ems, Baden-Baden, Bad Kissingen, Bad Orb, Bad Pyrmont, Bad Reichenhall, Bad Salzuflen, Bad Wildbad, Bad Kreuznach, Wiesbaden

Great Britain: Cheltenham, Droitwich, Leamington Spa, Llandrindod, Woodhall

Greece: Aedipsos, Icaria, Loutraki, Thermopylae

Hungary: Budapest, Hajdúszoboszló

Iceland: Hveragerdi

Israel: Hamme Zohar, Tiberias

Italy: Castrocaro Terme, Ischia Terme, Monetcatini Terme, Salice Terme, Salsomaggiore Terme

Jamaica: Milk River

Japan: Arima, Beppu, Hakone, Ibusuki, Ito, Kusatsu, Shiobara, Shirahama, Tamagawa

Luxembourg: Mondorf

Mexico: Ixtapán de la Sal, San José de Porúa, Tehuacán

New Zealand: Hamner Springs, Miranda Hot Springs

Peru: Chancos, Monterrey

Poland: Busko-Zdrój, Ciechocinek, Kolobrzeg

Portugal: Caldas da Rainha, Termas dos Cucos, Termas de Luzo

Romania: Băile Olănești

Russia: Essentuki, Sochi

Slovakia: Bardejov

Slovenia: Radenci, Rogaška

Spain: Arteojo, Caldas de Montbui, Caldas de Malavella, Fitero

Switzerland: Bad Scoul-Tarasp-Vulpera, Baden, Bex, Bad Ragaz, Rheinfelden, Yverdon-les-Bains

Turkey: Izmir-Balcova, Izmir-Çesme, Yalova

United States: Saratoga Springs, New York; Hot Springs, Arkansas; Desert Hot Springs and Palm Springs, California; Truth or Consequences, New Mexico; Glenwood Springs, Colorado; Thermopolis, Wyoming

GASES

Either one of two types of gas may appear in some mineral waters: carbon dioxide or radon. While at first glance, one would imagine that these waters are dangerous, they can be, in fact, highly medicinal.

CARBON DIOXIDE

Carbon dioxide is generally produced through the combustion, decomposition, or fermentation of carbon or its compounds. Carbon dioxide, a normal component of the air we breathe, is exhaled by the lungs, as well as through urine and perspiration. Once in the atmosphere, it is also used by green plants, which transform carbon dioxide into oxygen.

In small quantities (up to about 5 percent), carbon dioxide stimulates breathing. It also has the ability to help dilate the arteries, and it helps increase peripheral blood circulation.[1] In some spas in France, carbon dioxide gas (which is found naturally in wells) is injected subcutaneously. According to Dr. Michel Boulangé, this method has positive effects on the blood flow in the arteries that nourish the heart.[2]

The most respected French spa for the treatment of heart disease and circulatory problems is Royat-Chamalières, located in the Auvergne region. Its mineral waters contain a large amount of carbon dioxide, which is used therapeutically in bathing. The gas is also extracted from the springs to be used in injections and in carbon dioxide bagging, which involves placing an airtight plastic bag around an affected limb and injecting carbon dioxide and oxygen into the bag. Over the past 50 years, an extensive amount of research has been carried out to verify the therapeutic actions of the carbon dioxide at Royat-Chamalières, which include the following:

- vasodilating properties, the result both of bathing in the waters, and of regional vasodilation through subcutaneous carbon dioxide gas injections or through bagging with dry carbon dioxide gas

- an overall calming effect on the autonomic nervous system, which can reduce vascular spasms in particular

- a direct effect on the heart, both producing a slowdown of the pulse rate and strengthening heart contractions

- an ability to help the body produce new blood vessels, thus increasing blood circulation[3]

Carbon dioxide is found in many lightly mineralized waters, especially those containing bicarbonates. In addition to their light mineralization, these waters are carbonated, meaning that they are characterized by tiny bubbles of carbon dioxide, and tend to be cold rather than warm or hot. They are also popular for both drinking and bathing.

Perhaps the best-known springs in the United States containing carbon dioxide are those in Saratoga Springs, and treatments involving carbon dioxide waters have been popular for treating people with circulatory disorders.

Under the direction of Walter McClellan, M.D., who was appointed Associate Professor of Medicine at what was then the Albany Medical College, extensive research was carried out at Saratoga Spa on the effects of the carbon dioxide–rich mineral water on the human body. His studies found that Saratoga water was especially useful in treating people with arthritis and other joint diseases and also helped cardiovascular patients.

One of his first studies was undertaken in 1932 on the effects of mineral water baths and blood pressure of persons with hypertension. The results showed a significant drop in blood pressure after a series of mineral water baths. Other research followed. The cardiovascular benefits of Saratoga's waters were described by Grace Maguire Swanner, M.D., a former medical consultant to the spa, in her book *Saratoga: Queen of Spas:*

> This careful research has established the fact that the carbon dioxide gas in the mineral water, absorbed through the skin, has a cardiotonic effect on the circulatory system very comparable to that of digitalis. It was noted that cardiac patients, following the program of treatment at the Spa with carbon dioxide waters, showed clinical improvement in their ability to exercise without producing pain, or other evidence of coronary embarrassment. Clinical observations over the years support the conclusion, obtained in similar waters in Europe, that these patients do indeed experience real improvement.[4]

These findings led Simon Baruch, M.D., Professor of Balneology at the College of Physicians and Surgeons at Columbia University in New York City, and a medical consultant at Saratoga Spa, to develop a holistic program designed to treat patients with cardiovascular disease. His program was based on one used at Bad Nauheim in Germany involving bathing, diet, exercise, rest, and recreation.

The bathing phase of this treatment involved a 5-minute bath at 34°C (94°F) with a small amount of carbon dioxide in the water, which was regulated by adding warm water to the spring water and mixing it manually. After three baths, the bathing time was increased to 10 minutes at 15 to 20 percent carbon dioxide saturation. Toward the end of the course of therapy, which normally involved 18 to 20 baths, the bathing time was increased to 15 to 20 minutes at 30°C (86°F), and carbon dioxide saturation was increased to 40 percent. According to a brochure describing the cardiovascular cure at Saratoga:

> The cutaneous circulation is highly stimulated without provoking undesirable thermic reaction, congestion is relieved and the labor of the heart greatly lessened because of the better distribution and more active movement of the blood throughout the body. The skin is excited to increased eliminative and respiratory activity, thus lessening the labor of the kidneys.[5]

While the Saratoga cardiovascular cure is no longer available at the spa, one can still bathe in its carbon dioxide–rich waters. For those with cardiovascular and circulatory problems who wish to undergo spa therapy, balneologists recommend the following spas for the healing powers of their carbon dioxide waters, their medical facilities, and their competent medical staff: Royat-Chamalières in France, Balatonfüred in Hungary, Rogaška in Slovenia, and Pyatigorsk and Zheleznovodsk in Russia.

Some Springs Rich in Carbon Dioxide

Australia: Daylesford, Hepburn Springs
Austria: Bad Gleichenburg, Bad Tatzmannsdorf
Brazil: Lambari, Lindoia, São Lourenço
France: Balaruc-les-Bains, La Bourboulle, Châtel-Guyon, Royat-
    Chamalières, St. Honoré, Vichy, Vittel
Germany: Bad Ems, Bad Homburg, Bad Kissingen, Bad Orb, Bad
    Pyrmont, Bad Salzuflen, Bad Wildungen
Great Britain: Bath, Buxton
Hungary: Balatonfüred
Iceland: Hvergerdi
Italy: Agnano Terme, Chianciano Terme, Recoaro Terme
Japan: Narugo, Nikko Yumoto, Shirahama

Peru: Yura
Portugal: Termas da Curia, Pedras Salgadas, Termas de Vidago
Russia: Pyatigorsk, Zheleznovodsk
Slovenia: Rogaška, Šmarješke Toplice
Spain: Ledesma
Switzerland: Bad Scoul-Tarasp-Vulpera, Rheinfelden
United States: Saratoga Springs, New York; Vichy Hot Springs, California

RADON

Some hot springs have radioactive elements in their waters derived from trace amounts of radium. In Japan, for example, a spring is considered to have radio-activity if it contains over 8.25 Mache units (3×10^{-9} curies) of radon (radium emanation) per kilogram of water.

Radon is a radioactive inert gas that has a very short life. It is normally found in soil, rock, and water. In the United States today, radon is highly controversial. Easily absorbed by the body (especially by the respiratory passages, the skin, and the digestive system), radon is recognized as a carcinogen by the United States Environmental Protection Agency (EPA) and has been linked to lung cancer, especially among smokers. Many Americans test for radon in their houses, where it usually emanates from the soil and rock underneath the building. It is also found in well water and building materials.

Radon treatments were given by physicians in the United States and other countries before it was found to be carcinogenic. However, bathing in water containing small amounts of radon gas is used by many European spas to treat a wide range of health problems, including rheumatic diseases, gout, neuralgia, dermatosis, gynecological problems, and diabetes. Chronic digestive problems, gallstones, bronchial asthma, and fatigue have been treated by ingesting water or inhaling humid air or steam containing radon, which also has strong analgesic effects.[6,7]

One of the most unusual treatment centers using radon gas is at the Badgastein-Bockstein-Thermalstollen Spa in Austria, the home of the famous Gastein cure. After a thorough examination at a clinic known as the Stollen-kurhaus, patients don bathing suits and are transported by electric train through a former gold mine 2 miles within Radhaus Mountain. During the trip, the train passes through four chambers containing radon gas at progressively higher temperatures. Accompanied by a team of physicians, the passengers inhale the humid air and rest at different stages of the journey. This therapy is often combined with thermal bathing at the nearby spas of Bad Gastein and Bad

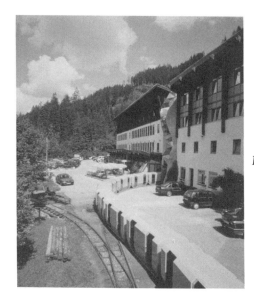

*The train to the Gastein curative
gallery, Bad Hofgastein, Austria.
Photo courtesy of Foto Wolkersdorfer,
Bad Hofgastein, Austria.*

Hofgastein. Indications for treatment at Bad Gastein include rheumatism, rheumatoid arthritis, ankylosing spondylitis, vascular diseases, diseases of the endocrine system, metabolic imbalances, diseases of the mouth, and geriatric conditions.[8]

According to Dr. Sigmund Forster, bathing in water containing radon is useful for treating a wide variety of health problems, including rheumatic disorders; arthritis; central nervous system and peripheral nerve diseases; posttraumatic, orthopedic, and postoperative disorders; gynecological disorders; skin diseases; and cardiovascular disorders. He recommends three to six baths weekly lasting 8 to 15 minutes each in water heated to 35–38°C (95–100°F), for 15 to 20 treatments per cure.[9]

Although radon treatments in Europe are normally approved by the respective Ministries of Health, more studies need to be done concerning the long-term safety of radon exposure in medicinal springs. If you have been subjected to long-term radon exposure in your home, or if you were given radon treatments as a child in the 1950s and 1960s, you may want to avoid bathing in radon springs.

Some Springs That Emit Radon Gas

Argentina: Los Molles, Pismanta
Austria: Bad Gastein, Bad Hofgastein, Warmbad-Villach
Brazil: Aguas de Prata, Araxá, Caxambú, Lambari, Lindoia, Serra Negra

Bulgaria: Hissarya, Pavel Banya, Velingrad

Colombia: Tabio

Croatia: Igalo, Topusco

Cuba: El Cedrón, Elegua, San Diego de los Baños

Czech Republic: Jáchymov

France: Aix-les-Bains, Amélie-les-Bains, Ax-les-Thermes, Bagnère-de-Bigorre, Bourbon-Lancy, Dax, Luchon, Luxeil, Plombières, Royat-Chamalières, St. Amand-des-Eaux

Germany: Baden-Baden, Kreuznach, Nauheim

Great Britain: Bath, Buxton

Greece: Icaria, Loutraki

Italy: Abano Terme, Bagni di Lucca, Fuiggi, Ischia Terme, Lurisia Terme

Jamaica: Milk River

Japan: Arima, Ibusuki, Masutomi, Misasa, Tamagawa

Mexico: Agua Hedionda, Ixtapán de la Sal, San José de Porúa

Portugal: Caldas do Geres, Curia, Felgueira, Luso

Turkey: Yalova

8

PELOIDS

P*eloid* is essentially a technical term for mud, and using thermal mud for medicinal purposes is known as pelotherapy and fangotherapy. The use of mud as a firming masque has been documented since ancient Egyptian and Roman times and continues to be practiced today. In addition to helping firm and soften the skin, mud helps remove toxins from the body, maintains heat in various parts of the body, and aids the absorption of minerals and other therapeutic elements by the skin.

Mud therapy is indicated for a wide range of health complaints. They include:

- rheumatic disorders and orthopedic complaints, including rheumatism, osteoarthritis, rheumatoid arthritis, sciatica, and neuralgia

- sequelae of (a condition resulting from) an accident or operation to a joint or vertebra

- vascular complaints, including disorders of the venous system such as phlebitis, Raynaud's syndrome, or varicose veins

- skin diseases such as psoriasis, eczema, dermatitis, and acne

- disorders of the peripheral nervous system

- gynecological problems, including inflammatory infections and hormonal problems

- digestive complaints, such as gastritis or constipation, as well as chronic disorders of the internal organs such as cholecystitis or gallbladder inflammation (In the French spas of Châtel-Guyon, Vichy, and Vittel, mud poultices are applied to the abdomen or the area over the liver as an adjunct treatment to the drinking cure.)[1]

In general, mud is made up of water and earth containing approximately one-third solids and two-thirds water. Either the mud itself may be plain mud, usually without a significant concentration of therapeutic substances, or it may naturally contain a variety of minerals (such as sulfur) as well as decomposed vegetable matter (including fungi, microflora, and algae) containing mineral and medicinal elements. Prolonged contact between the earth and mineral water (a process known as maturation) can produce a variety of chemical reactions within the mud itself and can contribute to its therapeutic properties.

As with the tremendous varieties of mineral waters found throughout the planet, the chemical composition of therapeutic mud varies from place to place. One of the best-known muds is at the Piešťany Spa in Slovakia, whose sanatorium can accommodate over 1,500 patients. According to *Spa Treatment in Czechoslovakia,* "The sulphur-bearing mud at Piešťany is formed by a remarkable natural process in which the alluvial deposits in a creek by the river Vah are mixed with the water of a sulfurous thermal spring (67°C) [152°F]."[2] Bacterial activity, in the presence of specific flora, gives rise to a unique chemical composition with excellent therapeutic properties. As a result, Piešťany ranks among the most important European spas for the treatment of nervous disorders and diseases of the locomotor system.

There are several main sources of therapeutic peloids. They include:

• peats, composed primarily of vegetable residue from peat bogs, or peat from the bottom of certain lakes

• moors, composed of minute amounts of inorganic substances as well as sulfur, iron, and sulfates

• bog earths, made up primarily of soil

• clay

A typical mud bath given at Calistoga, California, contains 50 percent local white volcanic ash and 50 percent peat moss, heated by geothermal water. While peloids such as those at Calistoga may result from a natural combination of water and earth, mud can also be prepared artificially by adding certain chemicals. Natural mud can also be chemically modified for specific therapeutic purposes and can be applied at different temperatures.

Mud is sometimes collected from an area at the spa itself; the mud used at the spas in Calistoga, for example, is mined within the city limits. When local mud is not available, it is transported to the spa and reconstituted for use.

Using reconstituted mud is a controversial issue among balneologists, because reconstituting the mud with different types of water can produce unwanted chemical changes. According to a brochure copublished by the Abano Terme and the Montegrotto Terme in the Euganean Basin in Italy:

The liquid component, that is the hyper-thermal salso-bromo-iodic water, plays a very important role in the maturing process, since its temperature and chemical components influence the development of its typical microflora. It is therefore impossible to expect therapeutic results from mud that is not mature, or that has been taken from the Euganean Spas, dried and taken to distant countries, as it has sometimes been attempted.[3]

Peat balneology is used extensively at the spa town of Héviz in Hungary, where peat is collected from the bottom of Lake Héviz, a sulfurous lake that is the largest thermally heated lake in Europe. It is later applied in the form of mud baths or mud packs to treat a wide range of health problems, including degenerative spine and joint illnesses, dermatological diseases, gout, and gynecological infections. Over 40,000 patients are treated annually with therapeutic peat at Héviz, and over 60 percent have reported high-grade improvement, 30 percent feel better, and 10 percent remain unchanged after peat balneotherapy.[4]

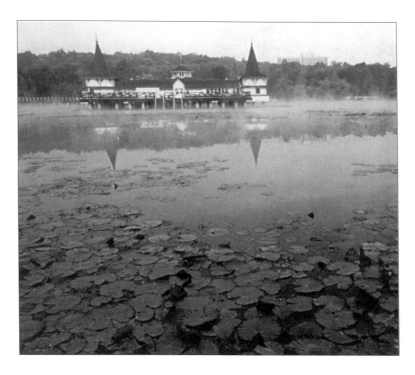

Lake Hévis and Hévis Spa, Hungary.
Reprinted courtesy of the Hungarian National Tourist Office.

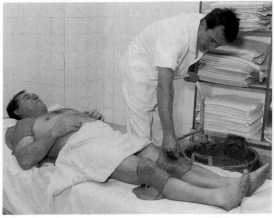

Patient receiving mud packs. Photo courtesy of the Hungarian National Tourist Office.

There are three basic methods of applying therapeutic mud. One is to apply mud packs to certain parts of the body. Those who use mud as a beauty mask are familiar with this method, as are people who have used mud on other parts of the body such as the joints of the arms and legs to relieve symptoms of rheumatism and arthritis. The warm mud (usually applied to a thickness of 10 centimeters at a temperature of 38–46°C [100–115°F]) is allowed to remain on the skin for approximately 20 to 40 minutes and then washed off with warm water. Sometimes the area of the body to which the mud has been applied is wrapped in cloth to help conserve body heat. By causing perspiration, this is believed to allow the body to eliminate toxins more efficiently.

Internal mud applications are applied vaginally or rectally to treat gynecological and urological disorders, respectively. Applied at a temperature of 45–52°C (113–126°F) for 15 to 30 minutes, they are given three to six times a week over an average of 4 weeks.[5]

Mud baths are also used in spas throughout the world, although they are rarely used as medical treatment. They involve immersing the body (except the head) in a tub filled with thermal mud. This unique experience, which has been compared to being immersed in a bath of warm gelatin, is often taken at a temperature of 37–45°C (99–113°F) for 15 to 30 minutes, depending on the individual. After a shower or bath to wash off the mud, the person is often wrapped tightly in blankets, put to bed, and allowed to perspire for another 15 or 20 minutes, which is believed to enhance the therapeutic benefits of the mud bath itself. Massage is often recommended following a mud bath or mud pack.

Ideally, mud baths should be taken on an empty stomach, allowing 3 to 4 hours to pass since one's last meal. In European spas, mud bath therapy is normally undertaken no more than once or twice a year, unless otherwise

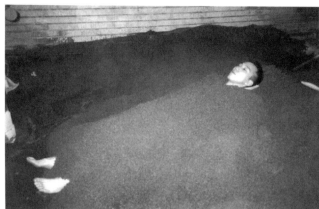

Enjoying a sand bath in Beppu, Japan.

recommended by a physician. A normal course of mud bath therapy lasts 1 to 2 weeks, involving a total of six to twelve sessions.

As opposed to mud packs, which can be safely enjoyed by nearly everyone, mud baths require caution. Because whole-body immersion in thermal mud increases body temperature, metabolism, and circulation, some balneologists suggest that a mud bath not be taken within 3 hours after a meal, before 10 o'clock in the morning, or within 2 hours of bathing in a thermal spring. You should conclude the mud bath immediately if you feel any physical discomfort, such as chest pain or difficulty in breathing.

Many of the contraindications for mud baths are the same as those for hot spring bathing. Women who are pregnant or persons who have acute rheumatic disorders, severe heart disease, kidney insufficiency, severe hypertension, or malignant tumors should avoid mud baths unless recommended to do so by a qualified health professional.

Closely related to mud baths are sand baths, popular in Japan. One of the most enjoyable experiences in researching this book was taking the famous sand bath (*sunayu*) in the city of Beppu, Japan. One sunayu is on a beach outside the city, where one can experience the bath in open air; another is in an old onsen in the city itself, which contains several hot mineral springs. Leaving your shoes at the door, you are directed to a large room (there are separate rooms for men and women), where the sand is thermally heated. After stowing your clothes in a locker and placing a small towel strategically around the genitals, you lie down face up on the coarse sand, and an attendant shovels hot sand onto your body until only your head and toes are exposed. The sand feels gritty and very warm. Like bathing in therapeutic mud, the sand bath is soothing and relaxing, and is especially helpful for the relief of sore joints. In Beppu,

10 minutes is considered adequate time for a sand bath, although trying to wash off the sand afterward with water poured from a small plastic bowl (provided by the onsen) takes nearly 10 minutes by itself!

Some Springs Known for Their Mud and Peat Treatments

Argentina: Copahué, Rosario de la Frontera
Austria: Bad Aussie, Bad Goisern, Bad Ischl, Bad Tatzmannsdorf, Salzburg
Belgium: Spa
Brazil: Araxá
Chile: Panimávida, Termas de Chillán, Termas de Puyehue
Croatia: Igalo, Topusco
Czech Repubic: Františkovy Lázně, Karlovy Vary, Mariánské Lázně, Lázně Poděbrady
Finland: Naantali, Tampere
France: Bagnères-de-Bigorre, Balaruc-les-Bains, Barbotan-les-Bains, Châtel-Guyon, Dax, Vichy, Vittel
Germany: Baden-Baden, Bad Bertrich, Bad Neendorf, Bad Pyrmont, Kreuznach
Hungary: Budapest, Bükfürdo, Héfiz
Israel: Ein Bokek, Ein Gedi, Hamme Zohar
Italy: Abano Terme, Acqui Terme, Agnano Terme, Castrocaro Terme, Chianciano Terme, Ischia Terme, Lurisia Terme, Montecatini Terme, Montegrotto Terme, Salsomaggiore Terme, Sirmione Terme
Japan: Beppu (mud and sand), Tamagawa
Luxembourg: Mondorf
Mexico: San José de Porúa
Poland: Busko-Zdrój, Krynica
Portugal: Termas dos Cucos
Romania: Băile Felix, Băile Herculane, Geoagiu Bai, Sovata
Russia: Essentuki, Kislovodsk, Pyatigorsk, Zheleznovodosk
Slovakia: Bardejov, Bojnice, Trenčianskě Templice, Pieštany
Slovenia: Čatež, Dobrna, Moravske Templice, Radenci
Spain: Alhama de Aragón, Archena, Caldes de Montbui, Fitero, Jaraba
Switzerland: Bad Scoul-Tarasp-Vulpera, Baden
United States: Calistoga, Desert Hot Springs, and Palm Springs, California; Saratoga Springs, New York; Hot Springs, Virginia
Venezuela: Las Trincheras

OTHER MINERALS

LIGHTLY MINERALIZED SPRING WATERS

Many of the hot springs and mineral springs around the world—whether thermal springs or not—do not contain strong concentrations of minerals, and are thus classified as lightly mineralized, or oligomineral, waters. When heated at over 35°C (95°F), these waters are popular because of their sedative and thermal properties, which help reduce stress, increase body temperature and general circulation, relieve muscle and joint pain, and aid in the relief of other rheumatic and locomotor disorders.[1, 2]

These waters are also good for drinking, and many have been bottled and sold commercially. Among the most famous are Evian, Fiuggi, Spa, Volvic, Vittel, and Contrexéville in Europe, and Arrowhead Spring, Naya, Poland Spring, Calistoga, Saratoga, and Vermont Pure in North America.

Water is, of course, essential for all body processes, and every cell, tissue, and organ in our body needs water to function. Water regulates body temperature, transports nutrients and oxygen to the cell, and is essential for the elimination of toxins. When sufficient water is lacking, symptoms can include fatigue, headache, and decreased physical performance; more severe symptoms can include muscle spasms, delirium, and kidney failure.[3]

Nutritionists suggest that most people need 8 to 12 cups of water daily (approximately 1 to 1½ liters) from drinking water and other beverages, in addition to the water in the food we eat. However, when we are exposed to extreme hot or cold, when we do strenuous work, when we have a fever or diarrhea, or when we eat a high-fiber diet, we need to be careful to ingest adequate amounts of water.

Some physicians, such as F. Batmanghelidj, M.D., believe that humans do not get enough water. In his controversial book *Your Body's Many Cries for Water,* Dr. Batmanghelidj claims that his clinical experience shows many common diseases—including colitis, dyspepsia, high blood pressure, depression, neck pain, headaches, allergies, asthma, and diabetes—to be the result of chronic dehydration. He stresses that the human body needs an absolute minimum of six to eight 8-ounce glasses of pure water a day.[4]

When the drinking cure with lightly mineralized waters is taken at the source, balneologists suggest consuming 600–1,200 milliliters of water on an empty stomach before breakfast. Since drinking this much water at once is not very pleasant, one can drink smaller amounts of water over four sessions, spaced 10 to 15 minutes apart. Mineral water can also be consumed throughout the day (500–750 milliliters is recommended).[5]

Contraindications to drinking large amounts of spring water include severe kidney disorders and edema. In any case, one should never drink more water at one time than feels comfortable; in addition, drinking should be a pleasant and leisurely process. Many of the most exclusive European spas have traditionally provided beautiful and quiet surroundings for drinking mineral water to enhance the spa-goer's relaxation and enjoyment.

Some Springs That Feature Lightly Mineralized Waters

Argentina: Pismanta, Rosario de la Frontera, Reyes
Brazil: Araxá, Cambuquira, Lindoia
Chile: Palguín, Puyehue
Croatia: Topusco
Cuba: San Miguel de los Baños
France: Bain-les-Bains, Evian, Thonon-les-Bains
Germany: Badenweiler, Bad Wildbad
Italy: Fiuggi, Lurisia Terme
Peru: Baños del Inca
Poland: Polanica-Zdrój, Potczyn-Zdrój
Portugal: Caria, Gerez, Luso
Romania: Băile Herculane
Slovenia: Čatež, Dobrna
Spain: Alhama de Aragón
United States: Hot Springs, Arkansas; Hot Springs, Virginia; Berkeley Springs, West Virginia
Uruguay: Termas de Arapey

IRON

Our blood depends on iron, which helps nourish it with oxygen and promotes the formation of red blood cells, which are essential for the immune system to

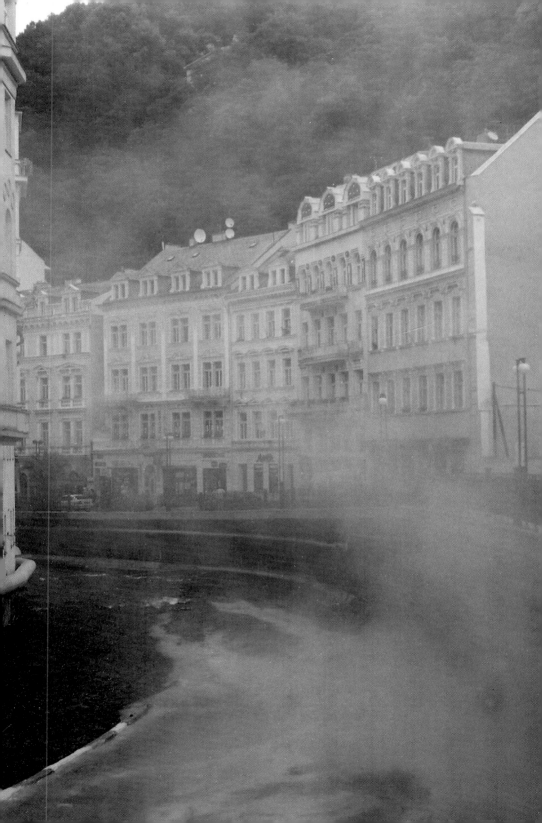

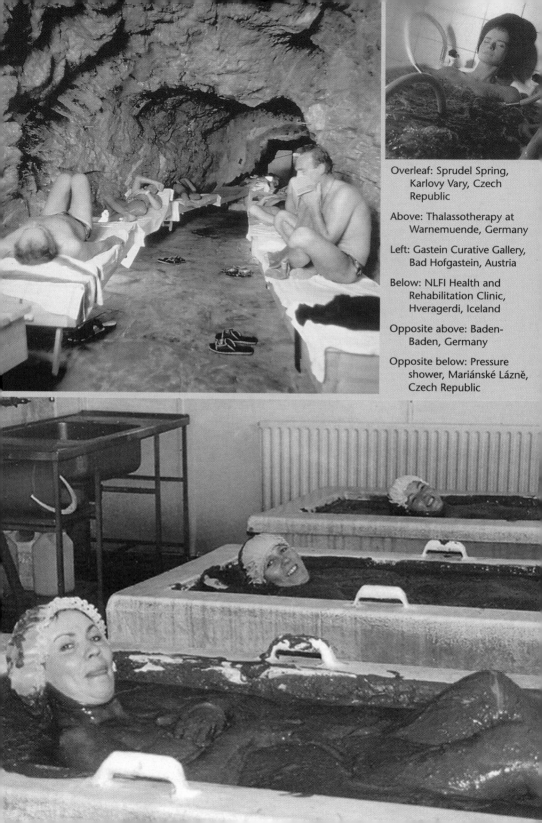

Overleaf: Sprudel Spring, Karlovy Vary, Czech Republic

Above: Thalassotherapy at Warnemuende, Germany

Left: Gastein Curative Gallery, Bad Hofgastein, Austria

Below: NLFI Health and Rehabilitation Clinic, Hveragerdi, Iceland

Opposite above: Baden-Baden, Germany

Opposite below: Pressure shower, Mariánské Lázně, Czech Republic

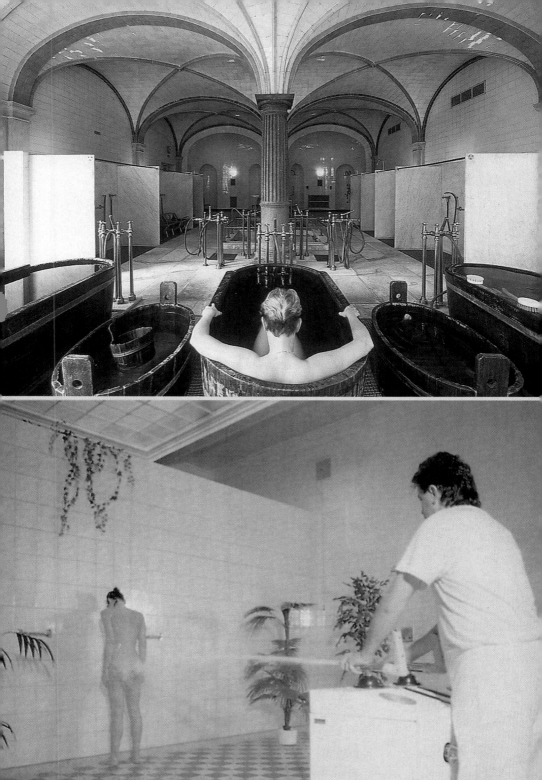

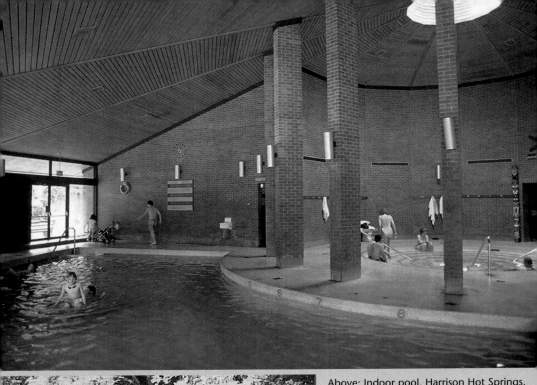

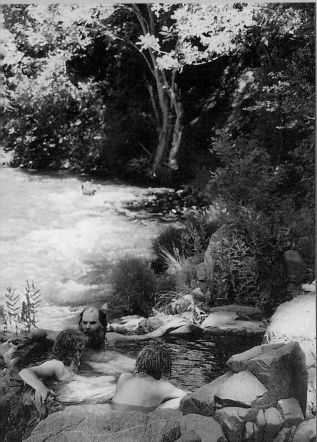

Above: Indoor pool, Harrison Hot Springs,
British Columbia, Canada

Left: Kosk Creek Hot Springs, California

Below: Mud bath at Indian Springs,
Calistoga, California

Opposite: Caracalla Terme, Baden-Baden,
Germany

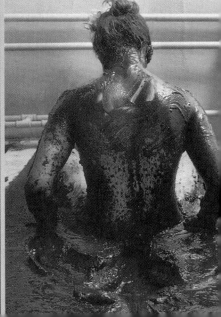

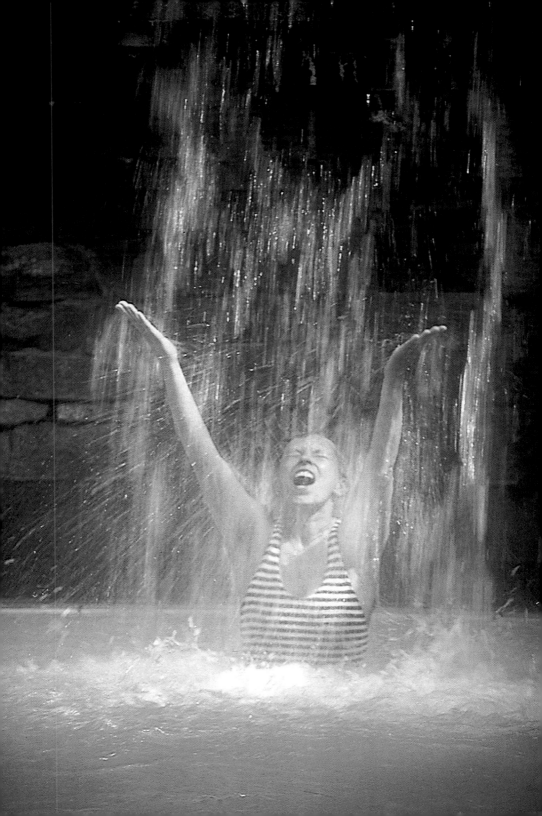

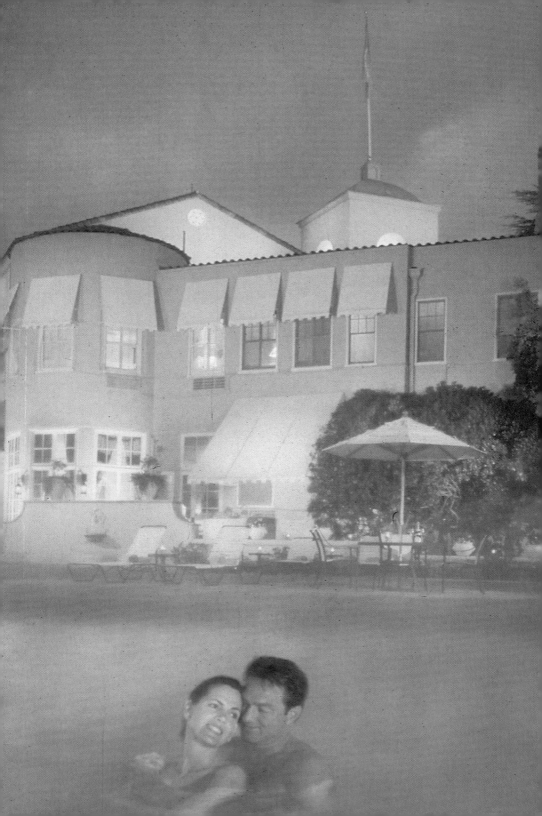

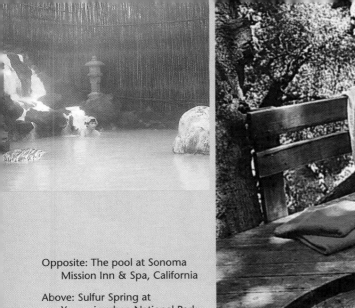

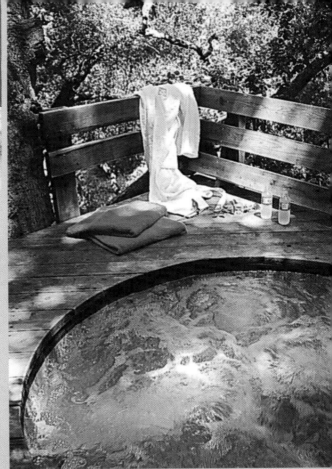

Opposite: The pool at Sonoma
    Mission Inn & Spa, California

Above: Sulfur Spring at
    Yangmingshan National Park,
    Taiwan

Right: Redwood tub at Sycamore
    Mineral Springs Resort,
    California

Below: Hydrotherapy massage at
    Vittel Spa, France

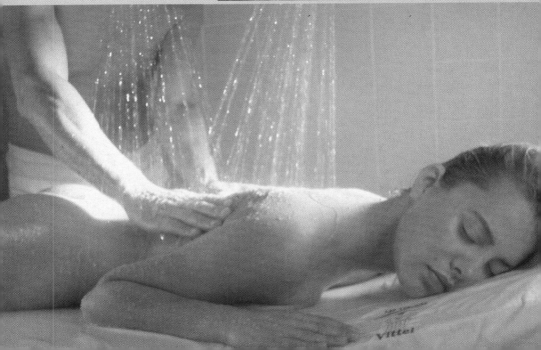

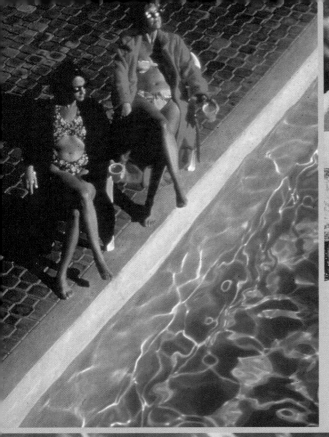

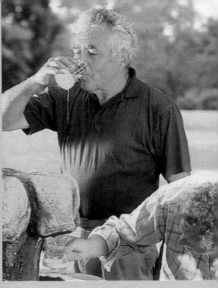

Above: Medicinal water at Bad
    Bellingen, Germany

Left: Chico Hot Springs, Montana

Below: The Warm Pool at Harbin
    Hot Springs, California

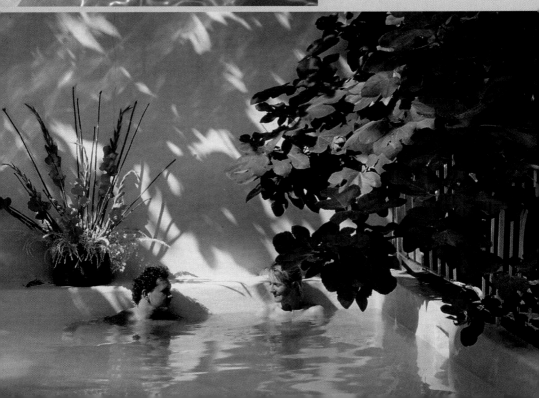

function. Iron also helps maintain the body's metabolism and better enables the body to resist disease. It is found in many vegetarian foods, including seeds, wheat, and oats; dried fruits such as raisins and apricots, and spinach and other leafy greens, as well as animal foods such as eggs and liver.[6]

Iron is found in many mineral springs around the world and is often responsible for their having a slightly brownish color. Iron springs are also known as ferruginous springs, whereas springs that are rich in other elements such as carbonate are classified as iron carbonate springs. The famous "golden waters" of the Arima Onsen in Japan are rich in iron, as is the large, light brown lake at Furnas in the Azores. Other well-known iron springs include Bagnères-de-Bigorre, Charbonnières, and Forages-les-Eaux in France, and Beppu, Togo, and Yashio in Japan, although the most famous is probably in Spa, Belgium.

Water from iron springs are used for both bathing and drinking. When ingested as a tonic, iron-rich water provides this essential mineral. Drinking water rich in iron is also prescribed therapeutically to help prevent and treat iron-deficiency anemia. While ingesting iron-rich water is also believed to help alleviate mental fatigue and calm the nerves, it is not recommended for people with indigestion or tuberculosis. Additionally, many persons, including postmenopausal women and most men, should avoid excessive iron intake.

Bathing in iron-rich springs is helpful for patients suffering from iron-deficiency anemia or excessive mental fatigue and stress-related conditions.

Some Springs Rich in Iron

Austria: Bad Tatzmannsdorf
Belgium: Spa
Brazil: Caxambú, Cambuquira, Poços de Caldas, São Lourenço
Czech Republic: Mariánské Lázně
France: Bagnères-de-Bigorre, Charbonnières, Barbotan-les-Thermes,
  Bourbon-Lancy, Forages-les-Eaux
Germany: Bad Orb, Bad Pyrmont, Bad Salzuflen
Great Britain: Buxton, Harrogate
Hungary: Bükfürdo
Ireland: Lisdoonvarna
Japan: Arima, Beppu, Kusatsu, Tamagawa, Togo, Yashio
Netherlands: Nieueschans
Poland: Kudawa-Zdrój
Portugal: Vidago, Furnas

Slovakia: Bardejov
Spain: Arteijo
Switzerland: Rheinfelden

CALCIUM

Calcium is an essential mineral that we often do not get enough of in the food we eat. Found primarily in cow's milk, enriched soy products, sea kelp, wheat germ, and green vegetables, calcium helps the blood to clot, builds bones and teeth (which are 99 percent calcium), regulates the permeability of the cell membrane, plays a role in normal liver function, and helps our muscles to contract and our heart to beat.[7]

Some Springs Rich in Calcium

Australia: Daylesford, Hepburn Springs
Austria: Baden bei Wien
Belgium: Spa
Canada: Harrison Hot Springs
Chile: Panimávida
Czech Republic: Františkovy Lázně, Karlovy Vary, Mariánské Lázně, Lázně Poděbrady
France: Bourbon-l'Archambault, Eugénie-les-Bains, Evian, Royat-Chamalières
Germany: Bad Homburg, Bad Nauheim, Bad Nenndorf
Hungary: Budapest, Bükfürdo
Iceland: Blue Lagoon
Israel: Hamme Zohar, Tiberias
Italy: Chianciano Terme
Japan: Tamagawa
Netherlands: Nieueschans
Peru: Yura
Poland: Kudowa-Zdrój, Polanica-Zdrój
Portugal: Caldas de Rainha, Curia, Monte Real
Romania: Băile Felix, Călimănești
Slovakia: Piešťany
Spain: Alhama de Aragón
Switzerland: Bad Ragaz, Bad Scoul-Tarasp-Vulpera, Leukerbad, Rheinfelden, Yverdon-les-Bains

Turkey: Bursa
United States: Thermopolis, Wyoming
Uruguay: Termas de Arapey

MAGNESIUM

Clinical studies have pointed to the importance of magnesium in helping reduce our risk of heart disease, although magnesium does much more than
that. It is an important part of more than 300 body enzymes that regulate the
body's functions. These include protein production, energy production, and
the proper functioning of the nerves and muscles, including the heart. Like
calcium and phosphorus, magnesium is essential for the formation of bones
and teeth.[8] Many American diets are deficient in magnesium.

Found primarily in legumes, nuts, whole grains, and green vegetables,
magnesium occurs in many mineral waters around the world in trace amounts,
although the commercial mineral waters with the largest amounts of calcium
are bottled in Europe, especially brands such as Badoit and Gerolsteiner. Magnesium can be easily absorbed by the digestive system by drinking magnesium-
rich mineral water, or it can be absorbed by the skin through prolonged hot
spring bathing.

Some Springs Containing Magnesium

Australia: Daylesford, Hepburn Springs
Belgium: Chaudfontaine
Brazil: São Lourenço
Canada: Radium Hot Springs, Miette Hot Springs
Czech Republic: Karlovy Vary, Mariánské Lázně
France: Bourbon l'Archambault, Eugénie-les-Bains, Evian
Hungary: Bükfürdo
Ireland: Lisdoonvarna
Israel: Hamme Zohar
Poland: Kudowa-Zdrój
Portugal: Caldas da Rainha, Curia
Romania: Călimăneşti
Russia: Kislovodsk
Slovakia: Šmarješke Toplice
Slovenia: Rogaška

Switzerland: Bad Ragaz, Bad Scoul-Tarasp-Vulpera, Leukerbad,
   Rheinfelden, Yverdon-les-Bains
United States: Hot Springs, Virginia
Uruguay: Termas de Arapey

POTASSIUM

Potassium, another important mineral, plays a role in numerous body functions, helping to transmit nerve impulses, regulate fluid and mineral balance
in the body, and maintain normal blood pressure. It is found in a wide variety
of foods, including fresh fruits and vegetables, meat, fish, and poultry. People
rarely become deficient in this mineral unless they are taking medication to
control blood pressure.[9] Like magnesium, trace amounts of potassium are found
in many mineral waters. A common element in many bottled waters, potassium can be absorbed either by the digestive system by drinking or by the skin
through prolonged hot spring bathing. Many mineral springs around the world
contain trace amounts of potassium. Those with the largest concentrations
include Termas de Huife in Chile, Vichy in France, Šmarješke Toplice in Slovenia,
and Shiobara in Japan.

LITHIUM

In its natural form, lithium is a silvery-white alkali metal that occurs in a variety of other compounds. Although a poison when ingested in excess amounts,
lithium carbonate has been used therapeutically in the treatment of manic
depression and can help stabilize psychological mood swings. Lithium can
also help correct sleep disorders in manic patients, possibly by suppressing the
rapid eye movements during sleep.[10]

Lithium is found in trace amounts in many hot springs around the world,
especially those rich in alkaline compounds. Although little is known about
the effects of trace amounts of lithium on normal individuals, many of those
who have enjoyed the lithium-containing waters at Rancho Río Caliente near
Guadalajara, Mexico, attest to its ability to help relax the mind and the emo-
tions. While the laid-back atmosphere and lack of radio, television, and tele-
phones at the spa may contribute to one's feelings of calm and relaxation, soaking in the hot springs several times a day may be a major factor by itself.

Some springs known for their lithium waters include Puyehue in Chile,
Tehuacán in Mexico, and Oostend in Belgium.

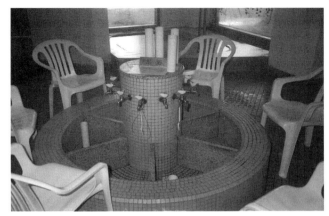

Footbath at Kusatsu Onsen, Japan.

ARSENIC

Arsenic has been known for centuries as a poison and has been widely mentioned in literature and folklore. Primarily as a byproduct of copper smelter dust, inorganic arsenic is considered much more toxic than the organic arsenic found in some mineral waters. When ingested over a long period of time, arsenic can contribute to lung and skin cancer as well as other diseases. An ingredient in pesticides and wood preservatives, arsenic finds its way into our bodies through air pollution and by seepage from hazardous waste dumps.[11]

However, arsenic is not all bad. Before penicillin was introduced, arsenic was used to combat diseases such as syphilis and amoebic dysentery for centuries. Arsenic springs are occasionally found. Although it is not recommended that we drink from such springs, they are helpful for helping the body heal venereal diseases and fungal infections. A small arsenic spring at Harbin Hot Springs is believed to cure athlete's foot and nail fungus; it is used primarily as a foot bath. I can personally attest to the value of arsenic waters: after I had soaked my feet in the arsenic foot bath at a Kusatsu kuahausu in Japan for several minutes, my case of athlete's foot healed within a matter of hours.

In times past, having an arsenic spring on the property was not always a blessing. In her book *Harbin Hot Springs,* Ellen Klages wrote about a man who effusively told all his friends how the arsenic-rich waters of nearby Witter Springs had cured his syphilis. Word about the miraculous waters soon spread, with unfortunate results:

> Its reputation for the curing of venereal diseases became so well known that the mere mention of the name "Witter" could produce ribald laughter among visitors on the springs circuit. A large hotel had been built on

the property, but, due to its dubious claim to fame, no one wanted to admit that they went to Witter Springs. The clientele dwindled, the resort declined, and the magnificent hotel never opened.[12]

Spas that feature arsenic waters sometimes have them set aside for soaking hands or feet. They include Puente del Inca in Argentina; Caxambú in Brazil; Harbin Hot Springs in California; Oostend in Belgium; La Bourboulle and St. Honoré in France; Levico and Roncegno in Italy; Kudawa-Zdrój in Poland; Darasun in Russia; Bad Nenndorf, Durkheim, Lindau, and Wiesbaden in Germany; Val Sinetra in Switzerland; and Kusatsu in Japan.

SILICA

Silica (silicon dioxide) is a compound that is widely distributed in the environment and is best known as beach sand. It is used industrially in the manufacture of glass and in the electronics industry, including the manufacture of semiconductors.

The body is composed of 0.05 percent silica, which is found in bones, skin, and all body organs. Silica is viewed as important in promoting cardiovascular health and plays a key role in both bone formation and bone remineralization. It also works synergistically with minerals such as calcium, magnesium, and potassium, as well as with ascorbic acid (vitamin C). Although normally found in foods, silica is often lost in food processing; people take silica as a nutritional supplement, and to restore health to aging skin, hair, and nails.[13]

Some springs whose waters contain silica are Hot Springs, South Dakota; the therapeutic springs at Desert Hot Springs and Palm Springs, California; Harrison and Radium Hot Springs in Canada; Los Molles, Pismanta, and Reyes in Argentina; Ax-les-Thermes in France; the Blue Lagoon in Iceland; Termas de Luso in Portugal; and Miranda Hot Springs in New Zealand.

BOTTLED WATERS

An estimated 700 brands of bottled water are sold in the United States and Canada today. Some, such as Poland Spring, Naya, and Calistoga, are derived from natural mineral springs; others, such as Alhambra, Aquafina, and Dasani, are purified tap water.

Water from a mineral spring is not inherently more pure than tap water. Chemical analyses of New York City water, which is derived from protected reservoirs in upstate New York and piped to the city through aqueducts, has shown a greater level of purity than that of many bottled waters. However, natural spring water is more likely to contain a higher quantity of essential minerals and to feature a more distinctive taste. Magnesium, for example, which is deficient in most American diets, protects us from heart diseases and plays an important role in body metabolism. It is found in small amounts in most American mineral waters and in much larger amounts in many European waters, especially brands such as Badoit from France and Gerolsteiner from Germany. In addition, new chemical elements are always being discovered; it is possible that waters from natural springs contain trace mineral elements that have not yet been discovered or are not able to be measured by present-day technology.

The following list contains a chemical analysis of several commercial mineral waters. Most are popular brands produced in the United States; others are bottled in Canada and Europe. They are listed by brand name and location of corporate office; the source of the water is included in the general description. For more information on bottled waters, consult one of the books listed in the resource section, or visit www.bottledwaterweb.com, an excellent source of information about water on the Internet.

ACQUA PANNA, Milan, Italy

ANALYSIS	MILLIGRAMS PER LITER
Bicarbonate	21
Calcium	3.6
Chloride	2.7
Magnesium	1.3
Potassium	4.1
Sulfate	1.5
Total dissolved solids (TDS)	41

The source is 3,700 feet high in the Tuscan Apennines of northern Italy on a natural 3,300-acre preserve 25 miles north of Florence. The water never comes in contact with the air or the environment, ensuring its purity.

ALHAMBRA WATER, Union City, California

ANALYSIS	PARTS PER MILLION
Calcium	0.7
Chloride	3.5
Magnesium	0.8
Sodium	3.8
Sulfate	3.4
pH 6.8	

Municipal tap water purified with ozone.

ARROWHEAD, Monterey Park, California

ANALYSIS	PARTS PER MILLION
Bicarbonate	124.44
Calcium	20
Chloride	7.2
Magnesium	5

Potassium	2.5
Silica	24.7
Sodium	3
Sulfate	4
TDS	129
pH	8.16

Natural spring water from the San Bernardino Mountains; ozonated and passed through ultraviolet light before bottling.

BADOIT, Evian, France

ANALYSIS	MILLIGRAMS PER LITER
Bicarbonate	1420
Calcium	222
Chloride	64
Magnesium	92
Potassium	11
Silica	39
Sodium	171
Sulfate	48
pH	6.1

A delicious, naturally carbonated mineral water from a source nearly 460 feet (153 meters) beneath the earth's surface, often served in European restaurants. The high amount of sodium bicarbonate is said to facilitate digestion. It is also one of the most magnesium-rich commercial bottled waters in Europe.

BLACK MOUNTAIN SPRING WATER, San Carlos, California

ANALYSIS	PARTS PER MILLION
Calcium	25
Chloride	10
Magnesium	0.73

Potassium	0.67
Sodium	8.3
TDS	44
pH 7.2	

Natural mineral water from a protected spring 25 miles south of San Francisco. The lightly mineralized spring water is filtered through sand and gravel, charcoal, and a micron filter and then is ozonated.

CALISTOGA, Calistoga, California

ANALYSIS	PARTS PER MILLION
Bicarbonate	130
Calcium	7
Chloride	250
Fluoride	9.5
Iron	0.1
Potassium	16
Magnesium	1
Nitrate	0.2
Sodium	150
Sulfate	12

Water from a protected geyser emerges at 100°C (212°F) and is then cooled to 4°C (39°F) for bottling. The bottler removes the hydrogen sulfide odor by filtering the water through green sand. The finished water is then ozonated for purity.

CAROLINA MOUNTAIN SPRING WATER, Cashiers, North Carolina

ANALYSIS	PARTS PER MILLION
Calcium	5.84
Sodium	4.83
Sulfate	9.3

TDS	60

pH	7.6

From a spring located near Terrapin Mountain within the Nantahala National Forest in North Carolina.

COBB MOUNTAIN SPRING WATER, Cobb, California

ANALYSIS	PARTS PER MILLION
Calcium	4.8
Chloride	1.2
Magnesium	1.6
Sodium	4.3
TDS	94
pH 7.3	

Cobb Mountain is an extinct volcano in Lake County, where a very large, cold spring surfaces at 3,000 feet above sea level. The water is ozonated and filtered through a 0.2-micrometer filter.

COLORADO CRYSTAL, Denver, Colorado

ANALYSIS	PARTS PER MILLION
Chloride	1.2
Sodium	1
Sulfate	2
TDS	95
pH 7	

Water is derived from a series of natural springs protected by a national forest, and piped by enclosed system to the bottling facility. The only processing is ultraviolet light and added carbonation from natural carbon dioxide wells in Colorado.

CORALBA, San Damiano Macra, Italy

ANALYSIS	MILLIGRAMS PER LITER
Calcium	15
Chloride	0.8
Hydrogen carbonate	240
Magnesium	18
Nitrate	2
Potassium	0.5
Silica	5.3
Sodium	0.4
Sulfate	9

A noncarbonated mineral water from a spring in the Italian Alps.

CRYSTAL GEYSER WATER COMPANY, Calistoga, California

ANALYSIS	PARTS PER MILLION
Calcium	12
Chloride	260
Magnesium	3.1
Potassium	8.7
Sodium	130
Sulfates	2.6
TDS	590

The aquifer of this water's source is 240 feet below the plant and surfaces at 60°C (140°F). Through a method of heat exchanges, the water is then cooled, filtered to remove sediment, ozonated, carbonated, and bottled.

CRYSTAL GEYSER NATURAL ALPINE SPRING WATER, Calistoga, California

ANALYSIS	PARTS PER MILLION
Calcium	27.4
Chloride	6.5
Magnesium	6
Potassium	2
Sodium	13
Sulfate	36.7
TDS	165
pH 7.9	

From a spring along the High Sierra mountain range, in the town of Olancha, California.

DIAMOND NATURAL SPRING WATER, Hot Springs, Arkansas

ANALYSIS	PARTS PER MILLION
Calcium	74
Chloride	7.2
Magnesium	3
Potassium	1.6
Sulfate	19
TDS	170
pH 7.58	

The source of this water is a deep aquifer made up of shale rock and Blakely lime-stone, where the water has been dated by the U.S. Geological Survey as being approximately 9,000 years old. It surfaces at 19°C (67°F) and has a distinct taste of iron. The water is processed by carbon filtration and ozonation, which removes the iron and sediment.

ﾠian, France

ANALYSIS	PARTS PER MILLION
Bicarbonate	357
Calcium	78
Chloride	2.2
Magnesium	23
Nitrates	3.8
Potassium	0.75
Sodium	5.5
Sulfate	10
pH 7.18	

The spring is Source Cachat, where the water emerges from a tunnel in the mountain at 11.5°C (53°F). The source is fed from the snowmelt and rainwater that filters from the Vinzier Plateau through glacial sand. The glacial sand is surrounded by clay, which protects the water from pollution. The water is bottled at a nearby bottling plant.

FIJI NATURAL ARTESIAN WATER, Palm Beach, Florida

ANALYSIS	MILLIGRAMS PER LITER
Bicarbonate	140
Calcium	17
Magnesium	13
Silica	83
TDS	160
pH 7.5	

Water is taken from an aquifer beneath volcanic highlands on the main island of Viti Levu in Fiji, and bottled at a state-of-the-art production facility. It was first bottled for use at the exclusive Wakaya Club, a resort on a 2,200-acre island in the Fiji Republic.

FOUNTAINHEAD WATER, Marietta, Georgia

ANALYSIS	MILLIGRAMS PER LITER
Calcium	9
Fluoride	0.41
Magnesium	0.3
Sodium	0
TDS	55
pH 7.5	

From a protected spring within Sumter National Forest, the water is naturally filtered through 500 feet of granite bedrock. Bottled at the source, the water has a light, soft, refreshing taste and is ozonated before bottling.

GEROLSTEINER, Gerolstein, Vulkaneifel, Germany

ANALYSIS	MILLIGRAMS PER LITER
Calcium	347
Carbonate	1807
Chloride	39.7
Magnesium	108
Sulfate	36.7
TDS	1577 ppm

Bottled since 1888, the water comes from a deep volcanic source in the heart of wooded highlands between the Rhine and Moselle River valleys. It is low in sodium, and high in magnesium and calcium, and is carbonated with its own natural gas.

GREAT BEAR, Greenwich, Connecticut

ANALYSIS	MILLIGRAMS PER LITER
Bicarbonate	5.5
Calcium	1.3
Chloride	1.4
Magnesium	1

Potassium	0.7
Sodium	1.7
Sulfate	5.3
TDS	24
pH	6.57

The spring is located in Chester County, Pennsylvania, where it is protected by woodlands and rock formations. The water filters through layers of gray and white sand and fine sandstone gravel, emerging at about 11°C (52°F). It is then processed through a carbon filter and passed under ultraviolet light. It has been bottled since 1888. Great Bear also produces a sodium-free purified water made from Allentown, Pennsylvania, municipal water that is carbon filtered, passed through reverse osmosis, and then deionized, filtered, and ozonated.

HAWAIIAN SPRINGS NATURAL WATER, Honolulu, Hawaii

ANALYSIS	MILLIGRAMS PER LITER
Bicarbonate	44
Calcium	6
Magnesium	3
Potassium	2
Sodium	6
Sulfate	4
TDS	80
pH	6.8

Water is naturally filtered through thousands of feet of lava rock and forms an underground water flow, where it is captured at the source in Kea'au (Puna District) on the slopes of the Mauna Loa volcano.

MATTONI, Karlovy Vary, Czech Republic

ANALYSIS	MILLIGRAMS PER LITER
Bicarbonate	541
Calcium	62.4
Chloride	12.9

Magnesium	18
Sodium	96.7

Bottled since 1872 in the famous spa town of Karlovy Vary, this water is the most popular carbonated water in the Czech Republic.

MOUNT OLYMPUS WATER, Salt Lake City, Utah

ANALYSIS	PARTS PER MILLION
Calcium	7.9
Chloride	5.9
Magnesium	2.4
Potassium	0.48
Sodium	3.4
Sulfate	8.8
TDS	56
pH 7.2	

The source is in Neff's Canyon, at approximately 5,000 feet above sea level on Mount Olympus in Salt Lake County. The spring is on federal reserve land and leased from the federal government. The company uses distillation, ozonation, reverse osmosis, carbon filtering, and deionization for its various water products.

MOUNTAIN VALLEY, Hot Springs, Arkansas

ANALYSIS	PARTS PER MILLION
Bicarbonate	238.05
Calcium	69.68
Magnesium	10.56
Potassium	1.13
Sodium	2.88
Sulfate	9.72

Bottled since 1871, the water emerges from an aquifer estimated to be at a depth of 1,600 feet below the earth's surface; the water filters through levels of shale, Blakely sandstone, and limestone. At the source, the water has a distinct iron taste, which is removed by micron filtration and ozonation.

NAYA, Mirabel, Québec, Canada

ANALYSIS	PARTS PER MILLION		
	MIRABEL (QC)	ST. ANDRÉ (QC)	REVELSTOKE (BC)
Calcium	45	42	50
Chloride	1	21	<1
Magnesium	22	21	18
Sodium	6	24	1
Sulfate	17	23	42
pH	7.5	7.7	7.8

Natural spring water is taken from protected springs in three locations in Canada: Mirabel and St. André springs in Québec, and Revelstoke spring at the floor of the Rocky Mountains in British Columbia.

PASSUGGER HEILQUELLEN, Passugg, Switzerland

ANALYSIS	PARTS PER MILLION
Bicarbonate	1,020
Calcium	286
Chloride	19
Iron	0.57
Magnesium	24
Potassium	3.4
Sodium	46
Sulfate	48

The naturally carbonated water emerges from a spring near Chur, Switzerland, at 8°C (46°F). Gravity flow brings the water into the bottling plant, where the water is recarbonated and bottled in silk-screened green bottles. The taste is a blend of carbonation with high mineralization, making the water a good digestive.

PEÑAFIEL, Tehuacán, Mexico

ANALYSIS	PARTS PER MILLION
Calcium	131
Chloride	131
Fluoride	0.51
Magnesium	41
Potassium	11
Sodium	159
Sulfate	130
TDS	880
pH .28	

Rainwater and snowmelt filter through volcanic strata, surfacing as warm mineral water. The water is bottled just outside the spa town of Tehuacán, and processed through sediment filtration, treated with ultraviolet light, and then carbonated. It is highly mineralized with strong carbonation, making it the most popular digestive water in Mexico.

PERRIER, Vergèze, France

ANALYSIS	MILLIGRAMS PER LITER
Bicarbonate	336.7
Calcium	145.3
Chloride	30.9
Magnesium	3.5
Nitrate	13.1
Potassium	1.1
Sodium	13.8
Sulfate	51.1
pH 6	

This water was first bottled in 1863. It is derived from a natural spring near the town of Vergèze and is then artificially carbonated.

POLAND SPRING, Poland Spring, Maine

ANALYSIS	MILLIGRAMS PER LITER
Bicarbonate	20
Calcium	8.3
Chloride	6.1
Fluoride	0
Magnesium	0.8
Potassium	0.5
Sodium	2.9
Sulfate	5
TDS	37

pH   6.4

The source is in a pine forest and is protected by 350 acres of preserved land that once included a famous spa. Rainfall and snowmelt percolate through a natural filter of sand and gravel into a 700-acre underground aquifer, and the water issues from a fissure near a crest of gneiss rock. Micron filtration is used to remove sediment, and ultraviolet light is used to ensure purity. Carbonation is added to Poland Spring sparkling water. The water has been bottled since 1893.

ROSPORT, Rosport, Luxembourg

ANALYSIS	MILLIGRAMS PER KILOGRAM
Bicarbonate	1043
Calcium	295
Chloride	76.1
Magnesium	119
Nitrate	0.3
Potassium	19.8
Sodium	66.1
Sulfate	405

A naturally carbonated mineral water from a protected spring in the Luxembourg countryside.

SAN PELLEGRINO, Milan, Italy

ANALYSIS	PARTS PER MILLION
Bicarbonate	225.65
Calcium	203.2
Chloride	67.26
Fluoride	0.58
Lithium	0.2
Magnesium	59.4
Nitrate	0.75
Potassium	4.1
Sodium	44.2
Sulfate	11.9
pH	7.25

The water's sources are in the mountains north of Milan. Three springs come from an aquifer 1,300 feet below the earth's surface, where limestone and volcanic rocks impart minerals and trace elements. The finished product has added carbonation, although the Aqua Limpia brand (available primarily in Europe) does not.

SARATOGA, Saratoga Springs, New York

ANALYSIS	PARTS PER MILLION
Bicarbonate	350
Calcium	93
Chloride	62
Fluoride	0.26
Magnesium	15.3
Potassium	4.3
Sodium	70
Sulfate	21.5

Bottled under the Saratoga brand for over 125 years, the water originally came from a hand-drilled well that went through 30 feet of sand and 150 feet of rock. Natural carbonation occurs in this pleasant-tasting water, although it is reinjected with additional carbonation during the bottling process. Carbonated Vichy water is also bottled at Saratoga.

SNOW VALLEY MOUNTAIN SPRING WATER, Annapolis, Maryland

ANALYSIS	PARTS PER MILLION
Chloride	2.6
Sulfate	3.7
TDS	30

The waters at this mineral spring are derived from snowmelt and rainwater. It is filtered through crystalline rock and surfaces at the source at 14°C (57°F). The water is transported from the holding tanks by tanker trucks to the bottling facility in Annapolis, where it is then put through a particle filter, which removes suspended solids such as sand. It is ozonated and bottled.

SPA, Spa, Belgium

ANALYSIS	PARTS PER MILLION
Bicarbonate	11
Calcium	3.5
Chloride	5
Magnesium	1.3
Nitrate	1.9
Potassium	0.5
Silica	7
Sodium	3
Sulfate	6.5
TDS	33

The source, known as Reine, or the Queen's Spring, is in the valley of the Ardennes. Rainwater and snowmelt percolate down through layers of clay, slate, flint, sand, and quartz, and it finally surfaces at 440 meters above sea level. This low-mineralized water is particle-filtered of unstable elements and then bottled with neither pasteurization nor sterilization.

TALKING RAIN, Bellevue, Washington

ANALYSIS	PARTS PER MILLION
Calcium	1.5
Iron	0.001
Magnesium	1.5
Potassium	0.05
Sodium	0.18
Zinc	0.001
TDS	200

Rainwater and snowmelt on 14,000-foot-high Mt. Rainier flows through underground streams, surfacing as an artesian spring, where the water is collected. It is bottled in Tumwater, where it is processed through 12 sets of filters and treated with ultraviolet light.

THEODORA QUELLE, Kekkut, Hungary

ANALYSIS	MILLIGRAMS PER LITER
Bicarbonate	1050
Calcium	220
Fluoride	0.8
Magnesium	76

Hungary's favorite naturally carbonated mineral water is taken from a protected spring in a national park near the shores of Lake Balaton.

UTOPIA SPRING WATER, Utopia, Texas

ANALYSIS	PARTS PER MILLION
Bicarbonate	284
Calcium	76
Fluoride	0.2
Magnesium	17
Sodium	8

Sulfate	34
TDS	284

This water surfaces from a spring at 20°C (68°F); the spring produces approximately 300,000 gallons per day, and the water is estimated to be 10,000 years old. The company also produces Utopia drinking water and Utopia purified water, using reverse osmosis processing.

VALSER ST. PETERSQUELLE, Bern-Liebefeld, Switzerland

ANALYSIS	PARTS PER MILLION
Bicarbonate	390.5
Calcium	436
Chloride	2.38
Fluoride	1.07
Iron	1.83
Magnesium	54.7
Sodium	10.1
Sulfate	988

St. Pierre Spring is in the town of Vals, and water emerges from a warm artesian well 3,200 feet deep. The water is highly mineralized but low in sodium. Carbonation from a well in Germany is added in the bottling process.

VERMONT PURE, Randolph, Vermont

ANALYSIS	MILLIGRAMS PER LITER
Calcium	41
Chloride	6.9
Magnesium	4.2
Nitrate	2.2
Potassium	1.1
Sodium	2
Sulfate	18

TDS	170
pH	7.2

Bottled from a spring in the Green Mountains of Vermont, the noncarbonated water is naturally filtered for up to 20 years through deep strata of rocks and minerals.

VICHY CÉLESTINS, Vichy, France

ANALYSIS	PARTS PER MILLION
Bicarbonate	3,000
Calcium	100
Chloride	220
Magnesium	60
Potassium	60
Sodium	1,200
Sulfate	130

The water emerges at 17°C (63°F) through strata of aragonite rock, which was formed by waterborne mineral deposits over millions of years. Rock layers of calcium carbonate have eroded over centuries, contributing to this water's unique natural carbonation and mineralization.

VITTEL, Vittel, France

ANALYSIS	PARTS PER MILLION
Bicarbonate	388
Calcium	181
Magnesium	37.7
Potassium	1.65
Sodium	3.76
Sulfate	277
TDS	816
pH	7.6

The source is an immense underground aquifer, where rock strata and sandstone charge the water with calcium, magnesium, and sulfates. The spring surfaces at 11°C (52°F) and is bottled in either the north or the south plant, depending on the type of packaging used.

ZEPHYRHILLS NATURAL SPRING WATER, Greenwich, Connecticut

ANALYSIS	MILLIGRAMS PER LITER
Bicarbonate	140
Calcium	58
Chloride	11
Fluoride	0.2
Magnesium	3.9
Potassium	0.2
Sodium	5.1
Sulfate	8
TDS	185
pH 7.7	

The water originates near the central Florida city of Zephyrhills (Polk County) from a deep limestone, sand, and silt aquifer that filters the water and provides its mineral balance. The spring water is then carbon filtered, passed under ultraviolet light, and ozonated.

PART III

LOOKING BETTER,
FEELING BETTER

THE HEALING
AND REJUVENATING
POWER OF WATER

Though healing springs are largely a secret in the United States and Canada, millions of Europeans and Japanese have discovered that bathing in them can have a profound effect on physical, mental, and emotional well-being. In addition to providing valuable minerals to the body, bathing in and drinking therapeutic waters can play an important role in both the prevention and the healing of disease.

Drawing from documented medical research from North America, Europe, and Asia, the following chapters focus on the therapeutic effects of hot springs and mineral springs on specific diseases such as arthritis, rheumatism, cardiovascular disease, gynecological problems, and skin disorders. In addition to a brief description of the diseases themselves, we examine the types of waters that best treat these common problems. Determinations are based on evidence taken from scientific journals, medical literature, and interviews with qualified health professionals from many parts of the world. As in the previous section, each chapter concludes with a list of springs where the reader can go for the prevention and treatment of the specific health conditions discussed.

SKIN DISEASES

The skin is made up of 15–40 percent water from the outer to the inner layers. Since the skin forms a protective barrier between ourselves and the outer environment, it is subject to several problems, including dermatitis. Dryness is often a factor in skin disease and is often related to aging, lack of sufficient drinking water, excessive perspiration, or living in a low-humidity environment.

Water plays an important role in treating skin diseases in the following ways:

- By hydrating the skin, it can affect the course of problems such as atopic dermatitis (dermatitis characterized by irritation, itching, and scratching) and ichthyosis (a condition in which the skin is dry and scaly).

- When used as a bath or in a compress, water can cool and cleanse.

- Water can serve as a vehicle for the enhanced delivery of active medicinal agents.[1]

Immersion in water produces mechanical, physical, and chemical effects on chronic skin diseases. A body in water weighs only a fraction of its actual weight, thus dissipating pain in cases of disease such as atopic psoriasis and scleroderma. Water can also be used to influence heat transmission and draw out the body's own water molecules to promote cleansing of tissues.

People have been taking the waters to relieve skin problems since the dawn of human civilization. The Dead Sea achieved fame as a healing center for skin diseases in pre-Biblical times, and clinics in Ein Bokek and Ein Gedi are renowned for dermatological treatment today. In ancient Greece, saltwater bathings were regarded by numerous physicians, including Hippocrates, as therapy for chronic inflammatory skin conditions. In Japan, the acidic waters of the famous thermal springs at Kusatsu have been used for nearly 1,000 years to treat a variety of skin problems, including atopic and neurodermatitis.

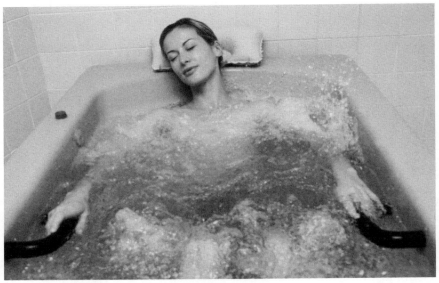

Whole-body bathing at the Vittel Spa, France. Photo courtesy of Thermes de Vittel.

Numerous European spas specialize in dermatological treatment today. One of the most important is La Roche-Posay, in the heart of the Poitou-Charentes region of France about 3 hours southwest of Paris. Over 10,000 patients (of whom 30 percent are infants and young children) visit the spa each year for the treatment of eczema, psoriasis, and scarring from accidents, surgery, and burns as well as for the prevention and treatment of gum disease. Therapies at La Roche-Posay include various types of filiform showers; underwater massage; facial, local, and whole-body mists; whole-body bathing; fangotherapy; irrigation of the mouth; and drinking the waters, which are rich in calcium bicarbonate, calcium, and silica. However, a unique aspect of the waters at La Roche-Posay is that they also contain small amounts of selenium, which is believed to promote DNA synthesis and cellular growth and also to fight cancer.[2]

Like many other spas, La Roche-Posay offers a wide range of recreational opportunities for adults, including concerts, movies, golf, horse racing, and casino gambling, as well as special activity programs designed for children. In addition, a clinical psychologist is on staff to offer short-term individual and family therapy.

Sulfur-rich waters are also useful in treating skin diseases. Dermatologists at the University of Florence and the University of Siena in Italy have found that sulfur in mineral water may interact with free radicals within the deeper layers of the skin, providing chemical compounds producing antifungal and antibacterial activity. This is why sulfurous waters are used for treating skin diseases such as acne, as well as infected leg ulcers, tinea versicolor (a type of fungus featuring yellow patches on the skin), tinea corporis (fungal infections on the body), and tinea capitis (scalp fungus).[3]

In addition, bathing in sulfur-rich water increases the proliferation of lymphocytes in the blood of patients with a variety of communicable diseases. Immersion in water rich in sulfur is able to regulate the skin's TH-1 and TH-2 lymphocyte levels. This is important, because some physicians consider atopic dermatitis to be the result of disregulation of lymphocytes in the blood and skin. Apparently, sulfur-rich water is able to work on the TH-1 lymphocyte, reducing the release of interleukin-2.[4]

Over the past few years, physicians have accumulated a large body of evidence that attests to the abilities of mineral waters to help the body heal itself of a wide range of skin diseases, including dermatitis, eczema, vitiligo, psoriasis, and hydrolipodystrophy. Balneotherapy has also been proved very effective in wound healing, in postoperative healing, and in the treatment of burns.

DERMATITIS

Dermatitis is a general term to describe itching and redness of the skin caused by irritants such as poison ivy or other allergens, including cold weather.

Atopic dermatitis, a common form of dermatitis, is characterized by irritation, itching, and scratching. Usually the cause is unknown. However, because it appears to run in families, it is thought to be genetic.

Dr. Kasuo Kabota and his colleagues at the Gumma University Hospital in Japan investigated the properties of balneotherapy at the Kusatsu spa on 100 adult patients with chronic atopic dermatitis that had resisted traditional treatment. The Kusatsu waters are highly acidic and contain aluminum, sulfates, and chlorides, with a pH of 2.0. Patients were given a 10-minute 40–42°C (104–107°F) hot spring bath once or twice daily from 46 to 75 days. This was followed by the application of white petroleum jelly. The physicians reported that "the skin symptoms of 79 of the 100 cases (79 percent) were improved through the balneotherapy and furthermore pruritus [severe itching] was improved in 55 of the 79 cases (70 percent)." They concluded that balneotherapy at Kusatsu could be useful for the treatment of stubborn cases of adult-type atopic dermatitis.[5]

Similar results were found in a later study with 70 teenagers and young adults, most of whom had had dermatitis since early childhood. They took a 10-minute bath in 42°C (107°F) spring water, and white petroleum jelly was later applied to the skin. Improvement occurred in 76 percent of cases. Research also revealed that Kusatsu hot spring water brought about a total or significant reduction in the number of *Staphylococcus aureus* in most of the patients whose skin improved, owing to the bactericidal activity of the manganese and iodide ions in the acidic hot spring water.[6]

The same researchers also made an unusual case study of addiction to hot spring bathing by a patient with chronic atopic dermatitis that had been resistant to traditional therapies, including steroids. The patient, a 21-year-old woman, began taking the very hot (47°C [117°F]) "time bath" *(jikan-yu)* at Kusatsu without medical supervision four times a day over a 30-day period. She found the baths so pleasurable that she could not stop taking them. After a month-long hospital isolation, the young woman was able to overcome her addiction. Dr. Kubota found that bathing in extremely hot water caused a transient rise in the plasma beta-endorphin levels, providing a feeling of physical and psychological well-being.[7]

ECZEMA

The Momin Prohod spa in Bulgaria is renowned for its thermal waters, which contain sulfates, sodium, fluorine, silica, and radon. Its success with patients with eczema is legendary, and many patients who do not respond to traditional medical therapy are referred here for treatment. During the 1960s, medical researchers studied 819 eczema patients who received a 3-week course of therapy at the spa that included bathing, drinking, and inhalations. Although balneotherapy was not successful for the patients with acute, paratraumatic, or infected eczema, 32.8 percent of patients were healed or greatly improved, 31 percent were moderately improved, 16.3 percent of patients were slightly improved, 17.2 percent were unchanged, and the conditions of 2.7 percent of patients deteriorated.[8]

Other studies on eczema patients have been carried out at the Swinoujscie health resort in Poland by dermatologists at the Medical University of Szczecin, which supervises therapy at the spa. One study carried out in the late 1970s involved a total of 1,141 patients with chronic eczema, hives, and atopic eczema. In addition to seawater baths and controlled solar irradiation, patients were only given emollients for their skin. Over 80 percent of the patients improved, the best results taking place in patients with atopic dermatitis.[9]

PSORIASIS

Psoriasis is a common form of dermatitis that may also be genetically related. It consists of itchy pink and dull-red skin lesions that take on the appearance of silvery scales. Although the symptoms tend to come and go, psoriasis is often chronic. While medications can provide comfort to the patient, there is no known cure.

Psoriasis responds well to bathing and mud baths, often in combination with sunlight, phototherapy, and medication.

Psoriasis is the most common skin disease among the 10,000 people who visit the Copahué Thermal Baths in Argentina each year. Considered Argentina's premier mineral spring, Copahué possesses a unique variety of cold and thermal sulfur-rich waters (in Aracuarian, *cope* means "sulfur" and *hué* refers to the place where it is found), as well as volcanic mud, algae, and vapors. Patients are treated under strict protocol conditions with balneotherapy, mud applications, and applications of cosmetics made from processed thermal products, for an average of 7 to 10 days. One physician who studied the Copahué patients commented that they "notice significant improvement in their eruptions . . . due to the keratolytic [loosening of the horny layer of the skin], antiinflammatory, antipruritic, antiseptic, and antiproliferative effects of the thermal compounds on psoriatic skin." Skin patch testing showed no allergic reactions and only rare cases of irritation.[10]

Psoriasis is also treated successfully at Bulgaria's famous Jagoda spa. Between 1984 and 1986, 54 patients (41 with psoriasis vulgaris and 13 with arthropathic psoriasis) were sent to the spa by dermatologists at the Medical University at Sophia for treatment. After a 3-week treatment protocol with the sulfate-rich and bicarbonate waters, 79 percent of the patients were discharged as either clinically healthy or having experienced major improvement.[11]

Bathing in salt water to alleviate skin problems has been practiced since pre-Biblical times. Because the saline content of the Dead Sea is approximately 30 percent (making it ten times as salty as the oceans), Dead Sea spas have long been important destinations for people with a variety of skin diseases. The Dead Sea area is also unique because it is the lowest point on earth, being 400 meters below sea level. Some dermatologists feel that the added distance screens out much of the damaging ultraviolet-B radiation, allowing for a higher concentration of ultraviolet-A radiation, having a favorable result in many skin diseases, particularly psoriasis. Approximately 10,000 patients travel to the Dead Sea each year, 8,000 of whom have psoriasis. Most are treated for 4 weeks with sunshine, Dead Sea water, sulfur baths, and mud.

At Ben Gurion University of the Negev, physicians studied the cases of 1,448 patients with psoriasis at the Mor Institute Dead Sea Psoriasis Clinic. Approximately 26 percent of the patients had more than 22 percent of skin involvement with the disease, while 10 percent had over 40 percent of their body surface involved. Treatment consisted of bathing in the Dead Sea for a maximum of an hour a day for 28 days, along with exposure to sunlight and the application of topical emollients. At the end of treatment, researchers observed a clearing of 80–100 percent in 88 percent of the patients treated, including almost 58 percent who experienced "complete clearing" of the disease. They concluded, "The overall response in a large cohort of psoriasis patients treated at the Dead Sea was excellent," and further investigation to determine the mechanisms of healing was recommended.[12]

At the Deutsches Medizinisches Zentrum, a German-run Dead Sea clinic in Jordan, all psoriasis medications used by patients are discontinued 4 weeks before therapy, which typically lasts 24 days. Once at the center, where the treatments are supervised by the Jordanian Dermatological and Venereological Society, patients are exposed to sunshine for 5 to 15 minutes twice daily. The exposure is gradually increased to a total of 6 to 7 hours a day. Patients bathe in Dead Sea water as well, beginning at 10 minutes twice daily and increasing to 45 minutes twice daily. Black mud is often applied to the body during the day, and creams and other lubricants are applied in the evening. The results of this type of therapy showed that approximately one-third of the patients enjoyed complete clearance of symptoms, approximately 40 percent of patients showed significant clearance, and approximately one-third had partial clearance.[13]

Several studies have been carried out at the Blue Lagoon in Iceland, a unique health care facility in a saltwater lagoon heated by a thermal spring. Physicians from the Department of Dermatology at the University of Iceland undertook a controlled 4-week study of 38 psoriasis patients: 21 were treated with bathing in the mineral-rich waters (sodium, silica, calcium, potassium) combined with five ultraviolet-B light treatments a week, while 17 took ultraviolet-B treatments alone. After 4 weeks, 20 of the 21 patients had an improvement rate of at least 75 percent in the combination group, while only 4 of the 17 patients taking the ultraviolet-B treatments alone showed improvement by at least 75 percent. The researchers concluded, "Bathing in the Blue Lagoon, with the addition of UVB light, is a useful alternative treatment of psoriasis, and better than UVB treatment given alone."[14]

At the University of Kiel in Germany, physicians in the Department of Dermatology tried to discover the actual healing mechanism of saltwater bathing for the treatment of psoriasis. Patients with psoriasis tend to have increased levels of protease elastase, an enzyme. Using 27 percent brine water from the Bad Bentheim spa near the Dutch border, the physicians investigated the progress of six patients with chronic psoriasis over a 30-day period. As the patients' conditions improved, the physicians measured their levels of protease elastase and found that it had fallen in all patients, especially during the first week of bathing. They concluded that "salt water therapy of psoriasis is able to diminish the skin content of potentially harmful protease elastase. [This phenomenon is] probably linked to the beneficial effect of salt water therapy."[15]

BURNS

It has been estimated that over 200,000 persons are severely burned each year; in 10,000 of them, the burns are either extensive or deep. In many cases, post-burn scarring can be severe and can present serious cosmetic defects. Among children in particular, scarring can inhibit normal tissue growth and the normal development of the jaw and face. Scarring can also cause psychological damage and can often lead to internal health disorders. Patients with severe burns often undergo many surgical procedures, thus risking infection.

We mentioned earlier that La Roche-Posay in France treats thousands of burn sufferers yearly, with a protocol that includes filiform showers, mists, and massage to help soften scar tissue and promote skin elasticity. As in its sister spas in Niederbronn-les-Bains and Saint-Gervais, these treatments have also been found to reduce inflammation and infection while promoting freer movement of the tendons and connective tissues.

At the Russian resorts at Sochi, a study was done involving over 6,531 patients (of whom 4,656 were children between 4 and 15 years of age) with burns on the face, neck, chest, and hands. They were treated with irrigations of sulfur-rich mineral water containing traces of strontium, barium, lithium, phosphorus, arsenic, and copper. Patients normally underwent a course of treatment involving 15 sessions of mineral water irrigations from specially designed hoses at different concentrations and pressures for 10 to 15 minutes. Many of these patients were referred to the clinic after traditional medications had failed to heal them.

Clinical findings on the patients revealed that treatment was effective in approximately 80 percent of the patients, with the best results manifesting in patients who received treatment within 7 to 10 days after their release from the hospital following plastic surgery. The researchers noted that in most patients skin microcirculation improved and the number of blood vessels in the scarred areas increased. Scars became smaller, and the skin became thicker and more uniform in texture. The researchers added, "Treatment as applied to the cicatrices [scars] results in diminution or complete cessation of itch and hurt, sensation of contraction. Functional disorders diminish, the amplitude and volume of movements in joints grow, so the need for further operational treatment not infrequently disappears."[16]

HYDROLIPIDYSTROPHY

Commonly known as cellulitis, hydrolipidystrophy primarily affects women. Cellulitis involves a modification of skin tissue caused by circulatory problems, retention of water and metabolites, and accumulation of fat in adipose tissue, primarily in the legs. Dr. Alberto López Rocha, a Spanish physician specializing in medical hydrology, found that a well-rounded program of balneotherapy can be very effective in controlling this problem. He recommended drinking 500–750 milliliters of mineral water on an empty stomach daily; bathing, involving partial or total immersion in warm mineral water; underwater massage; treatments with the Vichy shower, which involves a fine spray on the affected area, along with massage; pelotherapy, involving applying a layer of mud to the affected areas, which are then wrapped in cloth; steam baths; and the application of subaquatic ultrasound.[17]

Balneotherapy can serve both as an important alternative and as a complementary method of treating skin diseases. It is a natural and nontoxic modality that can be more effective than traditional drug therapy, and the pleasurable experience often adds to its inherent beneficial physical effects.

Some Springs That Are Known for the Treatment of Skin Diseases

Austria: Baden bei Wien
Bulgaria: Jagoda, Momin Prohod, Klustendil
Czech Republic: Mariánské Lázně, Smrdáky, Dolni Lipová
France: La Roche-Posay, St. Gervais, Sail-les-Bains, St. Christau, Avène-les-Bains
Germany: Bad Nenndorf, Bad Aachen, Bad Eilsen, Bad Bentheim
Greece: Icaria, Loutraki, Thermopylae
Hungary: Sarvar, Harkány, Hajdúszoboszló
Israel: Ein Bokek, Ein Gedi, Hamme Zohar

Italy: Abano Terme, Bagni di Lucca, Comano Terme, Lacco Ameno,
    Lurisia Terme, Sirmione Terme
Japan: Beppu, Kusatsu, Tamagawa, Shiobara, Nikko Numoto
Netherlands: Nieueschans
Poland: Busko-Zdrój, Ladek-Zdrój, Swinoujscie
Portugal: Taipas, Monfortinho, Amieria-Azenha
Romania: Băile Olăneşti, Herculane, Sovata
Russia: Pyatigorsk, Sochi
Slovenia: Moravske Toplice
South Korea: Bugok
Spain: Archerna, Arteijo, Ledesma

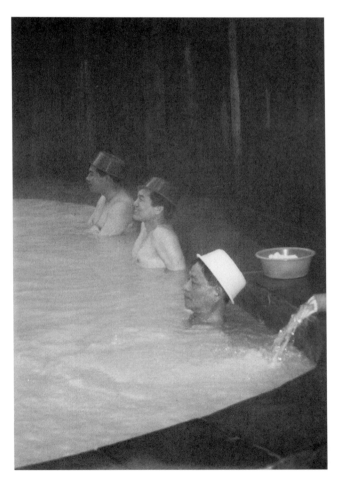

Sulfur spring bathing in the rain, Yangmingshan National Park, Taiwan.

JOINT AND MUSCLE DISEASES

Spa therapy has been used for joint and muscle diseases since the times of the ancient Greeks. Since then, an extraordinary amount of medical evidence, primarily in Europe and Japan, has revealed that different types of spa therapy—including bathing, hydrotherapy, pelotherapy, and drinking—can help the body heal itself of a wide range of joint diseases. These include inflammatory joint diseases such as rheumatoid and psoriatic arthritis, juvenile arthritis, and gout; connective tissue diseases such as scleroderma, spondylitis, and Reiter's disease; degenerative joint diseases such as osteoarthritis; and rheumatism, a general term used to describe acute and chronic soreness, muscle stiffness, and pains in the joints.

Many of the waters used to treat joint diseases are known as oligomineral waters because they contain small amounts of minerals such as sodium, calcium, magnesium, and chloride. Such waters are hypotonic because they have low osmotic pressure, allowing them to be easily absorbed into the intestine.

Spa therapy has been very popular among persons with joint and muscle diseases. In France alone, more than 250,000 patients a year undertake a 3-week course of treatment at spas to relieve lower back pain, osteoarthritis, and rheumatoid arthritis. Treatment may consist of thermal or cold spring water baths, mud baths, showers with jets of water directed at the joints, and underwater massage supplemented by drinking.

Over the years, researchers have found that many patients have often experienced a delayed-reaction to spa therapy, with lasting improvement manifesting after 3 or 4 weeks. For example, according to findings reported at spas throughout France, arthritis patients normally experience pain reduction, an improvement in joint mobility and quality of life, and less need for medication for a minimum of 6 months after treatment.[1]

LOWER BACK PAIN

Lower back pain very commonly affects adults and is considered a form of rheumatism. It is often treated with a variety of medications to relieve pain and inflammation, such as analgesics and nonsteroidal anti-inflammatory drugs, known as NSAIDs.

A controlled clinical trial study of 121 patients suffering from chronic low back pain was undertaken at the Institute of Hydrology at the Henri Poincaré University in Nancy, France, to determine whether spa therapy would lead patients to reduce their medication over a period of 3 weeks and 3 months. At the beginning of the trial, patients in the treatment group (which was given both drug therapy and spa therapy at Vittel, 6 days a week for 3 consecutive weeks) were taking larger doses of medications than those in the control group, who were given drug therapy alone. After 3 months, the results showed that "there was a statistically significant improvement of patient's health status in the treatment group compared with the control group. The functional disability, the pain duration, the pain intensity, and their finger to floor distance decreased in the treatment group. In the treatment group, overall health status of the back improved and drug consumption decreased significantly."[2, 3]

A controlled study of 38 patients with chronic lower back pain was carried out by researchers at the Reine-Hortense Hospital in Aix-les-Bains, France. The patients were divided into two groups: one group followed a water cure program for 5 months, while the other group did not; they were regularly examined by an independent physician with no connection to the spa. After the course of treatment, the treated group showed significant reduction of pain and stiffness, with increased flexibility. The researchers concluded, "The study findings tend to support the 4-month-delayed efficacy of a first spa treatment on functional impairment in patients with chronic low back pain."[4]

Hot springs therapy is also useful for treating postoperative conditions involving back pain. Rheumatologists undertook a 3-year-long study at Bourbonne-les-Bains in France, involving 52 patients who had undergone surgery to correct herniated discs and were still suffering back pain 1 year after surgery. The thermal waters at Bourbonne-les-Bains are rich in sulfates, chlorides, microminerals, and small amounts of radon. Patients were provided with a variety of spa therapies, including bathing in thermal water, a variety of massage techniques both with and without water, local applications of water under pressure, therapeutic exercises in water (hydrokinesitherapy), and local applications of thermal mud. Evaluations were made before and after each course of treatment, which was given once a year. Measurements made according to one scale of pain intensity showed improvement of 73 percent, and another measurement used to evaluate pain revealed improvement of 64 percent. Upon questioning by physicians, 14 patients reported that overall, they felt much better, 23 felt better, 12 felt the same while 3 felt worse.[5]

OSTEOARTHRITIS

Osteoarthritis is a painful degenerative disease affecting the joints. It involves the destruction of cartilage (which serves as a "shock absorber" to the joint), and overlapping of bone and the formation of spurs. It is said to affect 75 percent of the population over 60 years of age.

During World War II, a special research program of treatment under the direction of Walter McClellan, M.D., was carried out at the Veterans Hospital at Saratoga Spa in New York on 993 patients with arthritis and related disorders. In addition to bathing in the spa's famous carbonated waters and thermal mud packs, patients were given massage, whirlpool, and heat treatments. Over 92 percent of those treated showed definite improvement.[6] Although medical therapy is no longer offered at Saratoga, bathing in its waters continues to help many people with arthritis and other rheumatological complaints.

A double-blind placebo study of 62 patients at the Puspokladany Spa in Hungary, sponsored by the National Institute for Rheumatology and Physiology of Budapest, involved 18 treatments of 20 minutes each. The treatment group bathed in spa water (containing trace amounts of carbon dioxide, chloride, and iodine), while the control group received similar treatments in a pool containing heated tap water. Patients in both groups were also given standard doses of painkillers and NSAIDS. Clinical examination showed that the patients who had bathed in the mineralized thermal waters experienced a "significant" reduction in knee pain tenderness as opposed to patients who bathed in tap water.[7]

Despite the positive results obtained by this and other studies, doctors remain uncertain as to why patients improved. Some believe that the temperature of the thermal water has some effect; others believe that minerals such as chloride and sulfur may play a role. According to Daniele Fabiani, M.D., of the Institute of Internal Medicine of the University of Florence and his colleagues at other European medical schools, "These factors may interfere with diuresis and blood dilution and favor muscle relaxation, pain reduction, and joint motion." In addition, they suggest two primary actions: (1) anti-inflammatory action attributed to the drainage of extracellular fluids (with substances such as prostaglandin, histamine, and serotonin) and reduced tension of the structures, and (2) analgesic and relaxant actions caused by the release of analgesic substances by the body.[8]

A study of 50 patients with osteoarthritis of the knee joint was sponsored by Bulgaria's National Centre of Physical Therapy and Rehabilitation using hot compresses made of Dead Sea water. The patients were divided into two groups; one received compresses containing 1.5 grams per liter of salts, and the other group received compresses containing 300 grams per liter. After 20 days of treatment, which also included magnetotherapy and therapeutic exercises, researchers found both clinical and functional improvement. However, the group receiving compresses containing the higher concentrations of salts (which also contained magnesium, calcium, bromide, and others) did better. The researchers believed that the improvement may have been due to improved blood circulation caused by the sodium chloride and the antiallergic, relaxing, and anti-inflammatory effects of the other minerals.[9]

RHEUMATOID ARTHRITIS

Rheumatoid arthritis involves inflammation of the joints and includes pain, swelling, and stiffness. It also limits movement, sometimes so much that the patient requires a walker or a wheelchair to get around.

Bathing in warm mineral water, accompanied by special exercises, has been used in dozens of spas to help patients increase joint mobility. In addition, underwater massage with jets of water is helpful and provides many of the benefits normally associated with massage, such as improved muscle tone, pain relief, and increased blood circulation. In patients with advanced rheumatoid arthritis, mud packs may help increase movement as well.

A study was carried out at Caldas de Lugo in Spain, a spa that can trace its origins to Roman times. There, physicians from the University of La Coruña treated 645 patients with rheumatoid arthritis, a third of whom had been sent to the spa by their physicians. A 2-week program of thermal bathing with hydromassage, showers, and pelotherapy showed a marked reduction in pain. At the beginning of the therapy, 21.9 percent of the patients experienced intense pain, whereas at the end of the cure, only 4.6 percent felt intense pain. At the beginning of the therapy, 17.7 percent felt no pain, a figure which climbed to 82.6 percent at the end of the treatment.[10]

While immersion in warm water is the best-known form of balneotherapy for patients with rheumatoid arthritis, Japanese researchers have found that cold spring bathing is very effective as well. To help determine the mechanisms of healing, researchers at the Medical Institute of Bioregulation at Kyushu

University in Beppu analyzed patients at the Kan-no-jigoku cold sulfide spring in Beppu. Cold spring bathing brought about functional changes of the sympathetic nervous system as well as important and beneficial changes in the patients' health. After 3 weeks of bathing, patients reported a marked reduction in pain and morning stiffness, with increased mobility and grip strength.[11]

The Yangantau Sanitarium in Bashkiria, Russia, is renowned for its warm thermal vapors, which rise from a deep cavern. These vapors contain radon and nitrogen as well as trace amounts of minerals such as magnesium, iron, silica, and copper. A medical study of 207 patients found that a daily vapor bath lasting from 10 to 12 minutes, in conjunction with therapeutic exercise and massage, reduced inflammation and pain in 83.6 percent of the patients for 6 months or more after treatment. The researchers added that the treatment "possesses a favorable influence upon the course of immune reactions, the connective tissue system, [and] improves the conditions of the vegetative nervous system."[12]

PSORIATIC ARTHRITIS

This disorder is a type of arthritis that often accompanies psoriasis, an often chronic skin disease manifesting as scaly pink or red skin lesions that produce itching.

Several spa therapies have been found to be very effective in relieving the symptoms. In Italy, physicians at Abano Terme and other spas have introduced applications of mud containing large amounts of bacteria, algae, and protozoa that utilize sulfur; in some cases, bathing in waters rich in sulfur in combination with ultraviolet-B light has also been helpful.

At a clinic in Ein Bokek, Israel, researchers studied the effects of Dead Sea bathing and mud packs on 360 patients with psoriatic arthritis in 1992. Most patients had been taking NSAIDs. Treatment consisted of immersion in seawater with active mobilization of joints three to five times a day for 4 weeks, along with mud packs for 20 minutes a day, three times a week. The results showed that 86.6 percent of the patients experienced good results, which included being completely free of symptoms; or were almost free of symptoms (no drugs, no joint disability, very seldom slight pain), or were much improved, involving reduction of pain and drugs. The researchers concluded, "A four-week treatment at the Dead Sea represents an effective therapy for [psoriatic arthritis] by reducing in most of the cases pains, disability, and medications."[13]

What is it about thermal springs that help us heal from joint and muscle problems? Clinicians such as Czech physician Bohuslav Kocab, M.D., believe that bathing in thermal springs stimulates the activity of the pituitary gland, which secretes ACTH and cortisone, both pain inhibitors. In addition to producing an overall calming and relaxing effect on the body, heat also helps to relieve muscle spasm and suppress inflammation, thus allowing healing to take place.[14] Clinicians at the ORFI National Institute of Rheumatology and Physiotherapy in Budapest, Hungary, believe that the salts and other trace elements in mineral water improve recovery rates from injuries and reduce the quantity of painkillers needed.

A TYPICAL TREATMENT

The ORFI National Institute of Rheumatology and Physiotherapy, a 1,400-bed treatment center, is the world's largest health facility where physicians use healing waters in the treatment of muscle and joint diseases. The water used by the institute comes from two medicinal springs from the Császár Baths, which were discovered in the sixteenth century. Both springs have been found to be slightly radioactive; one contains calcium, magnesium, and hydrogen carbonate ions in different concentrations, and the other contains calcium, magnesium, hydrogen carbonate, alkalis, and fluorides.

A 3-week treatment is often recommended for patients with rheumatism. In addition to daily medicinal baths, the patient undergoes sessions of hydrotherapy (involving a strong jet of water that relaxes the muscles and dilates the blood vessels); since rheumatic pain often contracts the muscles, hydrotherapy is designed to relax them. This is complemented by treatments of electrotherapy, the application of small amounts of electricity to relieve pain. The weight bath calls for the patient to hang in the medicinal water supported by a neck collar, and weights are sometimes placed on the feet to lengthen the spine and increase the spaces between the vertebrae, which are often reduced by the rheumatism. Some patients are also given mud baths or mud packs made of mineral-rich mud heated to as high as 44°C (111°F). This treatment is considered very effective in relaxing joints and in relieving muscle pain. Massage and rehabilitative exercise are also an important part of the healing program. In addition to bathing in the healing waters, patients who also have stomach and gastric disorders drink them as well, with a recommended intake of 200 grams a day.[15]

While treatment will vary according to the individual, doctors at European spas generally prescribe simple baths in thermal waters (especially in water containing sulfur) followed by a period of rest. Bathing in springs containing hydrogen sulfide, iodine, bromide, and radon is also popular. Many European spas offer mud baths, high-pressure hosings with mineral water, and mud compresses as well, followed by bed rest in dry blankets. Physical therapy, remedial exercise, massage, and acupuncture all enhance the effects of the healing water. Individualized diets stressing high-protein foods and foods containing essential vitamins and minerals are often prescribed for people with joint and muscle problems, as well.

Some Springs with Healing Waters and Muds for Joint and Muscle Disorders

Argentina: Cachueta, Los Molles, Pismanta, Copahué
Australia: Daylesford, Hepburn Springs, Moree
Austria: Bad Aussie, Baddeutch-Altenburg, Baden bei Wien, Bad Gastein, Bad Gosern, Bad Schallerbach
Belgium: Spa
Brazil: Araxá, Caxambú, Lambari, Poços de Caldas, São Pedro, Serra Negra
Bulgaria: Velingrad, Pavel Banya, Kyustendl
Canada: Banff, Fairmont Hot Springs, Harrison Hot Springs
Chile: Termas de Chillán, Termas de Huife, Termas de Puyehue
China: Huanqing
Colombia: Paipa, Tabio
Croatia: Lipik, Topusco
Cuba: Ciego Montero, Elguea, San Diego de los Baños
Czech Republic: Františkovy Lázně, Jáchymov
Ecuador: Baños, El Tingo, Guapán, Papallacta
France: Balaruc, Neiderbronn-les-Bains, Bourbon-Lacy, Dax, Bagnères-de-Bigorre, Bourbonne-les-Bains, Bourbon-l'Archambault
Germany: Bad Griesbach, Baden-Baden, Bad Nenndorf, Bad Wildbad, Bad Kreuznach, Wiesbaden, Wiesenbad
Great Britain: Bath, Buxton, Harrogate, Leamington Spa, Llandrindod
Greece: Aedipsos, Icaria, Loutraki, Thermopylae
Hungary: Budapest, Bükfürdo, Eger, Hajdúszoboszló, Héviz
Iceland: Hveragerdi
Ireland: Lisdoonvarna
Israel: Hamme Zohar, Tiberias
Italy: Abano Terme, Acqui Terme, Agnano Terme, Bagni di Lucca,

Castrocaro Terme, Ischia Terme, Montegrotto Terme, Salsomaggiore Terme, Sirmione Terme

Jamaica: Milk River

Japan: Atami, Beppu, Dogo, Hakone, Ibusuki, Ito, Katsuura, Kusatsu, Narugo. Nikko Yumoto, Noboribetsu, Shiobara, Shirahama, Tamagawa, Unzen, Yugawara

Mexico: Agua Hedionda, San José de Purúa, Ixtapán de la Sal

New Zealand: Rotorua, Hamner Springs, Miranda Hot Springs

Peru: Baños del Inca, Monterrey, Yura

Poland: Busko-Zdrój, Ciechocinek, Cieplice Slaskie-Zdrój, Potczyn-Zdrój

Portugal: Caldas da Rainha, Furnas, Curia, Cucos, Luso, São Pedro do Sul

Romania: Băile Felix, Băile Herculane, Călimănești, Geoagiu Bai

Russia: Bashkiria, Pyatigorsk, Repino, Sochi

Slovakia: Bojnice, Piešťany, Trenčianskě Teplice, Čiz

Slovenia: Čatež, Dobrna, Moravske Toplice, Šmarješke Toplice

South Korea: Bugok, Onyang

Spain: Alhama de Aragón, Archena, Caldes de Montbui, Caldes de Malavella, Fitero, Jaraba, Ledesma

Switzerland: Bad Ragaz, Bad Schinznach, Baden, Leukerbad, Rheinfelden, Yverdon-les-Bains

Taiwan: Peitou, Chipen, Wulai, Yangmingshan

Turkey: Bursa, Izmir-Çesme, Pamukkale, Yalova

United States: Saratoga Springs, New York; Hot Springs Arkansas; Berkeley Springs and White Sulfur Springs, West Virginia; Hot Springs, Virginia; Calistoga, California; Glenwood Springs, Colorado.

Uruguay: Termas de Arapey

Venezuela: Las Trincheras, Aguas Calientes

GASTROINTESTINAL PROBLEMS

Thermal and mineral waters are often indicated for treating a wide range of gastrointestinal disorders, including problems with the stomach and duodenum, gastroenteritis, ulcer, and constipation. Karl Luhr, M.D., of the Evangelical Hospital in Gottengen, Germany, suggests that the appropriate therapies include balneotherapy, pelotherapy, and drinking of mineral waters.[1]

THE DRINKING CURE

The drinking cure is especially popular in relieving many gastrointestinal problems. Substances in the water are absorbed by the gastrointestinal tract and affect gastrointestinal functions. For example, research has shown that drinking salt spring water, as well as water rich in carbonic acid, increases gastric mucosal blood flow and enhances the ability of the stomach to eliminate toxins. When mineral water containing sodium bicarbonate and sodium sulfate is drunk before meals, it increases blood insulin levels and bile acid concentrations.[2] Drinking these waters also has an impact on the secretion of liver bile and on the motoric function of the gallbladder and large intestine. Drinking carbonate waters over a 4-week period has been found to normalize gastric secretions among patients with chronic gastritis and ulcer relapses, affecting both hyperacidity as well as anacidity.[3] Research carried out at the famous Olăneşti Spa in Romania showed that the mineral waters have an inhibiting effect on gastric secretions and stomach acidity, making the waters popular among patients with hyperacid gastroduodenitis (inflammation of the duodenum).[4]

According to the Czech balneologist Bohuslav Kocab, M.D., "The effect of the drinking cure is based on the action of the dissolved salts on the alimentary system, whose motivity, secretion, incretion, absorption and excretion are influenced. It has an anti-inflammatory and spasmolytic effect, abolished gastric and intestinal dyspepsia, normalizes the stools, creates good conditions for the restoration of impaired biliary and liver function (bile synthesis, evacuation of the gall bladder) and activates the pancreatic juice into the small intestine, regulates intestinal peristalsis and the antiseptic activity of bile acids."[5]

Founded by the Roman Emperor Flavius Vespasian during the first century, Caldas de Chaves is one of Portugal's oldest healing springs. People with gastrointestinal problems have been drinking its waters for nearly 1,900 years. Dr. Mario Gonçalves, Clinical Director of Caldas de Chaves, outlined the indications for drinking mineral water for gastrointestinal problems for the Ministry of Health in Galicia, Spain.

He found that waters rich in bicarbonate are indicated for disorders affecting the stomach, liver, and gallbladder. Waters rich in sodium bicarbonate are especially useful in treating gastritis and stomach ulcer. Drinking warm water is especially useful for persons with gastritis, and cold water helps stimulate gastric secretions. Waters that are rich in bicarbonate, calcium, and fluoride help calm intestinal spasm. Waters rich in calcium sulfate help relieve the symptoms of colitis and intestinal problems related to allergic reactions to food or medication.[6] Writing in the same publication as Dr. Gonçalves, Dr. Seraphin Pérez Pombo reported that drinking bicarbonate water and sulfated water helps relieve the symptoms of constipation; in fact, such waters should be avoided by patients with diarrhea.[7]

Researchers at the Tamagawa Hot Springs in Japan have found that drinking 100 milliliters of Tamagawa water (divided into three portions a day) is effective for treating several gastrointestinal complaints, including belching, nausea, gastritis, and heartburn, as well as anorexia. Despite the water's high acidity (pH 1.2), drinking Tamagawa water reduces the levels of gastric acid in patients with hyperacidity, while it raises gastric acid levels in those with hypoacidity. Researchers believe that these seemingly contradictory effects are due to the ability of this water to normalize gastric functioning.[8] Similar results were found in a study of 107 patients suffering from either constipation or diarrhea. After several weeks of bathing in and drinking Tamagawa water, normal functioning improved in both groups.[9]

A study on the value of mineral water in the complex treatment of stomach ulcer and gastritis was carried out at the Military Medical Academy in St. Petersburg, Russia. A group of 67 patients were given normal medical treatment with the addition of Ekateringofskaya mineral water, a bicarbonate water of low mineralization. The control group of 74 had the same diseases treated in a similar manner, but without mineral water. The treated group showed improvement of noncellular resistance, increased activity of mononuclear phagocytes, and a significant increase in tumor necrosis factor—all indicators of increased immune resistance. The treated subjects also experienced a normalization of interleukin-1b in comparison with the control group. The researchers concluded that Ekateringofskaya mineral water should be included in the complex treatment of gastritis and ulcer.[10]

IRRITABLE BOWEL SYNDROME

The Châtel-Guyon Spa is probably the most famous thermal establishment in France for the treatment of gastrointestinal disorders. A recent study by three physicians at Châtel-Guyon compared the quality-of-life responses of patients with irritable bowel syndrome who were treated with spa therapy at Châtel-Guyon with a control group of patients who received traditional medical therapy. Questionnaires were filled out by patients 1 month after therapy and again 6 months later.

The responses after the first month showed slight improvement in both groups, but it was not considered statistically significant. However, after the sixth month, the patients who had undergone the spa cure showed "significant" improvement as measured by quality-of-life responses. This led the researchers to conclude that the spa cure was "at least equivalent to conventional treatments."[11]

A TYPICAL PROTOCOL

Although persons taking the drinking cure should do so under the direction of a qualified health professional, the following general guidelines may be useful for normal, healthy individuals.

Generally speaking, the best time to begin drinking therapeutic waters is 30 minutes to an hour before meals.

Waters containing large amounts of salt, acid, radon, aluminum, or iron should be taken in small amounts or diluted with tap water.

The amount of water to be consumed during the day should be between 100 and 200 milliliters per session, and between 200 and 1,000 milliliters per day. Much will depend on the age, physical size, and sex of the individual; for example, women tend to retain water more than men, and this is taken into account when a balneologist prescribes a drinking cure.

For healthy individuals, contraindications to drinking spring water are few. However, avoid chloride water or waters rich in sodium sulfide if you have kidney disease, hypertension, or edema; avoid sulfate, bicarbonate, and sulfur waters if you suffer from diarrhea.[12]

FAVORITE PLACES FOR THE DRINKING CURE

Visitors to San Pellegrino, about 40 miles northeast of Milan, Italy, can experience the drinking cure as well as hydrotherapy, carbon dioxide baths, inhalation, paraffin baths, massage, and other treatments at the Cure Termali. The water is used to treat kidney and liver ailments as well as other digestive disorders. The high levels of sulfates and bicarbonates help control the acidic level of gastric juices and stimulate the digestive processes. San Pellegrino is one of the most popular of the premium carbonated mineral waters sold in the United States and Canada.

The famous thermal waters in Vals, Switzerland, were first noted in 1670 and have been ingested therapeutically for diuretic and purgative purposes. The Swiss have found Valser St. Petersquelle water effective in cases of heartburn and other digestive disorders. In addition to the water cure, the Hotel Therme in Vals offers a dietary program enhanced by mineral baths, sauna, physical therapy, and water gymnastics.

The spa at Vichy in the south of France dates back to the time of Julius Caesar, who had a health resort built there over 2,000 years ago. The Hall des Sources captures the elegant world of Emperor Napoleon III, who with his entourage of several thousand would make Vichy their primary summer resort. Vichy Spa is supplied by 12 springs, of which 6 are used for the drinking cure. The cold springs include Célestins, Parc, and Lucas, and the warm springs include Hôpital, Chomel, and Grande Grille. In addition to boasting two well-equipped thermal establishments, Vichy offers a convention center, a casino, ballet, concerts, plays, films, golf courses, a racing track, and facilities for tennis, volleyball, basketball, and horseback riding.

The source of Vichy Célestins, the most popular water used for drinking, emerges at 22°C (71°F) through strata of aragonite rock, formed by waterborne mineral deposits over millions of years. Layers of calcium carbonate have eroded over the centuries, contributing to Vichy's unique natural carbonation and mineralization. Vichy's low level of carbonation and high mineralization give it a taste that many associate with Alka-Seltzer. Vichy water has been used to treat stomach disorders, normalize biliary secretions, alleviate the symptoms of gastroesophagal reflux, provide relief from food and drug allergies, and reduce the symptoms of colitis. Thermal baths, thermal showers, mud therapy, steam baths, facials, thermal gas inhalation, and whirlpools are some of the other treatments used at Vichy for patients with gastrointestinal complaints. Vichy Célestins is bottled and enjoyed as a mineral water throughout Europe and parts of North America. Because of its rich sodium bicarbonate content, balneologists recommend that Vichy water be consumed after meals as a digestive.

We mentioned earlier that the thermal springs at Loutraki, source of the only natural mineral water in Greece that is recognized by the European community, are among the oldest in the world. Drinking therapy at Loutraki is carried out with either thermal or natural mineral water, depending on the patient's condition.

The Loutraki spa has five organized centers for drinking therapy, where visitors are treated for heart ailments, dyspepsia, disturbances of the nervous and circulatory systems, liver insufficiency, kidney stones, and gallstones.

The indications include digestive irregularities, chronic alkaline gastritis, irritations of the intestinal tract, simple chronic constipation, diarrhea, primary and secondary gastritis, duodenitis, nonspecific chronic proctitis, irregular movements of the bile ducts, gallstones, chronic inflammation of the gallbladder, kidney stones, chronic kidney insufficiency, metabolic disturbances of uric acid, and inflammations of the urinary tract.

Some Springs with Healing Waters for Gastrointestinal Problems

Argentina; Pismanta, Rosario de la Frontera, Termas de Reyes
Austria: Bad Gleichenburg, Bad Ischl
Belgium: Oostend
Brazil: Aguas da Prata, Caxambú, Lambari, Lindoia, Poços de Caldas, São Pedro
Bulgaria: Pavel Banya, Sophia, Velingrad
Chile: Panimávida
Colombia: Paipa
Croatia: Igalo
Cuba: San Miguel de los Baños, Santa Fé
Czech Republic: Karlovy Vary, Mariánské Lázně
Ecuador: El Tingo, Guitig
France: Vichy, Eugénie-les-Bains, Plombières, Châtel-Guyon, Vittel
Germany: Bad Bertich, Bad Homburg, Bad Kissengen, Bad Pyrmont, Hindelang

Great Britain: Cheltenham, Leamington Spa
Greece: Loutraki
Hungary: Budapest (Rác, Lukács, Széchenyi), Harkány, Balatonfüred
Ireland: Lisdoonvarna
Italy: Castellamare Stabia, Castrocaro Terme, Lurisia Terme, Montecatini
    Terme, San Pellegrino Terme
Japan: Atami, Beppu, Dogo, Narugo, Noboribetsu, Shiobara, Shirahama,
    Tamagawa
Mexico: San José de Porúa, Tehuacán
Peru: Chancos, Monterrey
Poland: Krynica, Kudowa-Zdrój, Polanica-Zdrój
Portugal: Caldas da Rainha, Caldas de Chaves, Caldas do Geres, Termas
    de Monte Real, Pedras Salgadas, Termas de Vidago
Romania: Băile Herculane, Băile Olăneşti, Călimăneşti
Russia: Essentuki, Pyatigorsk, Zheleznovodsk
Slovakia: Bardejov
Slovenia: Rogaška
Spain: Caldas de Malavella, Marmolejo, Fita Santa Fé, Mondariz
Switzerland: Bad Scoul-Tarasp-Vulpera, Vals
Turkey: Pamukkale, Yalova
United States: Saratoga Springs, New York; Truth or Consequences, New
    Mexico; Hot Springs, South Dakota

14

DISEASES OF THE LIVER, KIDNEYS, AND URINARY TRACT

The use of mineral water to treat diseases of the liver, kidneys, and urinary tract is among the oldest forms of spa therapy. Waters containing bicarbonate, sulfates, chlorides, and sodium facilitate the healing of a variety of liver complaints, including hepatitis, and also help improve liver and gallbladder function such as the synthesis of bile by the liver and its release by the gallbladder into the duodenum, or small intestine, which aids digestion.

HEPATITIS

Hepatitis is a serious viral disease affecting the liver, one of our body's most important and complex organs. It is sometimes accompanied by jaundice and liver enlargement. Although there is no known cure for hepatitis, it is controlled by medication.

Physicians at Olăneşti Spa, known as the "Carlsbad of Romania," have been treating hepatitis patients for more than 50 years. A major study done in 1960 focused on the effect of water from four of its springs—all rich in differing concentrations of sodium, chlorides, and trace minerals such as calcium and magnesium—on 150 patients with hepatitis and 250 patients with chronic cholecystitis (inflammation of the gallbladder). Improvement was observed in 133 of the hepatitis patients and 240 of the cholecystitis patients. Olăneşti also has a specialized children's sanitorium, which treats the sequelae of epidemic hepatitis approximately 6 months after the acute stage of the disease has healed. Treatment with waters from three of the springs reduced liver pain among 59 percent of the children treated.[1]

A medical research study in Russia focused on the effects of water rich in sulfides, chlorides, and sodium bicarbonate on individuals with chronic persistent hepatitis. Treatment consisted of sodium chloride baths, diet, and therapeutic physical training over several weeks. The therapy gave evidence of strengthening the body's immune system. The researchers concluded that bathing in water rich in sulfide, chloride, and sodium enhances the dynamics of the clinical and functional state of the liver and in the immune reactivity of the organism.[2]

Some Springs Whose Waters Are Used for Healing Liver and Gallbladder Disorders

Argentina: Cachueta, Copahué, Termas de Reyes
Austria: Baden bei Wien
Brazil: Caxambú, Lambari, Lindoia, Poços de Caldas, Serra Negra, São Pedro
Bulgaria: Hissarya
Chile: Panimávida
Colombia: Paipa, Santa Rosa de Cabal
Cuba: Santa Fé
Czech Republic: Karlovy Vary, Mariánské Lázně
Ecuador: Guitig
France: Châtel-Guyon, Brides-les-Bains, Eugénie-les-Bains, Plombières, Vichy
Germany: Bad Bertrich, Bad Homburg, Bad Kissingen, Bad Pyrmont, Hindelang
Greece: Loutraki
Italy: Castrocaro Terme, Chianciano Terme, Lurisia Terme, Montecatini Terme, San Pellegrino Terme
Japan: Atami
Peru: Chancos
Poland: Polanica-Zdrój
Portugal: Termas de Monte Real, Termas de Vidago
Romania: Băile Olăneşti, Călimăneşti
Russia: Essentuki
Slovenia: Rogaška
Spain: Caldas de Malavella, San Narciso, Mondariz, Marmolejo
Switzerland: Bad Scoul-Tarasp-Vulpera
United States: Glenwood Springs, Colorado; Truth or Consequences, New Mexico; Saratoga Springs, New York; Hot Springs, South Dakota

KIDNEY AND
URINARY TRACT DISORDERS

The first scientific evidence of the value of spa therapy for treating diseases of the urinary tract first appeared in 1943, when improved kidney function following the ingestion of alkaline sulfate waters was demonstrated. Since that time, physicians have confirmed the value of spa therapy—especially drinking, colonic irrigation, and physical therapy—as aspects of a holistic approach to treating kidney disease and related urinary tract disorders. Drinking mineral water, in particular, can alter the composition of urine and help dissolve kidney stones.[3, 4]

At the Czech spa of Mariánské Lázně, a study of 10,000 patients formed the basis of a scientifically planned method of treatment whose main component is the drinking cure. Many of the waters used in the drinking cure to treat kidney and urinary tract diseases are known as oligomineral waters because they contain small amounts of minerals such as sodium, calcium, magnesium, and chloride. Such waters are hypotonic because they have low osmotic pressure, allowing them to be easily absorbed into the intestine.

According to Joseph Mates, M.D., who served as head physician at the Research Institute for Physiology, Balneology, and Climatology at Mariánské Lázně, the different mineral waters produce specific physiological effects when consumed at the amount of 20 milliliters per kilogram of body weight:

- Simple natural carbonate waters are used as diuretics without changing the pH of the urine.

- Carbonated waters containing large amounts of calcium and magnesium are also good diuretics, and they raise the pH level of the urine to 7 (the neutral point).

- Waters containing calcium sulfate tend to be mildly diuretic and may lower the pH a small amount; such water is slowly absorbed into the bowel, while other types of water are more rapidly absorbed.

- Alkaline waters tend to reduce bladder irritation.

- Waters containing sodium sulfate influence the flora of the intestinal tract; they are strong diuretics and apparently produce diarrhea in some individuals.[5]

The scientific rationale behind his findings were substantiated by studies undertaken at the Edouard Herriot Hospital's Service of Renal Functional Research in Lyon, France. Three types of mineral water with varying compositions of sodium, chlorides, calcium, and magnesium were administered to six healthy subjects. Urinalysis was performed over an 8-hour period after the water had been consumed and revealed that the chemical findings corresponded to the type of water ingested. In addition, the amout of urine output differed according to the water's chemical composition. The researchers concluded, "These findings are a confirmation that when water is used therapeutically, both quantity and composition must be taken into consideration."[6]

Indications and recommendations of spa treatment for urinary tract infections are specific to the disorder. If the pH of the urine is low, alkaline waters are prescribed; if the urine is neutral or alkaline, alkaline earth and simple carbonated waters are recommended.[7] Contraindications include urinary tract obstruction, tumors of the genitourinary tract, and all conditions requiring restriction of water or sodium intake.

Although protocols for drinking mineral water are prescribed for each individual patient at many European spas, generally every patient drinks water on an empty stomach two to three times a day. Although it will not do any harm, drinking a glass or two of mineral water will not lead to permanent changes in one's health. Generally speaking, physicians recommend that drinking mineral water daily at the spa for 2 to 3 weeks is advisable in order to achieve more lasting effects.[8]

Dr. Bohuslav Kocab wrote specifically on the types of treatment given at Czech spas such as Mariánské Lázně and Trenčianské Teplice:

> The success of complex spa treatment consists in the effect produced on urine chemistry by the individually selected type of mineral water and by the diet, which affects the concentration of calculus-forming salts and substances inducing synthesis of organic acids, leading to stone formation, influence the reabsorption of calcium and phosphorus on the intestine and increase the solubility of calculus-forming substances. The beneficial effect is further potentiated by water intake and exercise.[9]

Some Springs Whose Waters Are Used for Healing Kidney and Urinary Tract Disorders

Argentina: Pismanta, Rosario de la Frontera
Austria: Baden bei Wein, Bad Gleichenburg
Brazil: Araxá, Cambuquira, Caxambú, Lambari, Lindoia, Poços de Caldas, São Lourenço, Serra Negra

Bulgaria: Hissarya, Pavel Banya, Sophia, Velingrad
Chile: Panimávida
Cuba: San Miguel de los Baños
Czech Republic: Mariánské Lázně, Trenčianskě Teplice
Ecuador: Tumbaco
France: Evian, Contrexéville, Eugénie-les-Bains, St. Nectaire, Vittel
Germany: Bad Wildugen, Bad Brukenau, Bad Ditzenbach
Italy: Agnano Terme, Chianicaino Terme, Fiuggi, Montecatini Terme, San Pellegrino Terme
Japan: Beppu
Mexico: Tehuacán
Poland: Krynica
Portugal: Termas de Curia, Termas de Luso, Pedras Salgadas
Romania: Călimăneşti, Băile Olăneşti, Tusnad, Slănic Moldova
Slovenia: Radenci, Rogaška
Spain: Jaraba, Solan de Cabras, Alzola, Castromonte, Borines
Switzerland: Bad Scoul-Tarasp-Vulpera
Turkey: Yalova
Uruguay: Termas de Arapey

15

HEART AND CIRCULATORY DISEASES

Individuals with cardiovascular problems have been taking the waters for thousands of years. Among the heart and circulatory diseases that respond to balneotherapy are arterial circulatory disorders, venous congestive disorders, high cholesterol, reflex dystrophy, hypertension, myocardial insufficiency, cardiac arrhythmia, lesions of the heart valves, angina, phlebitis, post myocardial infarction, impaired circulation in the lower limbs caused by diabetes, and autonomic cardiovascular disorders.

Clinical observations at spas around the world have shown that bathing in thermal spring water can affect the heart and circulatory system. Researchers at the British Royal Infirmary in Bristol, England, studied a group of eight men and women who were fed identical diets for several days. The subjects were immersed in water from the famous spa at Bath (a naturally thermal water rich in bicarbonate and sulfate) and on another day were immersed in ordinary tap water at a similar temperature. The researchers found that immersion in spa water at 35°C (95°F) resulted in a 50 percent increase in cardiac index. No such changes were observed when the subjects bathed in heated tap water.[1]

A study was carried out at the Paul Ribeyre Hospital in Vals-les-Bains, France, on 223 patients with cardiovascular problems, including 177 who also had diabetes. The goal was to evaluate the Vals-les-Bains 3-week treatment program, which included drinking water, hydrotherapy, diet, and blood sugar control. Extensive physical examinations and blood tests were done on all patients before, during, and after treatment. The researchers found a significant improvement in the fasting glucose, fasting insulin, and fructosamine values among the diabetic patients, even over a 120-day period, and improved blood pressures, both systolic and diastolic. Triglyceride and cholesterol levels fell significantly for all patients except those with insulin dependent diabetes mellitis.[2]

Medical studies in Japan on the effects of hot springs bathing on the circulatory system revealed beneficial effects. Whole-body bathing in thermal water produced a sharp, transient rise in blood pressure followed by a rapid fall, especially among individuals with hypertension whose blood pressure returned to prebath levels soon after bathing. Partial bathing in warm water rich in carbon dioxide caused blood pressure to fall gradually and remain at a lower level for "a fairly long time." Also, the effect of bathing on hemodynamics tended to become less intense during repeated treatments with partial bathing in water that was gradually warmed, especially in patients with hypertension.[3]

Intermittent claudication, a disorder that causes severe leg pain, is a result of inadequate blood supply to the legs from arterial spasm, atherosclerosis, or arteriosclerosis. Physicians at Royat-Chamalières, France, treated a group of 37 patients with this disease, using spa therapy and kinesitherapeutic readaptation; 15 patients in a control group were given only traditional medical treatment, primarily vasodilating drug therapy. Comparisons of the two groups after 18 days of treatment showed significant improvement in the experimental group; the control group showed no improvement.[4]

A study concerning the rehabilitation of patients who had recently had heart attacks was carried out at the Jaunkemeri Health Resort in Latvia. The research involved 207 patients who had suffered heart attacks 20 to 30 days before. Of 145 treated patients, 99 were given general bath treatment and the other 42 received local baths of the arms and legs only, with hydrogen sulfide baths. The control group of 62 patients did not undergo spa treatment. After extensive electrocardiographic and other cardiac testing, positive results were observed among those treated with spa therapy: the increase in blood volume in the treated patients was compensated by a decrease in the peripheral resistance of the blood vessels and an increase of the diastolic time. It was concluded that spa treatment with hydrogen sulfide water is useful for the early rehabilitation of patients after acute infarction of the myocardium.[5]

Hot springs bathing has also been found to help improve blood circulation in patients with severe diabetes. At the Institute of Physical Medicine, Balneology, and Medical Rehabilitation in Bucharest, Romania, 21 diabetic patients with arteriopathies of the lower limbs were studied. The researchers carefully evaluated the patients before, during, and after therapy with a battery of tests. Evaluations were made at the beginning, at the end, and a month after an 18-day treatment with sulfur-rich waters at the Călimănești Spa. By the end of the treatment period, all test results showed obvious improvement in blood circulation according to all testing parameters. Improvement remained constant after 1 month of treatment.[6] Related findings concerning spa therapy for the treatment of diabetes can be found in chapter 16.

Researchers at the spa at Aulus-les-Bains in France studied the effects of drinking spa water on cholesterol levels. The physicians selected 155 subjects whose cholesterol was between 2.20 and 3.40 grams per liter of blood; the participants were divided into two groups, with 65 patients receiving the drinking cure with Aulus water (which is rich in sulfates and bicarbonates, as well as trace minerals such as magnesium and iron). The other 50 participants drank ordinary tap water, which was taken from the water supply of the city of Toulouse. Participants consumed three glasses containing 200 milliliters of water in the morning and another three glasses in the late afternoon, with a 20-minute space between drinks per session. The results revealed marked improvements among those who took the water cure. Those who drank the Aulus water lost more weight than those who drank ordinary tap water, and their total cholesterol levels, HDL levels, and triglyceride levels fell much lower.[7]

In some cases, bathing in hot springs (especially very hot springs) can be dangerous. Researchers at the Gumma University School of Medicine in Japan have documented cases in which people bathing in very hot Kusatsu spa water (a 3-minute bath in 47°C [117°F] water) experienced sharp increases in the plasma level of plasminogen activator inhibitor 1 antigen within 15 minutes, which did not return to normal levels for another 6 hours. They believe that these changes were directly due to the bath's hyperthermal action, which decreased the fibrinolytic capacity of the blood (thus causing the blood to become more viscous), which could thus lead to coronary thrombosis in some individuals.[8] Bathing in 42°C (108°F) water for 10 minutes brought about transient changes in blood pressure, heart rate, blood viscosity, fibrinolytic activity, and platelet function induced by hyperthermal stress, which could lead to heart attack and stroke in individuals who are prone to these health problems.[9, 10]

Unless you suffer from heart disease, the news about contraindications to very warm spring baths is not all bad. In their studies on the effects of hot water bathing, the same researchers found that subjects who took the 3-minute time bath also had a threefold rise in plasma beta-endorphin levels, where "one feels an intoxicating sensation and desires to bathe more and more."[11]

As with other health problems, certain spas specialize in treating cardiovascular problems and have developed unique protocols and treatment programs. One of the most famous spas for heart and circulatory diseases is

Royat-Chamalières in France. Two thermal centers offer an extensive program, including carbon dioxide baths, underwater massage, arm and foot baths, leg baths, several types of shower baths, a special carbon dioxide bath involving walking against a water current, therapeutic swimming pools, and physical therapy. They also have a unique method for treating circulatory problems of the lower limbs by insufflating carbon dioxide gas into a nylon bag, which is placed around the affected limb. Royat is also the home of the Institute of Cardiovascular Research, which specializes in investigating the scientific basis and application of spa therapy for heart and circulatory disease. Cardiovascular treatments are supervised by eight cardiologists and two angiologists specializing in diseases of the blood vessels and lymphatic system.[12, 13]

THE CURES

Different cardiovascular diseases respond well to different types of balneotherapy. On the following pages can be found the primary forms of spa treatment, possible adjunct therapies, and possible contraindications to spa therapy. The information is based primarily on the recommendations of Dr. Victor R. Ott, Professor of Physical Medicine and Balneology at the University of Geissen in Germany.[14]

Arterial circulatory disorders

Treatment: Bathing in water rich in bicarbonate, iodide, and/or radon; baths in lightly mineralized thermal waters; Kneipp treatment

Adjunct therapies: Active exercise; connective tissue massage

Contraindications: Recent coronary thrombosis, gangrene, progressive inflammatory conditions

Venous congestive disorders

Treatment: Baths in water rich in bicarbonate, walking in thermal pools, Kneipp treatment

Adjunct therapies: Remedial exercise

Contraindications: Recent thrombosis, progressive inflammatory conditions

Reflex dystrophy

Treatment: Bathing in thermal exercise pools, Kneipp treatment

Adjunct therapies: Active exercise, massage according to individual needs

Contraindications: Acute stage

Essential hypertension
Treatment: Baths in water containing bicarbonate and/or iodide
Adjunct therapies: Nutrition, active exercise, stress reduction techniques
Contraindications: Heart failure with congestion, severe kidney problems, vascular fragility

Myocardial insufficiency
Treatment: Bathing in waters rich in bicarbonates
Adjunct therapies: Carefully prescribed exercise and dietary regimen
Contraindications: Congestive heart failure, marked right ventricular strain, progressive inflammation

Cardiac arrhythmias
Treatment: Varies widely and is designed for the individual patient

Lesions of the heart valves (including sequelae of valve operations)
Treatment: Bathing in waters rich in bicarbonates
Adjunct therapies: Supervised physical exercise, breathing exercises
Contraindications: Failure, severe mitral valve and aortic valve stenosis, right ventricular strain, progressive inflammation

Angina
Treatment: Bathing in water containing bicarbonates and/or iodide, Kneipp treatment
Adjunct therapies: Partial baths, exercise, connective tissue massage
Contraindications: Severe coronary insufficiency, imminent heart attack, acute myocardial infarction

Post myocardial infarction
Treatment: Bathing in water containing bicarbonates and/or iodide, Kneipp treatment
Adjunct therapies: Diet, exercise, "small" hydrotherapy (involving a single limb)
Contraindications: Severe coronary insufficiency, imminent heart attack, acute myocardial infarction

Autonomic cardiovascular disorders
Treatment: Bathing in bicarbonate saline waters, Kneipp treatment
Adjunct therapies: Exercise, "small" balneotherapy (involving a single limb)
Contraindications: Severe neurosis

KNEIPP TREATMENT

As mentioned earlier in chapter 1, the Kneipp treatment, or Kneipp kur, is a specialized program of hydrotherapy that also includes a natural foods diet, exercise, and herbs. Developed by German cleric Sebastian Kneipp during the mid-1800s, it features several specialized techniques, including ablutions of alternating hot and cold applications of mineral water, as well as washing the entire body with warm water every 20 or 30 minutes to induce perspiration.

Kneipp especially advocated the use of arm, leg, and foot baths and the application of various kinds of hot and cold packs and compresses to different parts of the body, such as the hips or calves. Kneipp techniques also include local affusions (pouring on of water) to various parts of the body; these may be given as pressure showers of differing temperatures and pressures, often followed by 10 to 15 minutes of exercise to increase circulation in the affected body region or part. Hot affusions may also be given to the back, neck, and buttocks to relieve muscle pain, or to the vertebral column to relieve disc complaints. Each affusion is applied according to a prescribed sequence; for example, all affusions begin at the point farthest from the heart. A contrast knee affusion may begin with a warm spray to the knees, right and left, followed immediately by cold water on both knees, and then repeating the hot and cold sprays once again.

Although there are over 50 Kneipp health resorts in Germany today, many other European spas use at least some of the Kneipp techniques to treat cardiovascular disorders. Writing in the textbook *Medical Balneology*, Dr. Kurt Franke described a typical morning program at a Kneipp resort:

> The most frequent prescription is for three partial applications a day over a period of four weeks. Treatment may begin between 6 and 7 A.M. with a small application in bed, such as an ablution of the trunk or a dry brushing of the skin followed by a cool after-ablution. Early morning treading on the dewy grass for one to five minutes, or treading in the snow in winter for one-half to one minute, stimulates the trophotropic para-sympathetic system. . . . During the forenoon, stronger applications are given in the hydrotherapy department; for example, a contrast foot bath or knee affusion at first and, later in the course, cold affusions to the upper thigh and back.[15]

In addition to the treatments themselves, visitors are given a plant-oriented diet that is rich in vitamins and low in fat, including whole wheat bread and an abundance of fresh raw vegetables. For overweight patients, a special reducing diet may be prescribed. In addition, visitors are encouraged to take walks, which are often on grounds that have been designed and posted according to distance and degree of inclination. Other activities, such as reading or working with arts and crafts, are encouraged to reduce stress and promote mental relaxation.[16] Kneipp techniques are continuously being updated and refined, and they remain an important part of many modern spa programs in Germany today.

CARBON DIOXIDE TREATMENT

Waters rich in carbon dioxide have been used therapeutically to treat circulatory diseases since the Middle Ages. These waters have vasodilating properties, which can be obtained by bathing in the waters as well as by regional subcutaneous carbon dioxide gas injections or bagging with dry carbon dioxide gas.

It also has an overall calming effect on the nervous system, which can reduce vascular spasms, and has a direct effect on the heart, both slowing the pulse rate and strengthening heart contractions. Bathing in carbon dioxide–rich waters also helps the body produce new blood vessels, thus increasing blood circulation, and can increase overall tone in the veins.[17]

MAGNESIUM IN DRINKING WATER

Magnesium has long been considered a factor in the prevention of heart disease. The relation between death from acute myocardial infarction and the level of magnesium in drinking water was examined using mortality registers and a case-control design, and was reported in *The American Journal of Epidemiology*. The study area comprised 17 municipalities in southern Sweden that have different magnesium levels in the drinking water. The study compared men in the area who had died of acute myocardial infarction with men of the same age living in the same area who had died of cancer during the same time period. In both groups, only men who consumed water supplied from municipal waterworks were included in the study. The subjects were divided into four groups according to the drinking water levels of magnesium and calcium and the quotient between magnesium and calcium. The results suggested that magnesium in drinking water is an important protective factor for death from acute myocardial infarction among men.[18]

SPA PROTOCOLS

Each spa features a distinctive approach to treating patients with cardiovascular disease. In addition, specific programs will be tailored for each individual, taking account of symptoms, the patient's age and physical condition, and the presence or absence of other diseases.

In the Czech Republic and Slovakia, the main constituent of complex balneotherapy for treating cardiovascular patients is carbon dioxide baths, given at different temperatures and pressures, usually no more than three times a week. According to *Spa Treatment in Czechoslovakia*, "The effect of complex spa treatment using carbon dioxide baths is revealed in more economic cardiac function, in increased systolic volume and cardiac output, prolongation of diastole, a slower pulse rate, improvement of coronary circulation, a decrease in diastolic pressure, and in hypertensives, a decrease in systolic pressure and an increased urine flow."[19] Carbon dioxide therapy is always supplemented with physical exercise, especially in the form of remedial exercises and prescribed walks. In addition to exercise, supplementary forms of physical therapy are often provided that improve physical resistance and adaptability.

The spa at Bagnoles-de-l'Orne in Normandy offers a comprehensive 3-week protocol for the treatment of phlebitis. The basic treatment is focused on the thermal water, which is administered daily at a temperature of 35–37°C (95–98°F) for 10 to 30 minutes, depending on the individual. Balneotherapies can include whirlpool baths, aeromassage and hydromassage, oxygen and gas applications, and vaginal douches. Treatment may also include physical therapy in thermal pools (especially walking), sitz baths, applications of thermal compresses and high-pressure applications of thermal water to affected areas, and applications of thermal mist.[20]

Dr. Victor R. Ott writes that the general principles in the treatment of cardiovascular patients include the following:

- Carbon dioxide baths are prescribed on alternating days or four times a week, often in bathtubs during the first half of the morning. However, some spas use swimming pools. The ideal temperature is 33–35°C (91–95°F).

- At the beginning of treatment, the baths are short, lasting 4–6 minutes; if they are well tolerated, they are gradually increased to 12–15 minutes.

- The first two or three baths are known as half baths: the water level reaches the lower part of the chest as the person is in a semireclining position. The person later moves on to three-quarter baths, in which the water reaches nipple level. Patients are generally advised not to breathe the carbon dioxide gas.

- In addition to bathing, patients are advised to rest at specified times of the day; they are also given specific forms of therapeutic exercise.[21]

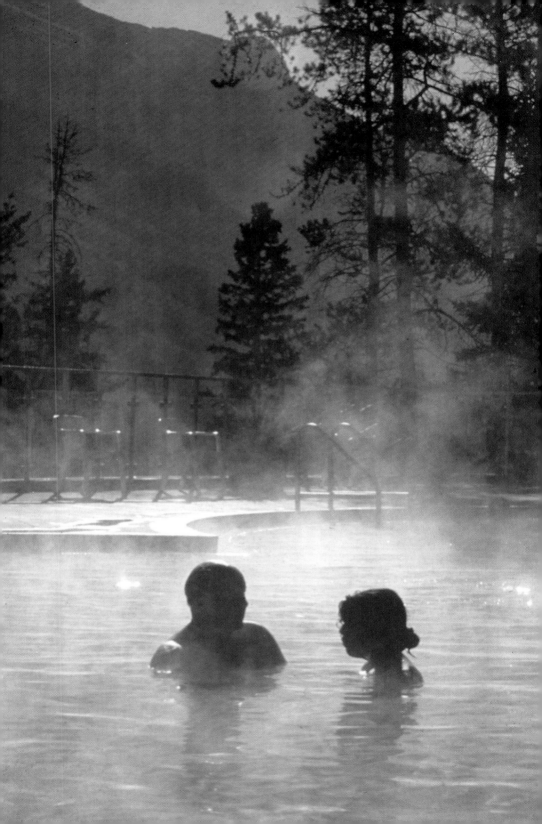

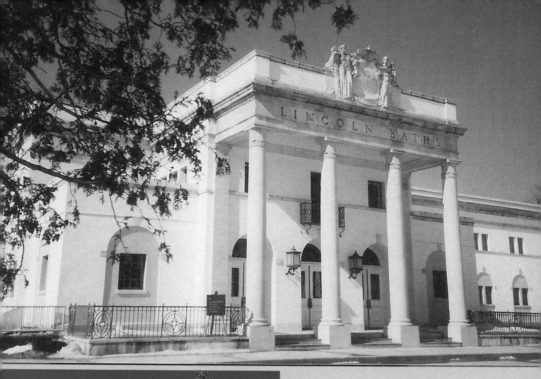

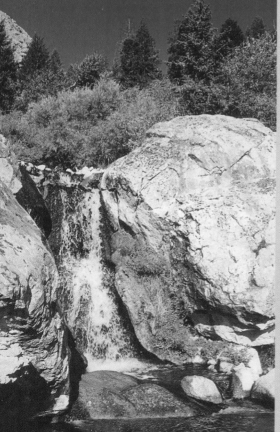

Overleaf: The pool at Banff Upper Hot Springs, Alberta, Canada

Above: Lincoln bathhouse, Saratoga Springs, New York

Left: Goldbug Hot Springs, Idaho

Below: Mud and mineral water, Köyceğiz, Turkey

Opposite: Montecatini Terme, Italy

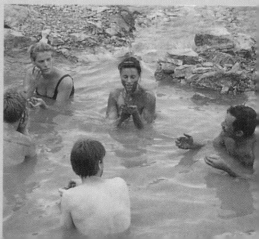

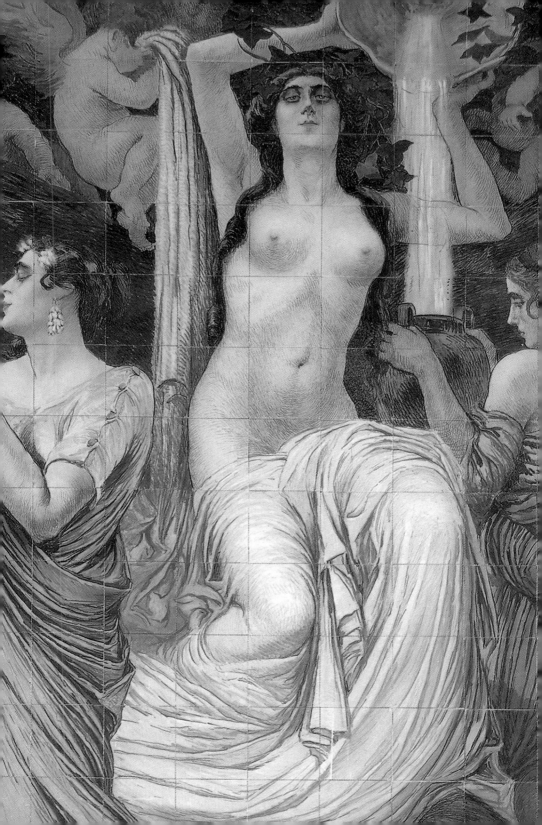

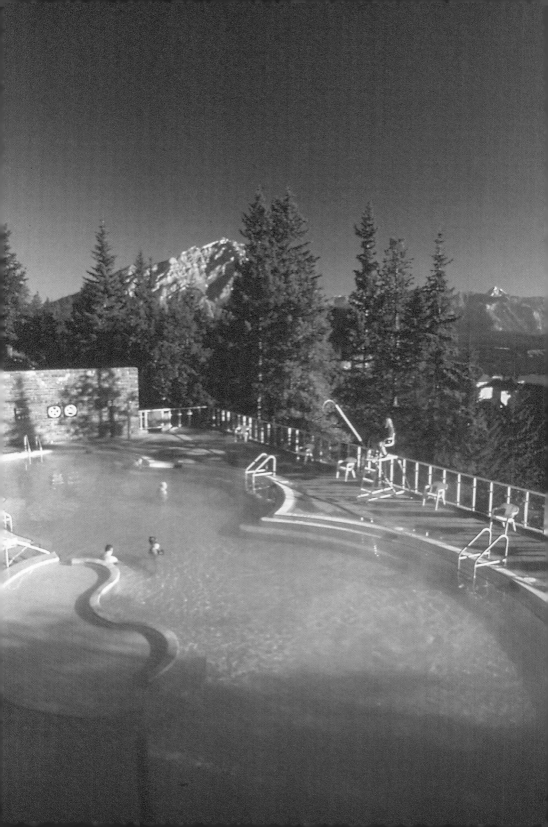

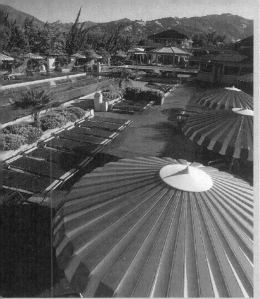

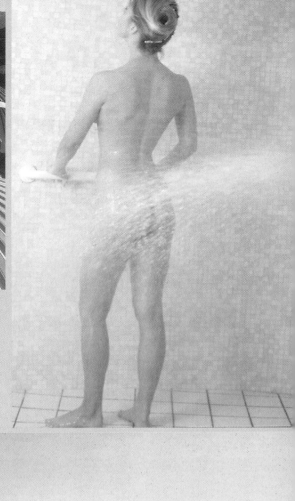

Opposite: Banff Upper Hot Springs, Alberta, Canada

Above: Outdoor mineral pool, Calistoga, California

Right: High-pressure hose treatment, Vittel Spa, France

Below: Thermal establishment, La Roche-Posay, France

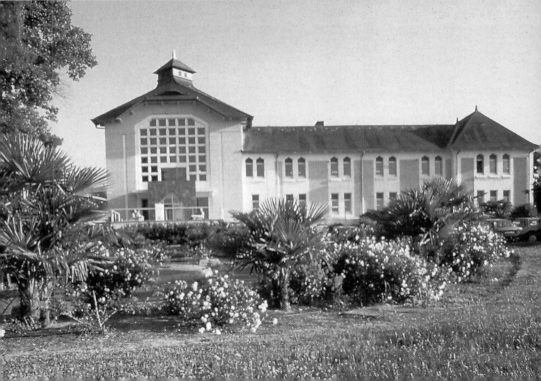

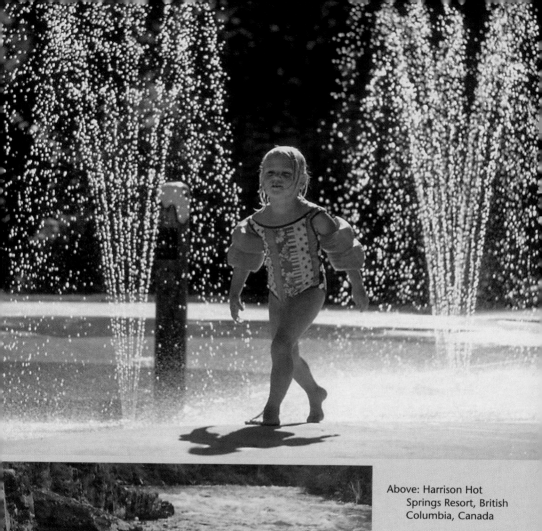

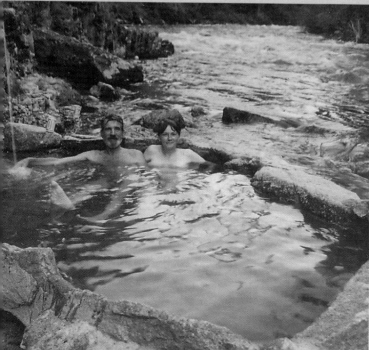

Above: Harrison Hot Springs Resort, British Columbia, Canada

Left: Soaking pool, Mile Sixteen Hot Springs, Idaho

Below: Winter bath, Yuzowa Onsen, Japan

Opposite: Terwilliger (Cougar) Hot Springs, Oregon

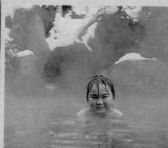

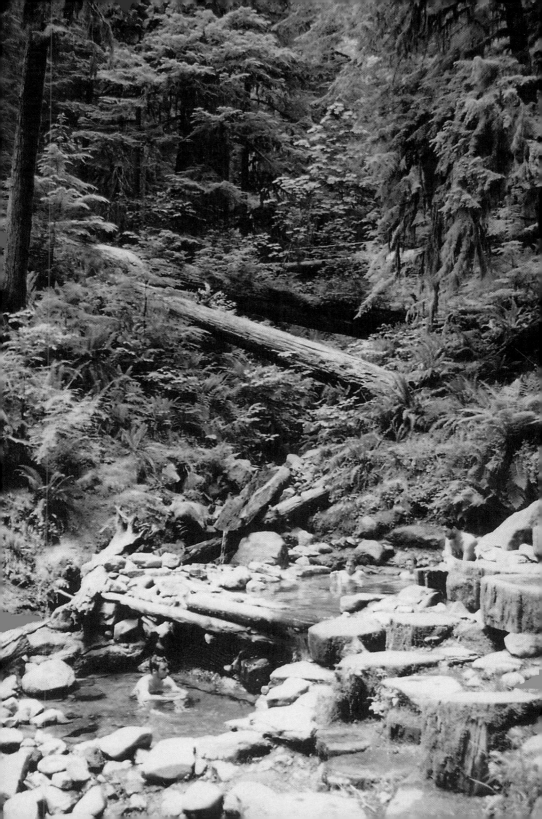

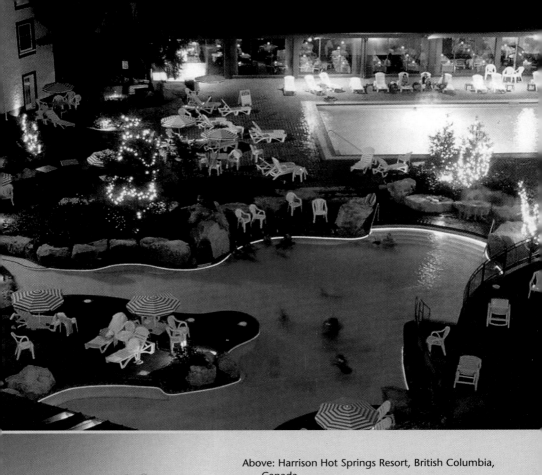

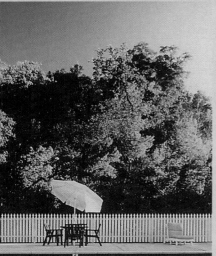

Above: Harrison Hot Springs Resort, British Columbia, Canada

Left: Vichy Springs, California

Below: Ruby Lakes Hot Springs, Nevada

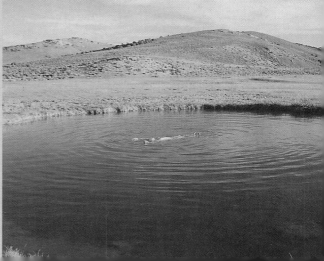

Finally, many spas provide a tranquil and beautiful natural environment, which helps distract the patients from the stresses of daily life.

Some Springs Whose Waters Treat Cardiovascular Disorders

Austria: Bad Hall, Bad Ischl, Bad Tatzmannsdorf, Warmbad-Villach

Bulgaria: Albena, Kyustendil

Czech Republic: Františkovy Lázně, Jáchymov, Konstantonovy Lázně, Lázně Poděbrady

France: Royat-Chamalières, Bain-les-Bains, Bourbon-Lancy

Germany: Bad Ems, Bad Nauheim, Bad Orb, Bad Pyrmont, Bad Salzuflen, Bad Wildungen

Hungary: Balatonfüred

Italy: Chianciano Terme, Ischia Terme, Montegrotto Terme, Salsomaggiore Terme

Japan: Arima, Zao (hypertension)

Poland: Busko-Zdrój, Ciechocinek, Kolobrzeg, Krynika, Kudowa-Zdrój, Polanika-Zdrój

Portugal: Caldas do Geres (hypertension), Termas de Luso

Romania: Băile Herculane, Sovata

Russia: Kislovodsk, Pyatigorsk, Repino, Sochi

Slovakia: Čiz (arteriosclerosis), Sliač

Slovenia: Radenci, Šmarješki Toplice

Spain: Jaraba

GYNECOLOGICAL PROBLEMS

Since pre-Roman times, women have been soaking in hot springs and mineral springs to help heal a variety of gynecological disorders. Although medication, hormone therapy, and surgery are most often used for treating gynecological complaints today, hot spring therapy is still popular in Europe for women who prefer more natural treatments that provide a minimum of adverse side effects. And while spa therapy may not cure all gynecological complaints (and, as we will see later on, some women with tumors and other conditions should avoid hot springs completely), balneotherapy—with its proven ability to soothe, disinfect, reduce pain, and normalize metabolic processes—can be an important part of a holistic approach to treating a wide variety of disorders particular to women.

Physicians at Luxeuil-des-Bains in France give several major indications for spa therapy. In France, approximately half the women who visit spas to treat gynecological problems suffer from various types of genital pain. The pain may be a result of infection after giving birth, suffering a miscarriage, or undergoing an abortion. It may also be the result of a sexually transmitted disease such as chlamydia, gonorrhea, or mycoplasma; postoperative pain as the result of a surgical procedure such as hysterectomy; cyclic pain related to menstruation (including premenstrual syndrome); or some other type of pain related to vaginitis, depression, poor circulation, accident or injury, stress, or some other cause.

Problems with conception also lead European women to seek treatment at hot and mineral springs. Balneotherapy is recommended for treating sterility caused by inflammation of the fallopian tubes, irregularities of the mucosal lining of the cervix, and hormonal problems that affect ovulation. Approximately 30 percent of women who visit French spas for gynecological complaints have one or more of these problems.

Menopausal difficulties include hot and cold flashes, feelings of weakness, and mental depression in some cases. Symptoms that sometimes affect post-menopausal women, such as vaginal dryness, vaginitis, circulatory complaints, osteoporosis, and urological and metabolic disorders, are often indications for gynecological treatment in European spas.

The following waters are often used to help treat gynecological conditions:

- mineral waters of low mineralization (such as those found in Luxeuil, Bagnoles de l'Orne, and Aix-en-Provence)
- waters rich in chlorides and sulfates (including those found at Challes, St. Sauver, and La Preste)
- springs with high concentrations of sodium chloride (Salies-de-Béarn, Salies-du-Salat, and Bourbon l'Archambault)
- waters rich in bicarbonate of chloride (Châtel-Guyon, Néris)
- springs rich in calcium chloride (Éveaux, Ussat)[1]

Some physicians suggest that waters having a slight amount of radioactivity are useful in gynecology for their sedative, decongesting, and anti-inflammatory properties.[2]

In addition to bathing and drinking, a wide range of water-related therapies are used in European spas for treating women with gynecological complaints. They include vaginal irrigation at differing pressures and temperatures, cervical-vaginal douches, external localized douches, and compresses made with thermal water or thermal mud.

We mentioned earlier that in France the government pays for up to 3 weeks of spa treatments annually that are prescribed by a physician, who often helps the patient select a spa that will provide maximum medical benefits. For example, while the spas at Luxeuil and Salies-du-Salat specialize in the treatment of gynecological complaints, a spa such as Balaruc or La Lechère may be recommended for women with gynecological problems who also have rheumatism or circulatory disorders.

In European spas, patients receive an individually designed program of spa therapy after a thorough examination by a resident physician. However, some Spanish balneologists state that a normal woman with mild to moderate gynecological complaints can safely bathe in mineral water at a temperature of 36–38°C (97–100°F) for 15 minutes to a half hour.[3]

Although spa therapy is well suited for women with a wide range of health problems, hot springs bathing should be avoided by women with tumors (especially cancerous tumors), severe infections, inflammation, obstructions of any kind, alterations in the position or structure of the uterus, or severe endocrine disturbances. Women who are pregnant should avoid hot springs bathing unless permitted to do so by a qualified physician.

Some Springs Whose Waters Are Used to Help Cure Gynecological Problems

Argentina: Los Molles, Cachueta, Río Hondo, Rosario de la Fronetra
Austria: Baden bei Wien, Bad Ischl, Salsburg
Belgium: Spa
Brazil: Aguas de Prata, Caxambú, Poços de Caldas, São Lourenço
Bulgaria: Blagoevgrad
Canada: Miette Hot Springs, Radium Hot Springs
Chile: Panimávida, Termas de Chillán
Colombia: Paipa
Croatia: Igalo, Topusco
Cuba: San Diego de los Baños
Ecuador: Guapán, Santa Elena, Tumbaco
France: Luxeuil-les-Bains, Salies-de-Béarn, Salies-du-Salat, Néris, Bourbon-l'Archambault
Germany: Baden-Baden, Bad Kissingen, Bad Nauheim, Bad Pyrmont, Bad Reichenhall, Bad Salzuflen
Greece: Aedipsos, Loutraki, Thermopylae
Hungary: Balatonfüred, Hajdúszoboszló, Harkány
Italy: Abano Terme, Agnano Terme, Bagni di Lucca, Ischia Terme, LurisiaTerme, Montecatini Terme, Montegrotto Terme, Salsomaggiore Terme, Sirmione Terme
Mexico: Ixtapán de la Sal, San José Purúa
Peru: Baños del Inca, Chancos, Monterrey, Yura
Poland: Krynica, Potczyn-Zdrój
Romania: Băile Felix, Băile Herculane, Băile Olăneşti, Călimăneşti, Geoagiu Bai, Sovata
Russia: Pyatigorsk, Sochi
Slovenia: Dobrna
Spain: Caldas de Montbui, Ledesma, Montemayor, Caldas de Bohui
Switzerland: Rheinfelden
United States: Berkeley Springs, West Virginia; Hot Springs, Arkansas; Hot Springs, Virginia; Glenwood Springs, Colorado; Truth or Consequences, New Mexico
Uruguay: Termas de Arapey

GLANDULAR AND METABOLIC DISORDERS

In this chapter, we will examine the effects of hot springs bathing and drinking on several common glandular diseases and metabolic diseases, including diabetes, obesity, gout, and prostatitis.

DIABETES

Most people think of controlling diabetes mellitus in terms of special diets or injections of insulin. However, several researchers in Europe and Japan have found that bathing in and drinking sulfurous mineral water can have a positive effect on patients with diabetes. The healing properties of the water are believed to penetrate the body both through the skin and when inhaled as vapor.

At the Medical Institute of Bioregulation at Kyushu University in Japan, the effects of cold spring bathing on diabetic patients were studied. Five elderly patients took two 15-minute baths a day for 12 days in the Kan-no-Jigoku spring. Located in the famous hot springs region of Beppu, Kan-no-Jigoku has been popular with people with asthma, skin diseases, and rheumatoid arthritis for hundreds of years.

Patients with a lower severity of the disease showed improved glucose tolerance and better energy utilization, and others reported improved appetite and greater ease of movement as therapy progressed. The conclusion was that "diabetic patients, especially patients with lower severity, showed a better control of diabetes after 12 days of Kan-no-Jigoku therapy," and the spring was recommended for helping patients control diabetes.[1]

Similar results were obtained by researchers at the Hokkaido University School of Medicine in a study of diabetic patients who exercised in a hot

(38°C [100°F]) pool for 30 minutes. Over several months, the patients' plasma glucose levels decreased significantly, and positive relationships on plasma glucose levels were observed before and after exercise. Lipid metabolism increased, the ratio of low density lipoprotein and high density lipoprotein cholesterol decreased, basal levels of plasma cyclic AMP decreased slightly, and plasma cyclic GMP increased significantly. The researchers added, "The tranquilizing function of hot springs is effective on psychological disturbance, diabetic autonomic and peripheral neuropathy."[2]

A team of Romanian researchers from the Institute of Internal Medicine, Balneology and Medical Rehabilitation in Bucharest studied the internal and external effects of the mineral waters at Călimănești on 40 diabetic patients over a period of 18 days and found consistently favorable effects. The researchers concluded the action of Călimănești spa water "an internal and external cure, to be advantageous [to] patients with diabetes mellitus, because of the favorable influence on some of the biochemical parameters involved in the development of both diseases and complications."[3]

The favorable results of the study led researchers to investigate the healing effects of Călimănești waters on arteriopathy of the lower limbs, a circulatory problem that is sometimes found among patients with advanced or chronic diabetes that can lead to gangrene and eventual limb amputation. Working in cooperation with the Clinic of Nutrition and Metabolical Diseases in Bucharest, researchers at the Institute of Physical Medicine, Balneology and Metabolical Rehabilitation in Bucharest studied 40 diabetic patients with arteriopathy of the lower limbs. Patients were treated for a total of 18 days at the spa, which including bathing, drinking, and walking under the direction of a physical therapist. A 140.9 percent increase in circulation was observed at the end of the cure, which was maintained at 30.3 percent after 1 month. A testing method called oscillometry was used to determine the degree of permeability of the main arteries. The researchers found that the increase of blood supply to the limbs showed an average increase of 83.33 percent over a 7-day period, which increased to 271.91 percent by the end of the 18-day cure period. They concluded that this type of therapy has "a favorable effect especially on the elements which theoretically have a potential of reversibility representing a useful method in the prophylaxis of gangrene."[4]

The possibility of using balneotherapy to help manage diabetes among patients with non–insulin-dependent diabetes mellitus was studied at the Hokkaido University School of Medicine. In addition to exercise, patients were treated with frequent hot springs water bathing over 4 weeks. The researchers found that daily changes in fasting plasma glucose, insulin, C-peptide, cortisol noradrenaline, and adrenaline indicated a "normalizing process of physiological functions" and found that metabolic and endocrine dysfunctions among the patients improved. They concluded that balneotherapy offers "a great advantage" in both treatment and prevention of the disease, and recommended that "careful" balneotherapy be used to help decrease the amount of medication (such as hypoglycemic agents and insulin) needed by diabetic patients.[5]

An interesting adjunct therapy to balneotherapy in treating elderly patients with diabetes is forest-air "bathing" and walking, known in Japan as *shinrinyoku*. Volatile components, such as negative ions emitted from the forest, have been found to possess certain chemical properties and can produce changes in physiological functioning in humans, including lowering blood pressure, increasing saliva secretions, decreasing the amount of cortisol, and balancing autonomic nervous system activity.[6] Walking in the forest is considered an "air bath" that is both healthful and enjoyable.

At the Hokkaido University School of Medicine, 48 non–insulin-dependent diabetic patients were studied; 11 were given only dietary and exercise therapy, while the other 27 were medicated orally, and 10 were given insulin. After careful examination of blood glucose levels, the participants were divided into two walking groups, with one group walking 3–4 kilometers and the other 6–7 kilometers. Blood samples were taken after the walk. Among patients taking the short walk, blood glucose levels dropped an average of 79 milligrams per deciliter, and levels among those taking the long walk dropped to a statistically similar 76 milligrams per deciliter. By contrast, when patients performed for 30 minutes on a cycle ergometer their blood glucose levels fell by only 13 milligrams per deciliter. Researchers concluded that exposure to negative air ions through forest walking enhances parasympathetic nervous activity, which can lead to decreased glucose levels.[7]

PROSTATITIS

Prostatitis is an inflamed condition of the prostate gland, often characterized by dull aching pain and a discharge from the penis. It is usually treated by antibiotics and other medications.

The clinic at La Preste-les-Bains in the Pyrenees Mountains of southern France specializes in the treatment of diseases of the urinary tract and metabolic disorders, as well as prostatitis and gynecological diseases. The waters are rich in sulfur and sodium sulfate, and they contain significant amounts of silica. They are recognized for their sterilizing, anti-infectious, and analgesic properties, particularly in the urinary tract. In addition to traditional balneotherapy (including bathing, douches, showers, and inhalations), the drinking cure is widely used at La Preste because of its direct effects on the kidneys and urinary tract.

Physicians at La Preste studied the effects of spa therapy in 53 men with recurrent acute prostatitis. After two courses of treatment at the clinic, 67.7 percent of patients were completely free of infection, and another 20.9 percent showed improvement by more than 50 percent. A 2-year follow-up of 23 patients showed that improvement stood at 72.3 percent. The researchers also noted a significant decrease in pain among 10 patients, testifying to the analgesic effects of the waters at La Preste.[8]

GOUT

Gout is a painful metabolic disease that includes acute arthritis and inflammation of the joints, especially the knees. It is caused by an excess amount of uric acid in the blood and deposits of urate of sodium in and around the joints.

Except in acute, gouty arthritis, spa therapy is well tolerated by patients with gout. Balneotherapy (involving both hot bathing and exercise), vapor baths, and pelotherapy (usually in the form of mud packs applied to the swollen joints) are also recommended by medical balneologists.[9] According to Dr. George D. Kersley of the Faculty of Medicine at the University of Bristol, England, "Patients with severe gout perhaps rely more on spa treatment than any other group of patients."[10]

WEIGHT CONTROL

Obesity is due to more than simple overeating: it is connected to disturbances in biological adaptation as well as psychological factors. Many European spas geared to weight loss offer comprehensive programs that include diet, exercise, and different types of hydrotherapy. Balneologists believe that the thermal and chemical properties of hot spring water (at approximately 40°C [104°F]) has a diuretic affect on the body, increases cardiac output, increases blood circulation, and stimulates the sympathetic nervous system. Such increases in body metabolism may lead to increased burning of calories, resulting in weight loss. Drinking hot spring water can also stimulate gastric function, leading to improved digestion, and drinking may also result in improved elimination of toxins from the body.

A 4-week-long study on obesity at the Russian Scientific Center of Medical Rehabilitation in Moscow involved 300 obese patients between 25 and 55 years of age, divided into treated and control groups. The treated patients were given a 1,300-calorie diet and hydrotherapy, which often involved contrasting hot and cold bathing in mineral water. The control patients were given diet therapy only. Because members of the treated group had different health levels, each person was given a custom-made hydrotherapy program.

After 4 weeks of treatment, the patients receiving balneotherapy showed a marked decrease in cholesterol and triglyceride levels. The control group actually showed a moderate increase in cholesterol and triglyceride levels. The average patient receiving diet therapy alone reduced weight by 7 percent, while the average patient who also received balneotherapy reduced weight by 14 percent.

The report of these findings described "improvement of the functional condition of the cardiovascular system. . . . The arterial pressure was normalized after the course of treatment without application of hypertensive drugs. A single contrast bath procedure reduced the body mass on an average of 200–240 [grams]" and concluded that treatment for obesity should be directed toward reducing body mass, normalizing body metabolism, and improving the functioning of the cardiovascular system—goals that all could be attained by a low-calorie diet coupled with supervised balneotherapy.[11]

Some Springs Noted for Treating Diabetes

Brazil: Araxá
France: Vichy
Luxembourg: Mondorf
Poland: Kolobrzeg, Krynica
Romania: Călimăneşti
Switzerland: Bad Schinznach

Some Spas Noted for Their Programs to Treat Obesity

Czech Republic: Mariánské Lázně
Finland: Naantali
France: Châtel-Guyon, Contrexéville, Vichy
Portugal: Caldes do Geres
Romania: Băile Olăneşti
Spain: Caldas de Malavella, Fitero

Some Springs That Treat Metabolic and Glandular Disease (Which Include Diabetes and Obesity)

Bulgaria: Banya, Hissarya

Czech Republic: Karlovy Vary

France: Evian

Germany: Bad Bertrich, Bad Kissingen, Bad Wildungen

Italy: Chianciano Terme, Fiuggi, Ischia Terme, Montegrotto Terme, Salsomaggiore Terme

Poland: Kudowa-Zdrój

Portugal: Termas dos Cucos

Romania: Geoagiu-Bai

Russia: Essentuki, Pyatigorsk, Kislovodsk

Slovenia: Radenci, Rogaška

Switzerland: Bad Scoul-Tarasp-Vulpera, Baden

Turkey: Yalova

18

RESPIRATORY PROBLEMS

Except for European and Japanese pulmonologists who have treated patients at spas, lung specialists tend to know little about the benefits of balneotherapy to treat lung conditions such as asthma and other bronchial diseases. Yet, by its very nature, mineral and thermal water provides an effective medium to infuse the lungs with heat and moisture as well as medicinal elements such as sulfates and chlorides to promote healing of the lungs and bronchial passages.

According to Armijo Valenzuela, M.D., a professor at the Complutense University Medical School in Madrid, mineral waters can have numerous medicinal effects on the respiratory tract. Especially, waters rich in sulfates have these properties:

- They have a positive effect on the integrity of the rhinopharyngeal, tracheal, and bronchial structures of the body.
- They are antiseptic, and make it difficult for certain germs to develop.
- They improve the ability of cells to receive nourishment.
- They relax muscular spasm in the bronchial tubes.
- They help regulate the muscle tone of the respiratory passages.
- They have been clinically demonstrated to reduce anaphylaxis, which involves strong allergic reactions of the body to certain substances, often resulting in shock.[1]

Waters rich in sodium chloride have a tonic and a bronchodilating effect on the respiratory passages, whereas waters containing mild radioactivity have decongestive, anti-inflammatory, and pain-relieving properties.[2]

As a result, spa therapy has a positive influence on the healing of a wide range of respiratory diseases, including sinusitis, chronic catarrh, adenoidal

infections, laryngitis, chronic bronchitis, pulmonary sclerosis, and acute catarrhal inflammation of the nasal mucous membrane.

ASTHMA

In Europe and Japan, the greatest amount of medical research has been devoted to asthma, a disease that obstructs the airways and causes breathing
difficulties, tightness in the chest, wheezing, and coughing. During an asthma
attack, the muscles of the airways that connect the mouth and throat to the
lungs tighten up. As the airways narrow, the flow of air both into and out of the
lungs becomes obstructed. An important feature of asthma is that these symptoms can be reversed, usually through the use of medications known as
bronchodilators. The onset of asthma symptoms is also controlled by avoiding
allergens (such as certain foods, dust, and pollen) and by taking steroids and
other drugs such as cromolyn sodium.

Swimming in a warm pool is often recommended for asthma patients. The
warm, moist environment of a heated pool provides adequate moisture to the
lungs and decreases the risk of an asthma attack. Whether the asthmatic person swims laps or enjoys water aerobics, a warm pool can be an excellent place
for such a person to exercise.[3]

Thermal bathing has long been considered an important factor in treating
asthma patients at the Sandanski Spa in Bulgaria, where patients with bronchial asthma have been studied. Bathing in thermal mineral springs was part of
a complex 28-day protocol involving breathing exercises, massage, outdoor
walking, and the inhalations of medications and vapor from mineral water.
Improvement was measured by a reduced use of steroids and bronchodilators,
as well as by the number of days taken off from work because of asthma attacks. In all patients, the symptoms diminished within 2 weeks of beginning
treatment, and the improvement often continued for up to a year after therapy
began. After 2 months, follow-up studies were done, and most patients continued to show "strong" improvement, with clinical remissions lasting from 2 to 12
months. Thirty-five patients (30.4 percent) experienced clinical remissions for
up to 2 months, while 5 patients (4.3 percent) had remissions for over a year.
Patients with infection-allergic and mixed asthma who were treated in the summer months averaged 166.3 days of post-treatment relief while those treated in
cool weather averaged 103.4 days of relief.[4]

The effects of swimming in a thermal pool on eight patients with intractable asthma were studied by researchers at the Okayama University Medical

School in Japan. Patients swam in a hot spring pool for 30 minutes a day, four times a week, for 4 months. Blood pressure, pulse rate, respiration rate, and lung sounds were checked before and after the swim sessions. After 1 week, the frequency and severity of asthma attacks decreased, and after 1 month, six of the eight patients were allowed to reduce their corticosteroid medication. The researchers added that symptoms were "clearly decreased" over the next several months. They concluded that "swimming training in a hot spring pool is one of the most beneficial ways for the treatment of intractable asthma, although the action mechanism of hot spring water on intractable asthma is not yet clear."[5] A related study involving five asthma patients showed improvements in ventilatory function. In that study, the researchers concluded that long-term swimming caused no significant decreases in function, despite the fact that medication was gradually reduced.[6]

This was followed up by a study involving 25 patients with intractable asthma. Although the results were similar to the earlier results, the researchers found that hot spring swimming was most effective among patients with type II (bronchiolar obstruction type) asthma, "rather" effective in type 1-b (bronchospasm + hypersecretion type) asthma, and least effective among patients suffering from type 1-a (bronchospasm type) asthma. They also found that overall, patients 41 years of age and older showed greater improvement than younger patients.[7]

A group of French researchers surveyed the effectiveness of the spa treatment at Allevard-les-Bains in France on patients with asthma and chronic bronchitis who returned to the spa every year over 5 years for 18 days of treatment per year. In addition to balneotherapy in sulfur-rich waters (which included bathing, drinking, and showers under pressure) the treatment included inhalations of vapor and treatment with nebulizers. The patients were asked if there was an improvement in overall quality of life after treatment, including the need to take less medication to manage their symptoms. Overall, most patients felt that their situation had improved because of the spa therapy. Among the respondents, most believed that the spa water, which is high in sulfates and bicarbonates, helped reduce bronchial infections, resulting in both an improved quality of life and less need for medication.[8]

OTHER RESPIRATORY DISORDERS

In Romania, Govora Spa has been renowned for the treatment of respiratory problems since the early 1800s. Some of the earliest systematic studies on the treatment of patients with nonspecific bronchopulmonary troubles were carried out by the Institute of Physical Medicine, Balneotherapy and Medical Recovery and revealed a 40–58 percent increase in breathing in half of the 50 patients tested. The researchers also noted decreases in bronchial secretions, white blood cells that fight infection, and the number of germs in the sputum. Follow-up research later showed similar results.[9]

A larger study of 17,800 people with diseases of the higher respiratory tract was carried out at Govora between 1963 and 1965. Patients were treated with the sulfurous waters at the spa, which brought about dramatic healing of throat dryness, coughing, nasal obstruction, edema, hyperemia of the mucous membrane, and pathological secretions. Doctors also applied ultrasonic aerosols, and water from the August 23rd Spring yielded improved breathing, especially among those whose breathing was deficient before therapy.[10]

RESPIRATORY DISEASES OF CHILDREN

In France, it is estimated that over 42,000 children receive spa treatment annually, which is covered by the national health care insurance system. Approximately 75 percent of these children have respiratory tract diseases that do not respond to conventional medical therapy. Among the most common complaints are asthma, recurrent bronchitis, spasmodic cough, seromucous otitis media, sinusitis, and refractory pharyngitis. Several types of waters have immunomodulating effects, especially those containing sulfur (beneficial to patients with chronic infections) and bicarbonate (beneficial to patients with allergy). The waters of Le Mont Doré and Luchon have specific effects on the immunostimulation of the submucous membranes of the nasal passages, and the waters of Allevard have been found to improve cellular immunity among children.[11]

In France, ten spas* specialize in the treatment of children's respiratory problems and offer a wide range of therapeutic modalities, usually administered over 18 to 21 days. Local techniques include gargling, pharyngeal douches, nasal baths and irrigations, tubal insufflations, and monosonic aerosol sprays. Inhalation therapies include collective inhalations in a steam room, specialized inhalations of warm vapors, and individual inhalations facilitated by a nebulizer. Hydrotherapy treatments include bathing, drinking, and showering in mineral and thermal waters. These therapies are also enhanced by

*La Bourboulle, Luchon, Allevard, Cauterets, St. Honoré, Le Mont Doré, Amélie, Challes, St. Gervaise, Gréoux.

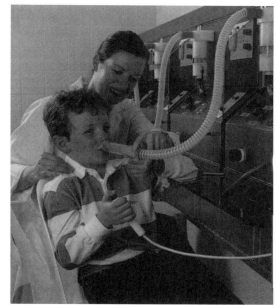

Patient being treated with monosonic aerosol. Photo courtesy of Thermes de La Bourboulle.

recreational and cultural activities as well as by educational programs dealing with the day-to-day management of asthma, for example. Since cigarette smoke is a major factor in precipitating asthma attacks, some spas offer special antismoking programs for the children's parents, who often partake of spa treatments as well.[12]

Statistical studies on the effectiveness of spa therapy in treating respiratory diseases among children have been carried out by the Service Nationale du Controle Medicale, a French government agency. A follow-up survey showed that significant clinical improvement occurred in 71 percent of patients who underwent a spa cure for their respiratory problems, but only in 26 percent who underwent traditional medical therapy.[13]

The contraindications to spa therapy for respiratory diseases include very grave or chronic conditions, accompanied by poor overall health. As with all forms of medical care, one should consult a qualified physician before attempting to treat any respiratory condition with balneotherapy.

Some Springs Whose Waters Are Used to Treat Respiratory Problems

Argentina: Los Molles, Cachueta, Rosario de la Frontera
Austria: Bad Aussi, Bad-Deutch-Altenburg, Baden bei Wien, Bad
    Gleichenburg, Bad Hall

Belgium: Spa

Brazil: Poços de Caldas

Bulgaria: Albena, Sandanski

Chile: Termas de Chillán, Termas de Puyehue

France: Allevard-les-Bains, Barzun, Eaux-Bonnes, Montbrun, St. Honoré, La Bourboulle, Luchon, Le Mont Doré, Amélie-les-Bains, Challes, Enghien-les-Bains

Germany: Bad Ems, Kreuznach, Bad Nauheim, Bad Nenndorf, Bad Reichenhall, Bad Salzuflen, Wiesbaden

Hungary: Budapest

Israel: Ein Gedi, Tiberias

Italy: Abano Terme, Acqui Terme, Agnano Terme, Bagni di Lucca, Ischia Terme, Lurisia Terme, Montegrotto Terme, Sirmione Terme

Japan: Tamagawa

Luxembourg: Mondorf

Mexico: Agua Hedionda

Peru: Chancos

Poland: Ciechocinek, Kolobrzeg

Portugal: Caldas da Rainha, Furnas, São Pedro do Sul, Vidago

Romania: Băile Olăneşti, Govora

Russia: Kislovodsk, Repino

Spain: Archena, Arteijo, Caldes de Montbui, Caldes de Malavella, Ledesma

Switzerland: Rheinfelden

Venezuela: Aguas Calientes

OTHER HEALTH PROBLEMS

In addition to the diseases addressed in earlier chapters, there are several health problems that do not fit neatly into a particular category. In addition to diseases such as cancer, they include depression, migraine, disorders of the nervous system, mouth diseases, and ear infections.

CANCER

Hot springs therapy is generally not recommended for cancer patients. However, some European spas offer rehabilitation programs for former cancer patients who have undergone surgery and/or radiation. A rehabilitation program at Bad Kissengen in Germany is especially geared toward helping survivors of breast cancer. In addition to medically supervised balneotherapy, the environmental factors and therapeutic programs offered at many spas can offer important physical, psychological, and social benefits that can increase the patient's ability to heal. Spa therapies such as massage, physical therapy, electrotherapy, therapy with alternating heat and cold, ergotherapy (work, such as gardening, used as a treatment for disease), and manual therapy may help heal scarring from surgery and radiation, reduce peripheral and central paralysis, relieve symptoms of edema, and increase joint mobility.[1]

MIGRAINES

For many years, migraine headache has been treated at the Vittel spa in France. Over a 30-year period, physicians at the spa have developed and refined a complex protocol that involves drinking mineral water and hydrotherapy treatments, including local showers, kinesitherapy (which focuses on the movement of certain muscles of the face and neck, with special attention given to the jaw and bite of the patient), and applications of thermal mud.

Although the exact protocol is designed according to the needs of each individual patient, water from the Source Hépar, a spring rich in magnesium, is consumed by the patient on an empty stomach upon arising in the morning: 100, 150, 200, and 300 milliliters are given at intervals spaced 20 to 30 minutes apart. Additional water is given before noon (two times) and in the afternoon (three times), providing a total water consumption of 2–3 liters over a 24-hour period. This is often supplemented by mineral water showers focusing on the neck and head, kinesitherapy sessions, and thermal mud applications on the face and neck to help the patient relax. The physicians at Vittel believe that a lack of adequate magnesium is a factor in migraine headache and that the success of the treatment is due in part to the high magnesium content of the water. They also believe that the showers, kinesitherapy, and thermal mud applications in a low-stress environment help promote deep relaxation of muscle groups, which may have an effect on the development of migraine.

Clinical research at Vittel has shown that the effectiveness rate of the cure increases with the number of times it is experienced. A 1976 study of 328 migraine sufferers revealed a cure rate of 31.6 percent, 202 patients who returned to Vittel for a second round of treatments had a 53.6 percent cure rate, and 104 patients who returned for a third time scored a 75 percent cure rate. A survey of 118 migraine patients reported by the French Hydrological Society revealed that 77.97 percent became completely free of symptoms after the cure, and 10.17 percent reported both a marked lower frequency and intensity of symptoms.[2]

Migraine patients are also treated successfully at the French spa at Vichy, which established a multidisciplinary center for treating migraine in 1978. The Migraine Center at Vichy is staffed by some 27 medical specialists, including internists, neurologists, psychiatrists, radiologists, and gastroenterologists. By 1990, over 7,500 migraine patients had been treated at Vichy with balneotherapy (including thermal bathing, showers, shower massage, and fangotherapy), psychotherapy, and relaxation techniques. A variety of studies of the Vichy cure showed positive results. One study of 171 subjects who underwent one cure program showed that 29 percent showed very good results (a year without migraines), 57 percent showed good results (6 months without a crisis), 11 percent had medium results (3 months without a migraine), and 3 percent showed no improvement.[3]

A 1988 study of 21 migraine sufferers between the ages of 8 and 15 showed that the Vichy cure produced very good results in 86 percent of the patients, while the remaining 14 percent had mediocre improvement or no improvement at all.[4]

DEPRESSION

Many people leave a hot springs bath feeling wonderful. This is due in part to the overall feelings of well-being associated with bathing in warm water, as well as the thermal and chemical effects that hot springs water (hot springs contain a large amount of negative ions) have on the production of endorphins—neurochemicals produced by the body that can increase feelings of well-being.

In Europe, several spas specialize in the treatment of depression with balneotherapy. In addition to bathing, drinking, exercise, and relaxation, patients are often given healthy diets and offered psychological counseling.

Physicians at the Medical Center at Divonne-les-Bains in France made a comparative study of 109 patients suffering from clinical depression. Of this group, 78 were given spa therapy and the other 31 served as control subjects. After a 6-month period, patients were evaluated for depression. The results showed a significant reduction in depression, a lower consumption of antidepressants, and a 20 percent reduction of benzodiazepines among the patients who were given spa therapy, when they were compared with the control group.[5]

Closely related to depression is psychalgia, which is mental distress or pain, especially in cases of melancholy. A physician at the Complutense University of Madrid has found that hydrotherapy and the local application of mineral water in baths and low pressure showers, along with supervised exercise in hyperthermal waters, bring about "subjective improvement in a high percentage of patients" suffering from psychalgia, which leads to more effective results from psychotherapy.[6]

NERVOUS SYSTEM DISORDERS

Disorders of the nervous system may be classified in two types: painful conditions of the nervous system that are primarily sensory, and nervous diseases that affect the locomotor system.

In former Czechoslovakia, several spas specialize in treating nerve-related disorders, including Mariánské Lázně and Jáchymov in the Czech Republic and Piešťany in Slovakia. The most common forms of treatment for painful conditions include therapies that have an analgesic, relaxing, and anti-inflammatory effect on the body, such as water and peloids rich in sulfurous and radioactive materials. Physical methods such as massage, electrotherapy, and spinal manipulation are also used. For conditions affecting the locomotor apparatus, physical therapy and exercise are paramount. For patients affected by spasticity, carbon dioxide baths, subcutaneous thermal gas injections, and peloid applications are used for their relaxing effects.[7]

PARKINSON'S DISEASE

No formal clinical studies have shown that hot springs bathing will cure Parkinson's disease, a chronic nervous disease characterized by tremor, muscle rigidity and weakness, and difficulty walking. However, some European balneologists believe that balneotherapy can help relieve some of the symptoms of Parkinson's disease by helping relax the muscles and reduce muscular rigidity. Immersion in thermal water may also help improve body coordination and mobility of the joints. Although it may be possible that the individual chemical attributes of mineral water may provide healing benefits as well, there have been no studies to evaluate them.

At the Fitero Spa in Navarra, Spain, patients with Parkinson's disease undergo a 15-day treatment that includes daily bathing in 38°C (100°F) mineral water (which is especially rich in sulfates) for 20 minutes. Treatment may also include exercise and hydromassage focusing on the limbs and spinal column, as well as steam baths at 43–45°C (109–113°F) for 10 minutes under medical supervision. In addition, pressure showers directed at the spinal muscles and other parts of the body, and mud packs applied to affected parts of the spinal column, are also administered according to the needs of each patient. A complex program of physiotherapy and therapeutic exercise, which is believed to complement the benefits of balneotherapy, is also given. While researchers describe their therapeutic program as bringing about "notable reduction of symptoms" in many Parkinson's patients, they hope to do broader studies in the future to provide more objective clinical findings.[8]

DISEASES OF THE MOUTH AND GUMS

Diseases of the mouth and gums, including gingivitis (gum disease), peridentosis (inflammation around a tooth), stomatitis (inflammation of the mouth) including stomatitis as the result of radiation therapy, keratosis (growths), leukoplakia (formation of white patches on the tongue), lichen (papillary growths), and glossitis (inflammation of the tongue) are indications for spa therapy in Europe.

Spa treatment for mouth diseases is part of the medical mainstream in many European countries, including France, where 13 designated thermal establishments specialize in treating mouth and gum disorders. Forms of treatment include spraying mineral water on affected areas of the mouth and gums with the goal of cleansing lesions and stimulating the gums. Mouth washing and gargling are also used. These treatments are often accompanied by counseling in proper dental hygiene.[9] Some spas, such as the Gellért (Budapest), Héviz, and Sarvar thermal centers in Hungary, have dentists on staff.

The most important thermal establishments for the treatment of mouth and gum diseases include Aix-les-Bains, Castéra-Verduzan, and St. Christeau in France; Salsomaggiore in Italy; and Rudas in Budapest.

EAR DISEASES

Clinical research was undertaken by physicians associated with the University of Milan and the Complutense University of Madrid on patients suffering from chronic otitis, a condition that often results in deafness.

Fifteen patients with chronic otitis were treated at the Saturnia Spa in Italy with a single daily insufflation of gas from sulfurous water over a 12-day period. This type of water was chosen for its antiseptic effects, its ability to improve mucosal trophism (a response to or a turning away from an external stimulus), its ability to restore cilia (the fine hairs projecting from epithelial cells located within the ear) and its ability to stimulate the production of immunoglobulin gamma A antibodies. Patients were evaluated both before and after therapy, using standard medical tests to measure hearing.

The researchers reported significant improvement in hearing as shown by audiometric levels with the best results taking place at frequencies which correspond to sounds of normal human conversation.[10]

DETOXIFICATION

With the growth of industrial and related pollution throughout the world, many people experience poisoning from heavy metals, such as cadmium and lead, which produce a variety of degenerative and nervous system diseases. At the same time, an increasing number are poisoned by illegal drugs as well as some prescribed and over-the-counter medications.

Both bathing in and drinking thermal and mineral water is seen as a simple and effective way to help the body's natural detoxification by stimulating the liver (whose job is to filter and cleanse toxins from the bloodstream), the circulatory system, and the digestive system, which helps removes toxins from the body. According to the text *Medical Hydrology:*

> They act partly by their heat and high solvent power and their hypotonicity. . . . They assist the solution and elimination of toxic material, and stimulate the intestinal and biliary secretions and the general circulation. They are, therefore, useful in cases of inactive liver, constipation and retention of toxins.[11]

Research evaluated at the National Center of Physical Therapy and Rehabilitation in Bulgaria has found that drinking water rich in sulfates has an antitoxic effect on persons with heavy-metal poisoning, while hypotonic waters and waters rich in calcium can help neutralize the ill effects of certain types of drugs. Waters rich in fluorides can play a role in neutralizing the effects of radionuclides (atoms that disintegrate by emission of electromagnetic radiation) that have accumulated in bones. Other research has shown promising results on individuals with radiation poisoning.[12]

USING MEDICINAL SPRINGS FOR WELLNESS

So far, we have focused on the healing aspects of medicinal waters and their use in treating a wide variety of health problems, including joint and muscle diseases, cardiovascular problems, endocrine disorders, gynecological problems, and skin diseases. Yet, the physical and psychological benefits of regular bathing in medicinal waters cannot be underestimated for their ability to reduce stress and strengthen the body's overall functioning, leading to a higher level of personal wellness. Although all the physicians I interviewed while writing this book were involved in treating sick patients with balneotherapy and related modalities, they emphasized the importance of hot springs bathing as an important factor in preventive health care. Here are some of the major ways that hot springs bathing can help us achieve and maintain our optimum health potential.

WARMING THE BODY

When we are ill, the "innate intelligence" that resides in our body often produces a fever, and since many germs and viruses cannot survive in a warm environment, they die. In addition, a fever helps increase blood circulation, which improves the delivery of oxygen and nutrients to the body's cells. Fever also stimulates white blood cell production, thus enhancing immunity. Finally, a fever helps the body to filter and eliminate toxins through increased perspiration, bowel movements, and urination. Because bathing in a hot spring gradually raises the body's temperature, it produces many of the health benefits provided by a fever without our feeling sick.

We mentioned earlier that most hot springs contain waters of differing temperatures. Cool springs, such as those at Saratoga Spa, are heated to ensure comfortable bathing. Others, such as those at Calistoga in California and Fairmont in Montana, are allowed to cool before being pumped into the pool. Generally speaking, 10 to 20 minutes is sufficient time for hot springs bathing. The cooler the temperature, the longer you can soak; you can always take a 10-minute break and enter the water again. However, some of the Japanese springs are so hot (sometimes exceeding 63°C, or 145°F) that no more than 3 to 5 minutes is permitted. In any case, no matter how long you soak, leave the water immediately if you feel dizzy, uncomfortable, or sick. And remember to drink lots of cool water after bathing in a hot spring to prevent dehydration.

UNDER PRESSURE

When we take a dip in a pool or hot tub, the weight of the surrounding water increases the hydrostatic pressure on our body. Although we aren't consciously aware of it, one of the major benefits of hydrostatic pressure is increased blood circulation.[1] The increased flow of oxygen-rich blood throughout the body enhances the nourishment to vital organs and tissues.

Hydrostatic pressure also improves cell oxygenation by increasing the amount of life-giving oxygen to the body's cells. This is important, because many of us are oxygen deficient. Whether through poor breathing, lack of exercise, environmental pollution, or eating foods that are low in oxygen (especially those that have been heavily processed, cooked, or preserved, or high-fat foods, meat, and dairy products), many of us do not get the oxygen our body needs. If the oxygenation process within the body is weak or deficient over the long term, the body cannot eliminate poisons effectively. In some cases, a toxic reaction can occur. The increase in oxygen-rich blood not only increases strength and vitality but also helps dissolve and eliminate toxins from the body.[2]

Sometimes people experience increased elimination (such as frequent urination and more frequent bowel movements with loose stools) after bathing in hot springs for several days. Elimination may increase even more when mineral water is consumed as part of a drinking cure. These symptoms should not be judged as "dirty" or "wrong" but rather be seen as a normal process of body cleansing. Although many of us feel uncomfortable when we experience occasional diarrhea, it is essentially a normal function of a body that is striving for health.

This is why many European hot springs establishments provide a spa diet that is rich in fresh fruits and vegetables, whole grains, herbal teas, and freshly pressed juices, along with plenty of rest and healthful exercise. Many actually custom-design a diet and exercise plan for each guest after a complete physical examination and interview. Some of the larger American hot springs resorts, such as the Sonoma Mission Inn and Spa in Boyes Hot Springs, California, the Homestead in Hot Springs, Virginia, and the Elms Resort and Spa in Excelsior Springs, Missouri, offer all-inclusive spa programs for guests that include diet and exercise.

BODY STIMULATION AND RELAXATION

In addition to an increase in body temperature, hot spring bathers often experience accelerated rates in heartbeat and breathing. After bathing in a hot spring, some find that they want to eat something or need to go to the bathroom. This is because bathing in thermal water increases body metabolism, which includes stimulating the secretions of the intestinal tract and the liver, aiding digestion. This may be one reason why many hot springs offer their visitors fresh fruit juices, herbal teas, and a wide range of healthy and delicious food. The restaurants at several hot springs resorts, including Sycamore Mineral Springs in San Luis Obispo, California, and French Lick Springs Resort and Spa in Indiana, are as well known as the healing springs themselves.

FINE-TUNING THE GLANDS AND THE NERVOUS SYSTEM

Earlier we showed how repeated hot spring bathing (especially over 3 to 4 weeks) can help normalize functions of the endocrine glands, such as the pituitary, thyroid, pineal, parathyroid, and adrenals.[3, 4] These important glands release hormones and secrete neurotransmitters directly into the blood or the lymph system to regulate body activities such as growth, sleep, sudden activity, feelings, and blood sugar for energy. This is why hot springs resorts are experienced by many people as among the most mellow places on earth and seem to be free of the stressful and frenetic energy found in many ordinary resorts.

Hot springs bathing also helps normalize the functioning of the body's autonomic nervous system.[5, 6] In this system, two sets of nerves, the sympathetic nervous system and the parasympathetic nervous system, generally work opposite each other to regulate homeostasis, or body balance. They are especially important in regulating the functions of the thymus gland and the spleen, which play an important role in proper immune system functioning.

NEGATIVE IONS

Over the past few years, scientists have discovered that mineral springs, such as waterfalls, forests, and gardens, contain high amounts of negative ions: electrically charged particles in the atmosphere that ease tension while leaving us full of energy.[7]

While visiting hot springs in Japan and Taiwan, I was surprised to find how quiet the bathing areas were, and I often noticed that some of the bathers were practicing deep meditation. Many of the North American hot springs establishments provide a meditative atmosphere for bathing. Nearly all discourage noise, and many provide restful music. Others offer private hot tubs and bathing tubs where you are left alone to enjoy peace and quiet. And several, such as Wilbur, Harbin, and Sierra hot springs in California, and Breitenbush hot springs in Oregon, are recognized as spiritual retreats. Several even have meditation rooms and quiet gardens for personal reflection and contemplation.

Atmospheres charged with negative ions offer a wealth of physical and psychological benefits: reduction of asthma and allergy symptoms and relief of seasonal depression, fatigue, and nervousness. They also help improve performance of voluntary movements, increase work capacity, and sharpen mental function. All hot springs contain high concentrations of negative ions, especially if they are located outdoors or contain natural fountains or waterfalls. While visiting Dr. Yuko Agishi at his renowned hot springs clinic at Arima Onsen in Japan, I accompanied him on a walk in a nearby cedar forest that was part of the hospital property. He explained that he was creating a series of walking paths in the forest for patients to increase their daily exposure to negative ions as a complement to the therapies they were receiving at the clinic, and to enhance the effects of the negative ions from the hot springs baths. Encouraging me to breathe deeply of the forest air, he explained that exposure to negative ions is vital to the healing process and that they increase energy and overall feelings of well-being.

MICRONUTRITION

Throughout this book, we've found that healing springs often contain a wide range of minerals and other elements, ranging from arsenic to manganese to zinc. When we bathe in a hot spring or mineral spring, small amounts of calcium, magnesium, iron, and lithium are absorbed by the body and provide healing effects to various body organs and systems.[8] They can stimulate the immune system, promote physical and mental relaxation, increase the production of endorphins (thereby reducing pain and bringing about enhanced feelings of well-being), and bring about glandular modulation, which is vital for proper body metabolism. As we have seen earlier, even the simple drinking of medicinal waters at the source can help eliminate toxins, nourish the body, and enhance normal functioning of the gastrointestinal system, urinary tract, kidneys, and other important body organs. Although hot springs bathing and drinking should never be a substitute for a healthy diet, it is a simple, comfortable, low-calorie way of allowing the body to absorb small amounts of minerals and other elements that are essential for good nutrition.

IN QUEST OF BABY SKIN

While doing research for this book, I had the good fortune to visit many hot springs around the world. In some places, I was (at 50 years of age) one of the youngest people in the springs. Yet, I noticed that many of the other bathers—who were in their sixties and seventies—had healthy, youthful skin.

In an earlier chapter we showed that bathing in certain types of mineral water, especially waters containing sulfur, sulfates, or sodium chloride, can have a therapeutic effect on diseases of the skin, including psoriasis, dermatitis, and fungal infections. While this is positive news for people with skin problems, it is also good for those of us who want our skin to retain a healthy, youthful appearance despite our chronological age. Many such springs are found in abundance in the United States and western Canada. Because prolonged hot spring bathing can produce dehydration, including skin dehydration, be sure to drink plenty of water after leaving the pool, and apply oil or lotion to your body after you dry off.

HEALTHY COMPLEMENTS

We mentioned earlier that the innate healing powers of hot and mineral springs are complemented by many of the services offered at spas for both relaxation and rehabilitation. These include balneotherapy (such as therapeutic showers and underwater massage); Swedish, shiatsu, and Watsu massage; acupuncture; therapeutic exercise; mud packs; steam baths and inhalations; and aromatherapy. Except for some family-oriented spas that are devoted primarily to recreation, most commercial springs offer a variety of complementary services, often by highly skilled therapists. Although a bath followed by an hour of simple relaxation can be highly beneficial for health and well-being, a good massage, herbal wrap, or mud treatment can enhance the bathing experience and provide lasting benefits for both body and soul.

When combined with the often beautiful surroundings of a natural mineral spring, the healthy food, and the slower pace (it is advised that when you visit a hot spring, you turn off your cell phone), the healing benefits of the waters can be powerful indeed. Finally, many modern spas offer educational programs and workshops in healthy eating, stress management, beauty enhancement, and physical fitness that can lead to positive lifestyle changes.

During a visit to the Szechenyi Thermal Baths in Budapest, Hungary, I was told one morning that I had just missed seeing their oldest client: a 107-year-old man who had been swimming in their famous Lido pool daily for the past 45 years. However, I did enjoy soaking in the hot springs with many other bathers, many of whom were well over retirement age. Several mentioned that they visited the hot springs on a daily basis, some even arriving before the doors opened at 7 A.M. While soaking in one of the sulfur-rich hot springs in Peitou, Taiwan, I got to talking with a doctor of traditional Chinese medicine, who was visiting from the city of Taichung, a 2-hour drive away. A man in his fifties who easily looked 20 years younger, he told me that regular hot springs bathing—along with a vegetarian diet—was vital to his personal health regimen, and added, "If I lived in Peitou, I would come here every day."

The gift of wellness care is perhaps one of the most important benefits that hot springs bathing can provide. The unofficial motto of the International Society of Medical Balneology and Climatology is "Die young, but live as long as possible." By utilizing the rejuvenating powers of healing springs, we can not only help heal ourselves of disease but remain young, healthy, and vital throughout our lives.

PART IV

A WORLD
FULL OF SPRINGS

Where to Find the Water

There are thousands of healing springs around the world, ranging from simple hot pools large enough for one person to luxury resorts that can accommodate thousands. The following pages introduce you to a variety of these healing springs. Selecting which springs to include was a difficult task. Considerations were given to choosing the largest or best-known thermal centers and the most important springs, as well as those that offer a variety of waters with a range of medicinal properties. In this way, you may have a small taste of the abundance of healing springs around the world.

However, the omission of a spring from this list does not mean that it is not significant, beautiful, or healing. For example, there are over a hundred commercial and noncommercial warm and hot mineral springs in California alone, may of which are well worth a visit. Many of California's commercial springs offer food and lodging, either on site or nearby. France has 107 recognized centers that offer bathing in thermal springs, along with medically approved treatments, food, and accommodations. Many of them are perfect vacation destinations, even if they are not listed here.

In the resource section of this book, we include several specialized guides to spas, hot springs, and mineral springs that may help you find the perfect healing spring destination. If you are planning to visit a particular state, province, or foreign country, a good local, regional, or country guidebook may have information about hot springs. Local or national tourist boards (many of which are listed in this directory) often offer special brochures or other types of literature highlighting their hot springs and mineral springs. The tourist boards of Spain and Portugal offer beautifully designed full-color guidebooks to their respective springs, along with information about lodging and local attractions.

The Internet is another good source for finding out about hot springs as well as tour companies that arrange spa tours. Several are mentioned in the

Resources section, although many individual mineral springs and spa towns have sites on the World Wide Web; their addresses can be located through major search engines by simply entering the name of the specific spa town (for example, Karlovy Vary or Montecatini). You can also enter the English words *hot springs* or *spas,* or *spas+Italy* for specific spas in Italy, as well as foreign-language keywords such as *thermes* or *bains* for French listings, *bad* for German listings, *terme* for Italian listings, *termas* for Spanish and Portuguese listings, or *onsen* for listings of hot springs in Japan. Many of the Web sites include text in several different languages, usually including English. It is often difficult to find information about hot springs from the Web sites of national tourist boards, probably because they focus on more general tourist information.

21

HEALING SPRINGS OF THE UNITED STATES AND CANADA

Many are surprised to learn that there are literally hundreds of commercial and noncommercial hot springs and mineral springs in the United States (mainly in the western states as well as Arkansas, New York, South Dakota, Virginia, and West Virginia) and in Canada, primarily in British Columbia and Alberta.

Space limitations do not allow a complete and detailed listing of the tremendous variety of healing springs in North America; here we will focus first on the active spa towns and resorts that balneologists and other scientists have considered to be among the most important for their size, their waters, or other distinguishing features. This will be followed by a listing of 50 of the "Top" healing springs in the United States and Canada, including a brief description of their facilities, healing waters, and adjunct therapies such as massage, aromatherapy, or mud packs, to give readers a sampling of some of the many healing spring possibilities that exist.

For additional information about how to find healing springs in the United States and Canada, consult the resource section.

MAJOR HEALING SPRINGS AND SPA TOWNS IN THE UNITED STATES

Arkansas

HOT SPRINGS NATIONAL PARK

Hot Springs has long been one of the major spa towns in the United States. The waters, which are weakly mineralized, come from a total of 47 springs and primarily contain sodium chloride. They have long been esteemed for their ability to help heal rheumatism, skin diseases, and stress-related disorders;

they are also believed to be useful during convalescence after accident, surgery, or illness. Although many of the original bath houses have closed, several provide a variety of spa services, including bathing, massage, beauty treatments, fangotherapy, and physical therapy. The mineral waters are also piped into several local hotels, which offer similar spa services. For more information, contact

Hot Springs Diamond Lakes Travel Association
P.O. Box 1500, Hot Springs, AR 71902
(800) SPA-CITY, (501) 321-1700
www.hotsprings.org

Publishes *Hot Springs Vacation Planning Kit.*

EUREKA SPRINGS

Located in the northwestern part of the state, Eureka Springs, founded in 1879, is considered one of the most charming towns in Arkansas and is known mostly for its restored downtown area filled with Victorian-era hotels, antiques shops, restaurants, and bed-and-breakfasts. The Palace Bath House, built in 1901, is the only facility where one can bathe in Eureka Springs mineral water. For more information, contact

Eureka Springs Visitor's Information Center
Highway 62 West
Eureka Springs, AR 72632
(501) 253-8737
www.eurekaspringsusa.com

Publishes *Eureka Springs Visitor's Guide.*

Palace Bath House
135 Spring Street
Eureka Springs, AR 72632
(501) 253-8400
www.eurekaspringsusa.com/lodging/palace.html

California

CALISTOGA

Although known to the Miwok peoples for centuries, the thermal springs in what is now Calistoga in the Napa Valley were first developed in the 1870s by the charismatic Samuel Brannan, who hoped to make Calistoga the "Saratoga Springs of California." Today, Calistoga is a charming community of 6,000 inhabitants in the heart of California wine country. The sulfurous waters, which have long enjoyed a reputation for treating rheumatism, arthritis, and stress-related problems, are piped into nine thermal establishments, many of them motel/spas, which offer swimming, bathing, steam baths, aromatherapy, and

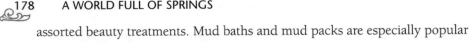

assorted beauty treatments. Mud baths and mud packs are especially popular here. For more information contact

Calistoga Chamber of Commerce
1455 Lincoln Ave., Suite 9
Calistoga, CA 94515
(707) 942-6333
www.calistogafun.com

Publishes *Calistoga Visitor's Brochure.*

DESERT HOT SPRINGS AND PALM SPRINGS

Desert Hot Springs is a small spa community in the Coachella Valley near Palm Springs, its more fashionable neighbor. Many of the more than 45 hotels and motels here pump the hot mineral water from underground wells for use in Jacuzzis and swimming pools. The waters, which are rich in sulfur as well as sodium, chloride, bicarbonate, and silica, have been known for their ability to treat arthritis and other joint diseases since the Cahuilla people inhabited the area hundreds of years ago.

Desert Hot Springs Home Page:

www.deserthotsprings.org

Palm Springs is a fashionable resort town in Riverside County known for its healthful climate and beautiful natural surroundings; it is also famous for its tennis courts, shopping, celebrity tours, and golf courses. Among its dozens of luxury resorts, some offer spas with thermal mineral water pumped from underground wells, similar to the waters at Desert Hot Springs. For more information contact

Palm Springs Desert Resorts Convention and Visitors Bureau
69-930 Highway 111, Suite 201
Rancho Mirage, CA 92270
(760) 770-900, (800) 417-3529
www.desert-resorts.com

Publishes *Palm Springs Desert Resorts Vacation Planner.*

Colorado

GLENWOOD HOT SPRINGS

Glenwood Springs is a large, historic hot springs resort that was known to Native Americans long before white settlers arrived in the area. The abundant waters (the main source, Yampah Spring, flows at a rate of over 3 million gallons a day) are rich in sodium chloride and calcium bicarbonate and have been popular for treating rheumatism, gastrointestinal disorders, and disorders of the nervous system for centuries. They are also used by those convalescing from accident, surgery, and illness.

In addition to lodging, dining, and nearby skiing, visitors can enjoy an enormous swimming pool more than two city blocks long, a smaller therapy pool, a vapor cave, and an athletic center. The resort also offers massage, chiropractic, and beauty treatments. For more information contact

Hot Springs Lodge and Pool, Inc.
P.O. Box 308
Glenwood Springs, CO 81602
(800) 537-7946, (970) 945-6571
www.hotspringspool.com

Montana

FAIRMONT HOT SPRINGS RESORT (ANACONDA)

The abundant thermal springs at Fairmont were first discovered by the Flathead, Nez Perce, and Shoshone peoples, who called the 12 hot springs Medicine Waters. The major minerals in the water include bicarbonates, calcium, magnesium, potassium, iron, manganese, and silica. Today, the resort includes two Olympic-size swimming pools and two mineral soaking pools, men's and women's steam baths, lodging for several hundred guests, restaurants, shops, and a conference center. A wide range of spa services is offered as well, including massage, reflexology, and beauty treatments. For more information, contact

Fairmont Hot Springs Resort
1500 Fairmont Road
Anaconda, MT 59711
(800) 332-3272, (406) 797-3241
www.fairmontmontana.com

New Mexico

TRUTH OR CONSEQUENCES

Named after the famous TV game show, Truth or Consequences was once an important healing center, with several hospitals and rehabilitation facilities. At present, at least four thermal establishments, including a municipal pool, offer swimming, bathing, massage, steam baths, and saunas. The abundant waters, which contain primarily sodium chloride, calcium chloride, and bicarbonate, were used to treat a variety of health problems, including rheumatism, arthritis, gastrointestinal problems, and neurological disorders. Once considered a bit rundown, many downtown establishments have been undergoing renovation. For more information, contact

Chamber of Commerce
P.O. Drawer 31
Truth or Consequences, NM 87905
(505) 894-3536, (800) 831-9487

New York

SARATOGA SPRINGS

Once considered the "Queen of American Spas," Saratoga Spa boasted the largest full-service thermal establishment in the world, containing three large treatment centers, a research laboratory, a bottling plant, a theater and a recreation complex. The waters, which have been compared to the best in Europe, have been used to treat cardiovascular diseases, rheumatism, gastrointestinal diseases, and functional nervous disturbances.

The only places where one now can bathe in the famous waters, which are rich in bicarbonates and sodium chloride, are the Lincoln Baths in Saratoga Spa State Park, [South Broadway, (518) 584-2011] and the nearby privately run Crystal Spa [120 S. Broadway, (518) 584-2556, www.crystalspa.com]. In addition to bathing, both facilities offer mud packs, massage, herbal wraps, and beauty treatments. There are also ten active springs throughout the park and eight in the city of Saratoga Springs that provide various types of mineral water for drinking. For more information, contact

Saratoga County Chamber of Commerce
494 Broadway
Saratoga Springs, NY 12866
(800) 526-8970, (518) 584-4471

Publishes *The Springs of Saratoga.*

Saratoga Spa State Park Administration
19 Roosevelt Drive
Saratoga Springs, NY 12866
(518) 584-2535

South Dakota

HOT SPRINGS

Few know that South Dakota's Black Hills are the home of eight warm mineral springs, including several that were used by the Sioux and Cheyenne as sacred healing sites long before the arrival of European settlers. By the 1890s, the settlers had taken over, and Hot Springs became a popular resort, replete with hotels, saloons, and numerous bath houses. Its abundant mineral waters, containing primarily calcium carbonate, sulfates, and silica, were found useful for treating liver and gallbladder problems, gastrointestinal tract disorders, rheumatism, and arthritis.

Today there are two major bathing establishments: Evan's Plunge, a large indoor pool built over several springs, and Springs Bathhouse, a small spa offering bathing, massage, and beauty treatments. Several public fountains provide mineral water for drinking. For more information, contact

Evan's Plunge
(605) 745-5165, (800) 325-6991

Springs Bathhouse
146 N. Garden Street
Hot Springs, SD 57747
(605) 745-4424, (888) 817-1972
www.gwtc.net/~bathhouse

Virginia

THE HOMESTEAD (HOT SPRINGS)

The healing waters at the Homestead, considered one of the premier resorts in North America, contain sulfur, magnesium, and 16 other minerals and have been enjoyed by people suffering from rheumatism, arthritis, gastrointestinal disorders, and stress-related problems since Thomas Jefferson's time. In addition to private marble soaking tubs and a magnificent swimming pool built in 1903, the resort offers a wide variety of health-related services, including hydrotherapy, steam baths, massage, aromatherapy, beauty treatments, and fitness and wellness programs. The Homestead also owns the Warm Springs Pools in nearby Warm Springs. These historic springs (Thomas Jefferson and Stonewall Jackson bathed here) are popular with day visitors and offer swimming pools for men and women in the nation's oldest working bathhouse. For more information, contact

The Homestead
P.O. Box 200
Hot Springs, VA 24445
(800) 838-1766, (540) 839-1766
www.thehomestead.com.

Warm Springs
(540) 839-5346

West Virginia

BERKELEY SPRINGS

Located in the extreme northern part of the state near Pennsylvania, the abundant waters at Berkeley Springs once served as a gathering place for Native Americans. George Washington first bathed here when he was 16, and he returned to the springs regularly as an adult. Some of the original trees he planted can still be found near the springs. The warm, lightly mineralized waters contain primarily carbonates and sulfates and have been used to treat rheumatism, skin diseases, and certain neurological disorders. They have also been found helpful to those recovering from accident, illness, and surgery.

The major bathing facilities, along with steam baths, massage, and physical therapy, can be found at Berkeley Springs State Park, although several other establishments offer mineral water baths and related health and beauty services. There are also nearby inns that provide accomodation, as well as several restaurants and shops. For more information contact

Travel Berkeley Springs
(304) 258-9147, (800) 447-8797
www.berkeleysprings.com

Berkeley Springs State Park
121 S. Washington Street
Berkeley Springs, WV 25411
(800) CALL WVA, (304) 258-2711

THE GREENBRIER (WHITE SULPHUR SPRINGS)

The Greenbrier is a large (6,500 acres) and historic luxury resort in the mountains of West Virginia. Once enjoyed by the Shawnee peoples, its three medicinal springs, which are rich in sulfates and hydrogen sulfide, have long been appreciated by people with rheumatism, gastrointestinal and liver problems, gallbladder disease, and stress-related disorders. In addition to such amenities as golf courses and tennis courts, the resort has a separate new mineral bath and spa building, where one can partake of bathing, Swiss showers, Scotch sprays, sauna, steam rooms, and massage. The hotel offers a wide range of beauty treatments and fitness programs. For more information, contact

The Greenbrier
White Sulphur Springs, WV 24986
(800) 624-6070
www.greenbrier.com

Wyoming

THERMOPOLIS

Thermopolis, whose name in Greek, means "hot city," is considered one of the largest hot springs in the world. The waters, which are rich in bicarbonate, sulfate, chloride, calcium, and sodium, flow from at least eight hot springs at a rate of some 15 million gallons a day and are believed to be therapeutic for people suffering primarily from rheumatism and stress. Several establishments offer indoor and outdoor swimming and bathing as well as water slides, steam baths, sweat wraps, and massage, with the local Holiday Inn offering the most complete spa services. There is also a steam cave at the historic Star Plunge. For more information, contact

Thermopolis-Hot Springs Chamber of Commerce
P.O. Box 78
Thermopolis, WY 82443
(800) 786-6772, (307) 864-3192

Publishes *Thermopolis Hot Springs Visitors Guide.*

State Bath House
Hot Springs State Park
220 Park Street
Thermopolis, WY 82443
(307) 864-2176

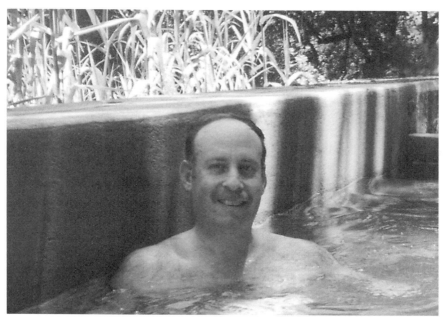

Author enjoying Gilroy Hot Springs, California.

NORTH AMERICA'S
"TOP 50" HEALING SPRINGS

Most of the springs in the listings that follow have not been the focus of medical research, although many, such as those described in the preceding section, are known for their healing waters. Because of the dearth of medical data, you will not find specific health problems mentioned here. The waters will be described, however, and you may wish to refer to the chapters in parts 2 and 3 for guidance on what health conditions these waters address.

The vast majority of these springs welcome day visitors at a nominal fee (usually between $10 to $20), although some offer their facilities exclusively to overnight guests. Please keep in mind that the entries in this list were chosen based on the size of the facility, its accessibility by road, and the range of services provided; a spring that is not included is not inherently less pleasurable or healing!

CANADA

Alberta

BANFF UPPER HOT SPRINGS

Waters: Sulfate, bicarbonate, calcium, magnesium.

Facilities and services: Large outdoor hot pool in major resort for swimming and bathing, plunge pool, steam room, aromatherapy, massage, beauty treatments; dining, picnic area. For more information, contact

Banff Upper Hot Springs
P.O. Box 900
Banff, Alta. T0L 0C0
(403) 762-1498, (800) 787-1611
www.worldweb.com/ParksCanada-Banff/springs

MIETTE HOT SPRINGS

Waters: Sulfate, bicarbonate, calcium, magnesium.

Facilities and services: Modern facility offers bathing and swimming in hot and cool pools; massage; hiking and nearby camping. For more information, contact

Miette Hot Springs
P.O. Box 2579
Jasper, Alta. T0E 1E0
(780) 866-3939, (800) 787-1611

British Columbia

AINSWORTH HOT SPRINGS RESORT

Waters: Sulfates, calcium carbonate, sodium carbonate, silica.

Facilities and services: Luxury resort offering unique hot springs cave, swimming pool, cold plunge; lodging, dining. For more information, contact

Ainsworth Hot Springs Resort
P.O. Box 1268
Ainsworth Hot Springs, B.C. V0G 1A0
(250) 229-4212, (800) 668-1171
www.hotnaturally.com

FAIRMONT HOT SPRINGS RESORT

Waters: Chlorides, sulfates, bicarbonate, silica, radium.

Facilities and services: Major resort with huge public pool for swimming and soaking; private soaking pools, swimming pool; massage, beauty treatments; lodging, dining. For more information, contact

Fairmont Hot Springs Resort
P.O. Box 10
Fairmont Hot Springs, B.C. V0B 1L0
(250) 345-6311, (800) 663-4979
www.fairmontresort.com

HALCYON HOT SPRINGS

Waters: Sodium, lithium, magnesium, calcium, radon.

Facilities and services: Country spa offers soaking pools, swimming pool; hiking, horseback riding; lodging, camping, RV hookups, dining. For more information, contact

Halcyon Hot Springs
P.O. Box 37
Nakusp, B.C. V0G 1R0
(250) 265-3554, (888) 689-4699
www.halcyon-hotsprings.com

HARRISON HOT SPRINGS RESORT

Waters: Sulfate, sodium, chloride, calcium, silica.

Facilities and services: Luxury resort offering soaking pools, swimming pools for overnight guests only; full-service spa offers hydrotherapy, massage, aromatherapy, and beauty treatments; boating, fishing, tennis; lodging, dining.

Harrison Hot Springs Resort
Harrison Hot Springs, B.C. V0M 1K0
(250) 796-2244, (800) 663-2266
www.harrisonresort.com

Note: The healing waters at the resort can also be enjoyed at the nearby indoor public swimming pool administered by the village of Harrison Hot Springs: (250) 796-2244.

RADIUM HOT SPRINGS

Waters: Sulfate, bicarbonate, calcium, magnesium, silica.

Facilities and services: National park with huge outdoor pool for swimming and a hotter pool for bathing; spa offers massage, foot baths, reflexology; lodging and camping nearby. For more information, contact

Radium Hot Springs
P.O. Box 40
Radium Hot Springs, B.C. V0A 1M0
(250) 347-9390, (800) 787-1611

Note: This spring, Banff, and Miette are all located within the Canadian Rockies and are managed by a special division of Parks Canada. Information on all three springs can be obtained through

Canadian Rockies Hot Springs
P.O. Box 900
Banff, Alta. Y0L 0C0
(403) 678-0966, (800) 767-1611

UNITED STATES

Alaska

CHENA HOT SPRINGS RESORT

Waters: Sulfate, chloride, sodium bicarbonate.

Facilities and services: Historic hot spring offers indoor soaking pools and whirlpools, outdoor swimming pool, massage; fishing, rafting, dog sledding, hiking; lodging, camping, RV hookups, dining. For more information, contact

Chena Hot Springs Resort
57 Chena Hot Springs Road
P.O. Box 73440
Fairbanks, AK 99707
(907) 452-7867
www.alaskaone.com/chena

Arizona

EL DORADO HOT SPRINGS

Waters: Calcium, chloride, bicarbonates, silica, sulfates.

Facilities and services: Country day spa offers soaking pools; reflexology, aromatherapy. For more information, contact

El Dorado Hot Springs
Indian School Road, P.O. Box 10
Tonopah, AZ 85354
(623) 393-0750
www.el-dorado.com

California

BEVERLY HOT SPRINGS

Waters: Naturally hot alkaline mineral water from a 2,000 foot depth.

Facilities and Services: Luxury day spa offering soaking pools; shiatsu massage, saunas, acupressure, beauty treatments; dining. For more information, contact

Beverly Hot Springs
308 N. Oxford Ave.
Los Angeles, CA 90004
(323) 734-7000
www.beverlyhotsprings.com

GLEN IVY HOT SPRINGS

Waters: Sodium chloride, calcium carbonate, fluoride.

Facilities and services: Luxury day spa offers soaking pools; massage, aromatherapy, beauty treatments. For more information, contact

Glen Ivy Hot Springs
25000 Glen Ivy Road
Corona, CA 92883
(909) 277-3529, (888) CLUB-MUD
www.glenivy.com

HARBIN HOT SPRINGS

Waters: 4 springs: sulfur, iron, magnesium, arsenic.

Facilities and services: New Age retreat and workshop center offers 5 soaking pools, swimming pool; massage (Swedish, Watsu, shiatsu), reflexology, acupressure, aromatherapy, beauty treatments; hiking; lodging, camping, dining, general store, meditation room. For more information, contact

Harbin Hot Springs
P.O. Box 72
Middletown, CA 95461
(707) 987-2477
www.harbin.org

MERCEY HOT SPRINGS

Waters: Carbonates, calcium, sodium, chlorides, silica.

Facilities and services: Rustic country resort offers hot tubs, outdoor swimming pool; lodging, RV hookups. For more information, contact

Mercey Hot Springs
62964 Little Panoche Road
Firebaugh, CA 93622
(209) 826-3388
www.merceyhotsprings.com

MONO HOT SPRINGS

Waters: Bicarbonates, chlorides, sulfates, silica, calcium, sodium.

Facilities and services: Rustic resort offers hot tubs, outdoor pool, Jacuzzi, massage; lodging, café. For more information, contact

Mono Hot Springs
General Delivery
Mono Hot Springs, CA 93642
(559) 325-1710
www.monohotsprings.com

SIERRA HOT SPRINGS

Waters: Sulfur, silica, lithium.

Facilities and services: New Age retreat and workshop center offers indoor and outdoor soaking pools; massage; lodging, camping, dining, kitchen. For more information, contact

Sierra Hot Springs
P.O. Box 366
Sierraville, CA 96126
(530) 994-3773
www.sierrahotsprings.org

SONOMA MISSION INN AND SPA

Waters: Calcium, sodium, magnesium, manganese, lithium.

Facilities and services: Luxury historic resort offers soaking pools; massage (Swedish, aromatherapy, Watsu, reflexology), Rolfing, acupuncture, meditation, bodywork, weight control counseling; golf; lodging, dining. For more information, contact

Sonoma Mission Inn and Spa
18140 Sonoma Highway
Boyes Hot Springs, CA 95476
(707)-938-9000, (800) 862-4945
www.sonomamissioninn.com

SYCAMORE MINERAL SPRINGS RESORT

Waters: Bicarbonates, calcium, magnesium, sodium.

Facilities and services: Historic luxury resort and bed-and-breakfast with 20 hot tubs, soaking pools; massage, facials; lodging, dining. For more information, contact

Sycamore Mineral Springs Resort
1215 Avila Beach Drive
San Luis Obispo, CA 93401
(805) 595-7302, (800) 234-5831
www.sycamoresprings.com

VICHY SPRINGS

Waters: Bicarbonates.

Facilities and Services: Historic resort offers soaking pools, swimming pool, hiking, walking; massage, beauty treatments; lodging, dining, picnic area. For more information, contact

Vichy Springs
2605 Vichy Springs Road
Ukiah, CA 95482
(707) 462-9515
www.vichysprings.com

THE SPA AT WARNER SPRINGS

Waters: Sulfur, magnesium, sodium, selenium, zinc, arsenic.

Facilities and services: Historic desert resort features soaking and swimming pools, massage, aromatherapy, beauty treatments; golf, equestrian center, tennis; lodging, dining. For more information, contact

The Spa at Warner Springs
Highway 79
P.O. Box 399
Warner Springs, CA 92086
(760) 782-4255
www.warnersprings.com

WILBUR HOT SPRINGS

Waters: Chloride, sodium, carbonic acid, potassium, sulfate, silica.

Facilities and services: Acclaimed holistic retreat offers soaking tubs, sitting pool, sauna, massage; lodging, dining, camping. For more information, contact

Wilbur Hot Springs
3375 Wilbur Springs Road
Wilbur Springs, CA 95987
(530) 473-2806
www.wilburhotsprings.com

Colorado

COTTONWOOD HOT SPRINGS AND SPA

Waters: Lithium, boron.

Facilities and services: Historic hot spring features 3 soaking pools; massage (deep tissue, chair, Watsu, aquamassage); lodging, dining. For more information, contact

Cottonwood Hot Springs and Spa
18999 Country Road 306
Buena Vista, CO 81233
(719) 395-6434, (800) 241-4119
www.cottonwood-hot-springs.com

FILOHA MEADOWS

Waters: Bicarbonate, chloride, sulfate, calcium, magnesium, sodium.

Facilities and services: Christian resort with mineral soaking pools; massage, physical therapy, counseling, wellness living program; lodging, dining. No day use. For more information, contact

Filoha Meadows
14628 Highway 133
Redstone, CO 81623
(970) 963-3566
www.fourcorners.com/hotsprings/filoha

INDIAN SPRINGS RESORT

Waters: Calcium, fluoride, iron, magnesium, sodium, silica, sulfates.

Facilities and services: Historic full-service resort offers cave baths, soaking pools, swimming pool, Jacuzzi; massage, beauty treatments, mud baths; lodging, camping, dining. For more information, contact

Indian Springs Resort
302 Soda Creek Road, Box 1990
Idaho Springs, CO 80452
(303) 989-6666
www.indianspringsresort.com

MT. PRINCETON HOT SPRING

Waters: Carbonate of lime, magnesium, potash; chloride, sulfate.

Facilities and services: Historic modernized hot spring offers indoor soaking tubs, outdoor swimming pools, water slide; lodging, dining, picnic area. For more information, contact

Mt. Princeton Hot Spring
Highway 162
Nathrop, CO 81236
(719) 395-2361, (888) 395-7799
www.mtprinceton.com

TRIMBLE HOT SPRINGS

Waters: Sodium, calcium, manganese, silica, lithium, magnesium.

Facilities and services: Historic hot spring offers soaking pools, swimming
pool; massage; lodging (private apartment). For more information, contact

Trimble Hot Springs
6475 County Road 203
P.O. Box 9201
Durango, CO 81301
(970) 247-0111
www.fourcorners.com/hotsprings/trimble

VALLEY VIEW HOT SPRINGS

Waters: Lightly mineralized (trace amounts of many minerals).

Facilities and services: Soaking pools, swimming pool, sauna; lodging,
camping. For more information, contact

Valley View Hot Springs
Country Road GG
P.O. Box 65
Villa Grove, CO 81155
(719) 256-4315
www.vvhs.com/soak

WIESBADEN HOT SPRINGS

Waters: Magnesium, potassium.

Facilities and services: Historic resort offers hot springs cave with soaking
pool, outdoor swimming pool, Jacuzzi, sauna; massage; lodging, dining,
picnic area. For more information, contact

Wiesbaden Hot Springs
P.O. Box 349
Ouray, CO 81427
(970) 325-4347

Idaho

LAVA HOT SPRINGS

Waters: Calcium carbonate, magnesium sulfate, sodium bicarbonate,
sodium chloride, silica.

Facilities and services: Large day resort, operated by Lava Hot Springs
State Foundation, offers soaking pools, swimming pools, massage. For
more information, contact

Lava Hot Springs
P.O. Box 69
Lava Hot Springs, ID 83246
(208) 776-5221, (800) 423-8597
www.lavahotsprings.com

RED RIVER HOT SPRINGS

Waters: Lightly mineralized, including lithium.

Facilities and services: Rustic hot spring resort offers hot tubs, private baths, swimming pool; lodging, dining. For more information, contact

Red River Hot Springs
Red River Road
Elk City, ID 83525
(208) 842-2589
www.redriverhotsprings.com

Indiana

FRENCH LICK SPRINGS RESORT AND SPA

Waters: 22 minerals, including sulfur, chlorides, sulfites, carbonates, lithium.

Facilities and services: Historic full-service resort offers soaking pools, swimming pools, steam rooms, saunas; massage, aromatherapy, mud therapy, reflexology, beauty treatments, exercise classes; golf, tennis; lodging, dining, convention center. For more information, contact

French Lick Springs Resort and Spa
8470 West State Road 56
French Lick, IN 47432
(812) 936-9300, (800) 457-4042
www.frenchlick.com

Missouri

THE ELMS RESORT AND SPA

Waters: "Sulfo-saline."

Facilities and services: Historic resort and conference center offers soaking pools, whirlpools, Swiss and Vichy showers, sauna, steam rooms; massage, mud therapy, beauty treatments, fitness room, golf, biking, walking, classes in meditation, t'ai chi, yoga. For more information, contact

The Elms Resort and Spa
401 Regent Street
Excelsior Springs, MO 64024
(816) 630-5500, (800) 843-3567
www.elmsresort.com

Montana

BOULDER HOT SPRINGS

Waters: Sodium, potassium, calcium, magnesium, silica.

Facilities and services: Historic hot spring offering indoor hot pools, outdoor swimming pool; steam rooms; lodging, dining. For more information, contact

Boulder Hot Springs
P.O. Box 930
Boulder, MT 59632
(406) 225-4339
www.boulderhotsprings.com

CHICO HOT SPRINGS RESORT

Waters: Calcium, magnesium, sodium, silica.

Facilities and services: Historic hot springs offers soaking and swimming pools; massage, beauty treatments; gardens, horseback riding, fishing, hiking, cycling, cross-country skiing; lodging, dining. For more information, contact

Chico Hot Springs Resort
1 Chico Road
Pray, MT 59065
(800) HOT-WADA
www.chicohotsprings.com

CHICO HOT SPRINGS LODGE

Waters: Calcium, magnesium, sodium, silica.

Facilities and services: Historic hot springs ranch with two pools, private hot tubs, Jacuzzi; boating, fishing, cross-country skiing; lodging, dining. For more information, contact

Chico Hot Springs Lodge
P.O. Drawer D
Pray, MT 59065
(406) 333-4933
www.montanacyberzine.com/chico

SYMES HOT SPRINGS HOTEL

Waters: Carbonates, sulfates, silica, sodium, potassium.

Facilities and services: Historic inn offers indoor tubs, outdoor pools; massage (Swedish, Watsu), reiki, therapeutic touch, beauty treatments; lodging, dining. For more information, contact

Symes Hot Springs Hotel
209 Wall Street, P.O. Box 651
Hot Springs, MT 59845
(406) 741-2361
www.ronan.net/~hscofc/symes.htm

Nevada

CARSON CITY HOT SPRINGS

Waters: Lightly mineralized, manganese.

Facilities and services: Historic hot spring with 10 private baths, outdoor soaking pools, swimming pools; massage; lodging, RV parking, dining. For more information, contact

Carson City Hot Springs
1500 Hot Springs Road
Carson City, NV 89706
(775) 885-8844

WALLEY'S HOT SPRING RESORT

Waters: Sulfate, chloride, calcium, potassium.

Facilities and services: Luxury resort offers 6 mineral pools, freshwater pool, steam, sauna, weight room, tennis; massage, full range of beauty treatments; lodging, dining. For more information, contact

Walley's Hot Spring Resort
2001 Foothill Road
Genoa, NV 89441
(775) 782-8155, (800) 628-7831

New Mexico

FAYWOOD HOT SPRINGS

Waters: Bicarbonates, calcium fluoride, magnesium, potassium, sodium.

Facilities and services: Country resort offers soaking pools, private hot tubs, massage therapy (Swedish, polarity, acupressure); horseback riding, hiking; lodging, camping, dining. For more information, contact

Faywood Hot Springs
165 Highway 61, HC 71, Box 1240
Faywood, NM 88034
(505) 536- 9663
www.faywood.com

JEMEZ SPRINGS BATHHOUSE

Waters: Sulfates, phosphates, magnesium, calcium, sodium, potassium, arsenic, lithium.

Facilities and services: Indoor soaking tubs, massage, herbal wraps, beauty treatments; picnic area. For more information, contact

Jemez Springs Bathhouse
P.O. Box 105
Jemez Springs, NM 87205

(505) 829-3303
www.jemez.com/baths

OJO CALIENTE MINERAL SPRINGS

Waters: Iron, lithium, sodium, bicarbonates, arsenic.

Facilities and services: Country resort offers several soaking pools; massage therapy, acupuncture, body treatments, skin care; lodging, dining. For more information, contact

Ojo Caliente Mineral Springs
50 Los Banos Drive, P.O. Box 68
Ojo Caliente, NM 87549
(505) 583-2233, (800) 222-9162
www.ojocalientespa.com

North Carolina

HOT SPRINGS SPA AND RESORT

Waters: Bicarbonates, sulfates, silica.

Facilities and services: Country spa offers 12 outdoor hot tubs; massage; camping, food. For more information, contact

Hot Springs Spa and Resort
315 Bridge Street, P.O. Box 428
Hot Springs, NC 28743
(828) 622-7676, (800) 462-0933
www.hotspringsspa-nc.com

Oregon

BREITENBUSH HOT SPRINGS RETREAT AND CONFERENCE CENTER

Waters: Sulfates, chlorides, sodium, silica.

Facilities and services: Holistic retreat offers hot tubs, soaking pools, steam room; massage (Swedish, Watsu), hydrotherapy, reiki; lodging, dining, sanctuary. For more information, contact

Breitenbush Hot Springs Retreat and Conference Center
P.O. Box 578
Detroit, OR 97342
(503) 854-3314
www.breitenbush.com

KAH-NEE-TA RESORT

Waters: Lightly mineralized, bicarbonates.

Facilities and services: Luxury resort, administered by the Warm Springs Indian reservation, offers soaking pools, swimming pools, water slide;

massage; golf, fishing, tennis, cycling; lodging, dining. For more information, contact

Kah-Nee-Ta Resort
P.O. Box K
Warm Springs, OR 97761
(541) 553-1112

Texas

CHINATI HOT SPRINGS

Waters: Lithium, boron, arsenic.

Facilities and services: Desert hot springs offers soaking pools, creek bathing; lodging, camping, dining, picnic area, workshops. For more information, contact

Chinati Hot Springs
Candelaria Road, Box 67
Marfa, TX 79843
(915) 229-4165

Utah

CRYSTAL HOT SPRINGS

Waters: Chloride, sodium, calcium, sulfate, potassium, magnesium.

Facilities and services: Historic hot springs with world's largest natural hot and cold springs, 50 feet apart. Olympic swimming pool, hot soaking pools, hot tubs, lap pool, waterslide; camping, RV hookups, picnic area. For more information, contact

Crystal Hot Springs
8215 North Highway 38
Honeyville, UT 84314
(435) 279-8104, (801) 547-0777

THE HOMESTEAD

Waters: Calcium.

Facilities and services: Luxury hotel and resort offers unique enclosed swimming pool, in natural mineral dome known as "The Crater," hot tub; sauna, fitness room, tennis, cycling, golf; lodging, dining. For more information, contact

The Homestead
700 North Hempstead Drive
P.O. Box 99
Midway, UT 84049
(800) 327-7220
www.homestead-ut.com

MYSTIC HOT SPRINGS

Waters: Sodium, calcium, chloride, nitrate, sulfate, bicarbonate, silica, iron.

Facilities and services: Rustic hot springs with travertine soaking tubs; massage, workshops, concerts; lodging, camping, store. For more information, contact

Mystic Hot Springs
475 East 100 North
Monroe, UT 84754
(888) 527-3286
www.mystichotsprings.com

PAH TEMPE MINERAL HOT SPRINGS

Waters: Calcium, magnesium, sodium, bicarbonate, sulfate, chloride.

Facilities and services: Rustic bed-and-breakfast offers 5 natural pools, swimming pool; massage, beauty treatments; lodging, dining, retreat center, RV hookups, picnic area. For more information, contact

Pah Tempe Mineral Hot Springs
825 North 800 East 35–4
Hurricane, UT 84737
(435) 635-2879, (888) 726-8367
www.infowest.com/pahtempe

Washington

CARSON HOT SPRINGS RESORT

Waters: Sulfate, phosphate, potassium, sodium, calcium, magnesium.

Facilities and services: Historic hot spring resort offers mineral pools for men and women; massage; lodging dining, private hot tub (with suite). For more information, contact

Carson Hot Springs Resort
1 St. Martin Road, P.O. Box 1169
Carson, WA 98610
(509) 427-8292, (800) 607-3678

SOL DUC HOT SPRINGS RESORT

Waters: Silica, bicarbonate, sulfate.

Facilities and services: Country resort offers soaking pools, swimming pool; massage; lodging, RV hookups, dining. For more information, contact

Sol Duc Hot Springs Resort
P.O. Box 2169
Port Angeles, WA 98362
(360) 327-3583
www.northolympic.com/solduc

22

HEALING SPRINGS OF LATIN AMERICA AND THE CARIBBEAN

ARGENTINA

CACHUETA (MENDOZA)
Waters: Several springs; sodium chloride, sulfate, bicarbonate.
Facilities and services: Swimming, balneotherapy, inhalation.
Indications: Stress, rheumatism, skin diseases, gastrointestinal problems, gynecological disorders, liver diseases.

COPAHUÉ (NEUQUÉN)
Waters: 3 springs; sulfur, sulfate.
Facilities and services: Swimming, bathing hydrotherapy, mud baths, drinking.
Indications: Gastric disturbances, rheumatism, arthritis, skin diseases, stress.

LOS MOLLES (MENDOZA)
Waters: Sulfate, bicarbonate, sodium chloride, silica; radon.
Facilities and services: Bathing, hydrotherapy.
Indications: Rheumatism, skin diseases, gynecological disorders, catarrhal conditions.

PISMANTA (SAN JUAN)
Waters: Sulfate, bicarbonate, silica; radon.
Facilities and services: Bathing, hydrotherapy, drinking; grape cure.
Indications: Rheumatism, gout, urological disorders.

TERMAS DE REYES (JUJUY)

Waters: 3 springs; calcium, sodium sulfate, silica.
Facilities and services: Bathing, hydrotherapy, drinking.
Indications: Locomotor disorders, rheumatism, gastric disturbances.

TERMAS DE RÍO HONDO (SANTIAGO DE ESTERO)

Waters: 8 springs; bicarbonate, sulfate, sodium chloride.
Facilities and services: Bathing.
Indications: Locomotor diseases, stress.

ROSARIO DE LA FRONTERA (SALTA)

Waters: 7 springs; chlorides, sulfates, bicarbonates.
Facilities and services: Balneotherapy, swimming, inhalations, mud baths,
    drinking.
Indications: Gastrointestinal problems, genitourinary and gynecological
    problems, rheumatism.

BRAZIL

There are more than 30 major hot springs and mineral springs in Brazil, including the following:

AGUAS DA PRATA (SÃO PAULO)

Waters: 4 springs; carbon dioxide, radon.
Facilities and services: Bathing, hydrotherapy, inhalation, swimming.
Indications: Gastrointestinal and genitourinary tract diseases, gynecological
    disorders, liver and kidney diseases, rheumatism.

ARAXÁ (MINAS GERAIS)

Waters: 2 springs; sulfur; radon.
Facilities and services: Major spa offers bathing, hydrotherapy, pelotherapy,
    swimming, bathing, inhalation, physiotherapy.
Indications: Metabolic diseases, rheumatism, diabetes, skin diseases,
    diseases of the urinary tract.

CAMBUQUIRA (MINAS GERAIS)

Waters: 9 springs; iron, alkali, radon.
Facilities and services: Bathing, swimming, drinking.
Indications: Genitourinary and gastrointestinal tract disorders, anemia.

CAXAMBÚ (MINAS GERAIS)

Waters: 10 springs; bicarbonate, iron, carbon dioxide, radon.

Facilities and services: Major spa offers swimming, bathing, hydrotherapy, drinking.

Indications: Gastrointestinal and urinary tract diseases, gynecological disorders, rheumatism, convalescence.

LAMBARI (MINAS GERAIS)

Waters: 4 springs; carbon dioxide; radon.

Facilities and services: Swimming, bathing, hydrotherapy, physical therapy, inhalation.

Indications: Digestive disorders, urinary tract diseases, rheumatism, hypertension, skin diseases.

LINDOIA (SÃO PAULO)

Waters: 3 springs; radon.

Facilities and services: Swimming, bathing, hydrotherapy, physical therapy, drinking.

Indications: Genitourinary tract diseases, gynecological disorders, arthritis, arteriosclerosis.

POÇOS DE CALDAS (MINAS GERAIS)

Waters: 6 springs; bicarbonate, sulfate, iron, radon.

Facilities and services: Major spa offers swimming, bathing, hydrotherapy, inhalation, physical therapy.

Indications: Rheumatic disease; anemia; diseases of the eyes, nose, and skin; urinary tract disorders; gynecological disorders.

SÃO LOURENÇO (MINAS GERAIS)

Waters: 6 springs; carbon dioxide, bicarbonate, alkaline, magnesium, iron, sulfide, radon.

Facilities and services: Major spa town with several thermal establishments that provide bathing, swimming, inhalation, drinking.

Indications: Digestive and urinary tract diseases, gynecological disorders, iron deficiency diseases, rheumatism.

SÃO PEDRO (SÃO PAULO)

Waters: 3 springs; sulfur, bicarbonate.

Facilities and services: Major spa offers hydrotherapy, balneotherapy, physical therapy, inhalation, drinking.

Indications: Rheumatism, gastrointestinal and hepatobiliary tract disorders, skin diseases.

SERRA NEGRA (SÃO PAULO)

Waters: 1 spring; chloride, sulfate, radon.
Facilities and services: Swimming, bathing, inhalation, physical therapy.
Indications: Diseases of the kidney, liver, and skin; arthritis; arteriosclerosis.

CHILE

PANIMÁVIDA (COLBUN)

Waters: Sulfate, chlorides, calcium.
Facilities and services: Major resort features bathing, hydrotherapy, steam baths, mud baths and packs, massage, drinking.
Indications: Circulatory problems; gynecological disorders; liver, kidney, and urinary tract disorders; skin diseases; arthritis.

TERMAS DE CHILLÁN (CHILLÁN)

Waters: Bicarbonates, sulfate.
Facilities and services: Major resort features bathing, mud baths, inhalation, steam, massage.
Indications: Rheumatism, arthritis, gynecological problems, respiratory disorders.

TERMAS DE HUIFE (PUCÓN)

Waters: Sodium, potassium, sulfides, chlorides.
Facilities and services: Modern resort offers swimming, bathing, hydromassage.
Indications: Stress, arthritis, rheumatism, skin conditions.

TERMAS DE PALGUÍN (VILLARICA)

Waters: Lightly mineralized, sulfate, chloride.
Facilities and services: Rustic spa resort offers swimming and bathing.
Indications: Rheumatism, stress.

TERMAS DE PUYEHUE (VILLARICA)

Waters: Lightly mineralized; chloride, sodium, lithium.
Facilities and services: Full-service resort offers swimming, bathing, hydrotherapy, mud baths and packs, massage, beauty treatments.
Indications: Rheumatism, arthritis, neuralgia, gynecological disorders, respiratory problems, skin diseases, nervous system disorders.

COLOMBIA

PAIPA (BOYACÁ)
Waters: 3 springs; sulfates, chlorides, bicarbonate.
Facilities and services: Thermal resort offers swimming, bathing, hydrotherapy.
Indications: Rheumatism, skin diseases.

TABIO (CUNDINAMARCA)
Waters: 3 springs; sulfates, radon.
Facilities: Swimming, bathing.
Indications: Skin diseases, rheumatism

COSTA RICA

AGUA CALIENTE (CARTAGO)
Waters: 2 springs; sulfates, chlorides.
Facilities: Outdoor pools for swimming, bathing.
Indications: Rheumatism, stress.

CUBA

The Republic of Cuba is slowly beginning to redevelop its hot spring resorts, primarily to attract foreign tourists. In October 1999, Cuba was the site of "Cubater 99," the first national conference on spa medicine.

AMARO (LAS VILLAS)
Waters: 3 springs; chlorides.
Facilities and services: Swimming.
Indications: Liver diseases, stress.

CIEGO MONTERO (LAS VILLAS)
Waters: 5 springs; chloride, sulfate.
Facilities and services: Swimming, bathing, drinking.
Indications: Rheumatism, skin diseases, stress.

EL CEDRÓN (SANTIAGO DE CUBA)
Waters: Sulfates, calcium, radon.
Facilities and services: Bathing, swimming.
Indications: Rheumatism, skin diseases, stress.

ELGUEA (LAS VILLAS)

Waters: 5 springs; chlorides, sulfates, radon.
Facilities and services: Bathing.
Indications: Rheumatism, skin diseases, stress.

SAN DIEGO DE LOS BAÑOS (PINAR DEL RÍO)

Waters: 6 springs; sulfates, radon.
Facilities and services: Swimming, bathing, hydrotherapy.
Indications: Nervous system disorders, skin diseases, gynecological
    diseases, rheumatism.

SAN MIGUEL DE LOS BAÑOS (MATANZAS)

Waters: 2 springs; bicarbonates.
Facilities and services: Bathing, hydrotherapy, drinking.
Indications: Metabolic and glandular problems; gastrointestinal, kidney,
    and urinary tract disorders.

SANTA FÉ (ISLA DE PINOS)

Waters: 2 springs; calcium bicarbonate.
Facilities and services: Swimming, bathing, hydrotherapy.
Indications: Metabolic and glandular problems, gastrointestinal and liver
    problems.

ECUADOR

BAÑOS (AZUAY)

Waters: Sodium chloride.
Facilities and services: Bathing, drinking, hydrotherapy.
Indications: Rheumatism.

EL TINGO (PICHINCHA)

Waters: 3 springs; bicarbonates, chloride.
Facilities and services: Bathing, drinking.
Indications: Cardiovascular disorders, rheumatism, gastrointestinal problems.

GUAPÁN (CANAR)

Waters: 1 spring; sodium chloride, bicarbonates.
Facilities and services: Bathing, hydrotherapy.
Indications: Gynecological disorders, rheumatism, skin diseases, metabolic
    disorders.

GUITIG (PICHINCHA)

Waters: 2 springs; bicarbonate, chloride.
Facilities and services: Bathing, drinking.
Indications: Gastrointestinal problems, disorders of the hepatobiliary system.

TERMAS DE PAPALLACTA (QUITO BAEZA)

Waters: Sulfate, alkaline.
Facilities and services: Rustic new resort provides swimming, bathing,
    drinking.
Indications: Rheumatism, arthritis, stress.

SANTA ELENA (GUAYAS)

Waters: Chloride.
Facilities and services: Swimming, bathing.
Indications: Circulatory problems, gynecological disorders, rheumatism,
    stress.

TUMBACO (PICHINCHA)

Waters: Chloride.
Facilities and services: Bathing, drinking.
Indications: Gynecological and genitourinary tract disorders, neurological
    disturbances.

JAMAICA

MILK RIVER (CLARENDON)

Waters: Chloride, radon.
Facilities and services: Bathing, drinking.
Indications: Rheumatic diseases.

MEXICO

Hot springs and mineral springs have been used in Mexico since pre-Columbian
times. Today, Mexico offers a wide variety of places to enjoy healing springs
ranging from modest balnearios to first-class and luxury resorts.

AGUA HEDIONDA (MORELOS)

Waters: Sulfur, chlorosulfates, radon.
Facilities and services: Public pool offers swimming, bathing.
Indications: Arthritis, rheumatism, respiratory problems, nervous disor-
    ders, skin diseases.

IXTAPÁN DE LA SAL (MEXICO)

Waters: Many springs; chloride, bicarbonate, sulfate, radon.

Facilities and services: Major resort features swimming, bathing, hydro-therapy.

Indications: Arthritis, skin diseases, rheumatism, gynecological and nervous disorders.

SAN JOSÉ DE PORÚA (MICHOACÁN)

Waters: 2 springs; bicarbonates, chlorides, radon.

Facilities and services: Established resort offers swimming, bathing, pelo-therapy.

Indications: Rheumatism, skin diseases, gastrointestinal, gynecological and circulatory problems.

TEHUACÁN (PUEBLA)

Waters: Several springs; bicarbonate, sulfate, chlorides, lithium.

Facilities and services: Known for their bottled water, simple balnearios offer bathing, drinking.

Indications: Gastrointestinal disorders, diuresis.

PERU

There are over 150 hot springs and mineral springs in Peru, including the following:

BAÑOS DEL INCA (CAJAMARCA)

Waters: 2 springs; low mineralization.

Facilities and services: Bathing, swimming.

Indications: Rheumatism, gynecological disorders.

CHANCOS (ANCASH)

Waters: Chlorides, bicarbonate.

Facilities and services: Bathing, inhalation.

Indications: Respiratory, gastrointestinal, hepatobiliary and gynecological disorders.

MONTERREY (ANCASH)

Waters: Chlorides, bicarbonate.

Facilities and services: Swimming, bathing.

Indications: Rheumatism, gastrointestinal problems, gynecological disorders.

YURA (AREQUIPA)
Waters: Calcium, sodium bicarbonate.
Facilities and services: Swimming, bathing, drinking.
Indications: Cardiovascular diseases, rheumatism, gynecological problems.

URUGUAY

TERMAS DE ARAPEY (SALTO)
Waters: Bicarbonate, calcium, magnesium.
Facilities and services: Swimming, bathing, hydrotherapy.
Indications: Rheumatism, neuralgia, urinary tract disorders, gynecological
   problems.

TERMAS DE DAYMÁN (SALTO)
Waters: Thermal.
Facilities: Swimming, bathing.
Indications: Rheumatism, stress.

VENEZUELA

There are dozens of hot and mineral springs in Venezuela, including several
near the city of Merida. One of my most pleasant experiences was soaking in a
small thermal pool after hiking in the mountains about an hour from a Merida
suburb. The two most important spas in Venezuela are these:

AGUAS CALIENTES (TÁCHIRA)
Waters: 9 springs; sulfur, sulfates.
Facilities: Swimming, bathing.
Indications: Rheumatism, respiratory problems, skin diseases.

LAS TRINCHERAS (CARABOBO)
Waters: 3 major springs; hydrogen sulfite, sodium bicarbonate.
Facilities: Swimming, bathing, steam baths, mud baths.
Indications: Rheumatism, arthritis, skin problems.

23

HEALING SPRINGS OF EUROPE

AUSTRIA

Austria contains a multitude of mineral springs along with a rich spa history dating back to the Romans and the Celts. Many of the historic spas have been modernized and expanded, and they offer a wide range of spa and related services that rank them among the finest in the world. As in some other European countries, spa treatments are supervised by medical professionals, and many are covered by European health insurance plans.

BAD AUSSIE (STYRIA)
Waters: Sodium chloride.
Facilities and services: Full-service spa features brine bathing, hydrotherapy, mud baths, inhalations.
Indications: Rheumatology, gynecology, respiratory problems, pediatric conditions.

BAD-DEUTCH-ALTENBURG (LOWER AUSTRIA)
Waters: Sodium, calcium sulfate, bicarbonate.
Facilities and services: Full-service spa features bathing, hydrotherapy, mud packs, drinking; research institute for rheumatology.
Indications: Rheumatology, nervous disorders, upper respiratory tract diseases.

BADEN BEI WIEN (LOWER AUSTRIA)
Waters: Sulfur, calcium, sodium, sulfate, chloride.
Facilities and services: Several thermal establishments offer bathing, hydrotherapy (including douches and inhalations), drinking; rehabilitation hospital; research institute for rheumatology.

Indications: Rheumatology, diseases of the locomotor system, skin diseases, gynecological diseases, respiratory diseases, metabolic disorders, stones, paradentosis.

BAD GASTEIN (SALZBURG)

Waters: Sodium sulfate, bicarbonate, radon.

Facilities and services: Home of the famous Gasterin curative gallery located within a mountain, Badgastein offers numerous full-service thermal establishments providing all types of balneotherapy, including bathing, drinking, steam, douches; research institute.

Indications: Rheumatism; collagen disorders; diseases of locomotor, vascular, and endocrine systems; geriatric conditions.

BAD GLEICHENBURG (STYRIA)

Waters: Sodium bicarbonate, chloride, carbon dioxide.

Facilities and services: Full-service spa features bathing and hydrotherapy, inhalation, physiotherapy, drinking.

Indications: Respiratory and cardiovascular problems, disorders of the urinary passages and gastrointestinal tract.

BAD GOISERN (UPPER AUSTRIA)

Waters: Bicarbonate, sulfate, sodium.

Facilities and services: Resort features bathing and hydrotherapy, mud packs, inhalation, drinking.

Indications: Rheumatology, sequelae of inflammatory problems.

BAD HALL (UPPER AUSTRIA)

Waters: Sodium chloride, iodide.

Facilities and services: Several thermal establishments offer bathing, hydrotherapy, drinking; physical therapy, gymnastics; research institute.

Indications: Cardiovascular disorders, rheumatology, endocrine and gynecological disorders, diseases of the peripheral nervous system, respiratory tract disorders.

BAD HOFGASTEIN (SALZBURG)

Waters: Sulfate, bicarbonate, radon.

Facilities and services: Several thermal establishments offer balneotherapy and hydrotherapy, including bathing and drinking, physical therapy; unique inhalation cave; sports medicine; medical research and training institute.

Indications: Rheumatology; diseases of the locomotor system; vascular, endocrine, and metabolic diseases; geriatric conditions.

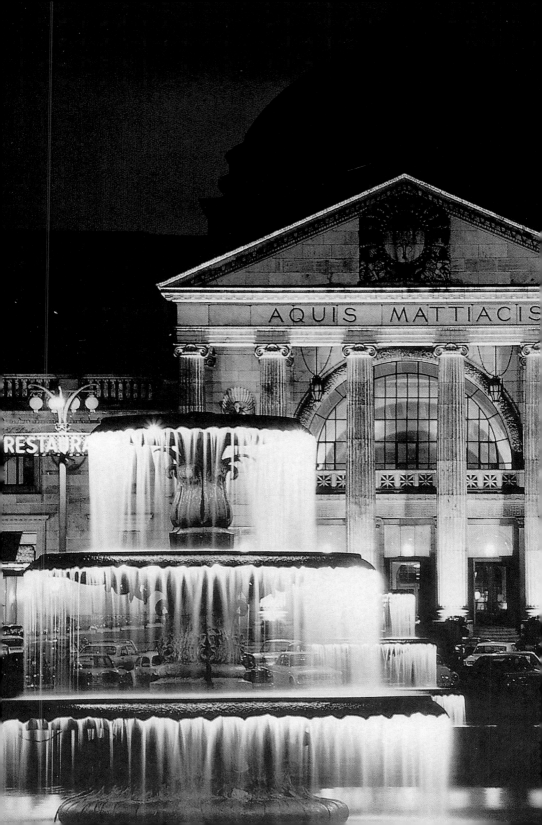

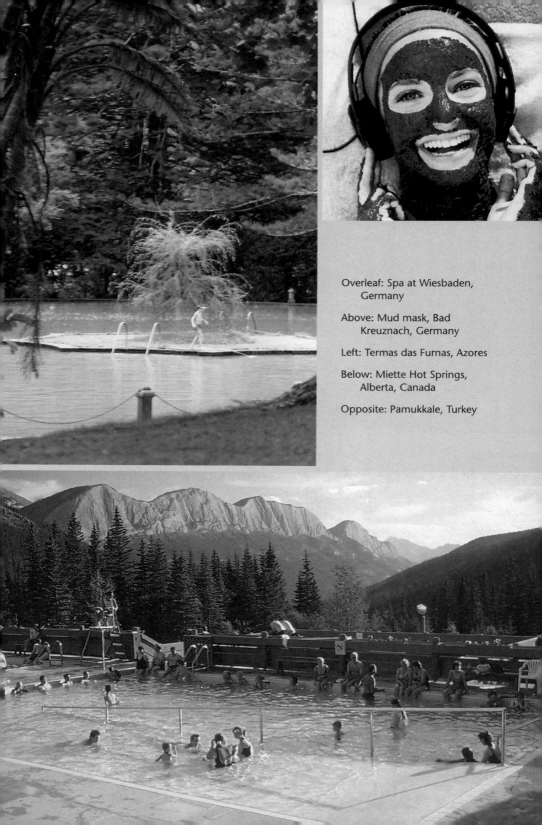

Overleaf: Spa at Wiesbaden, Germany

Above: Mud mask, Bad Kreuznach, Germany

Left: Termas das Furnas, Azores

Below: Miette Hot Springs, Alberta, Canada

Opposite: Pamukkale, Turkey

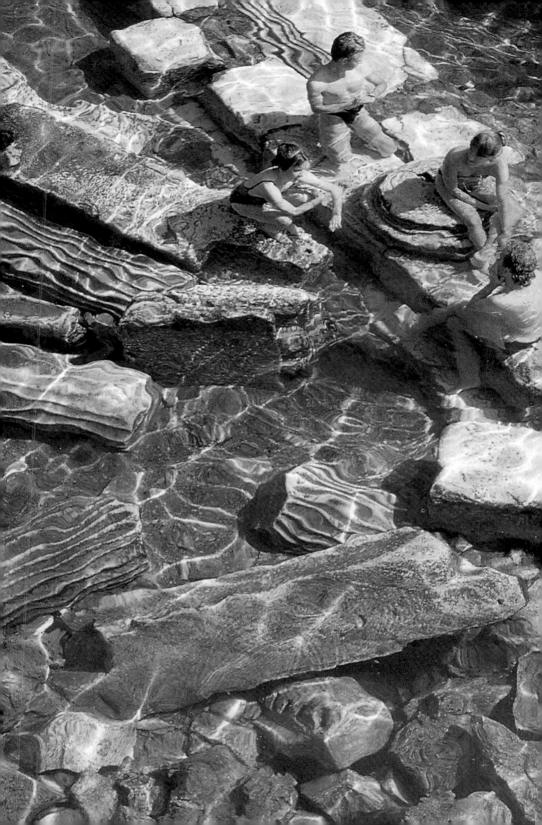

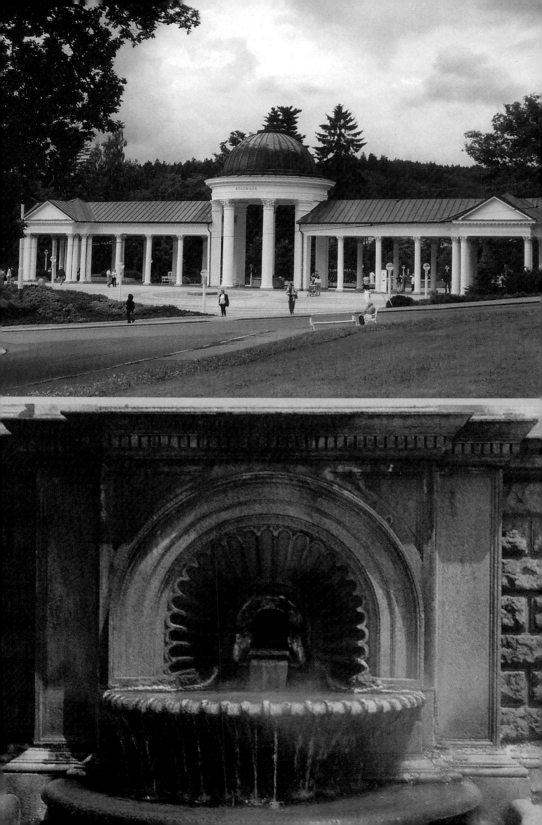

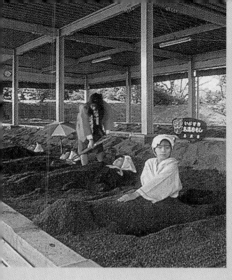

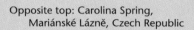

Opposite top: Carolina Spring,
    Mariánské Lázně, Czech Republic

Opposite bottom: Bollente hot spring,
    Acqui Terme, Italy

Above: Sand bath, Beppu, Japan

Right: Bath at Spring Hotel, Peitou,
    Taiwan

Below right: Yeşil Yayla Springs, Bursa,
    Turkey

Below left: Winter bathing, Hokkaido,
    Japan

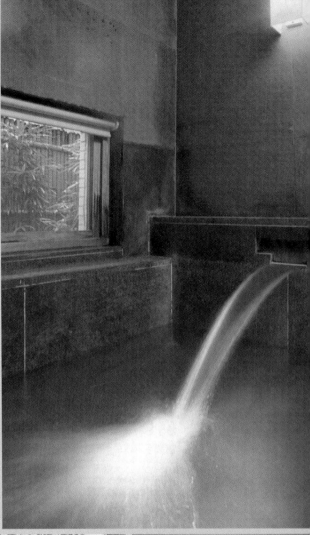

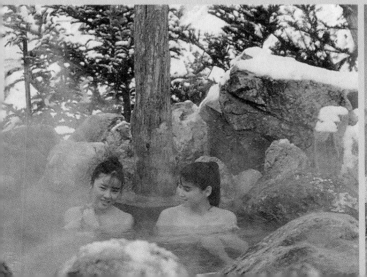

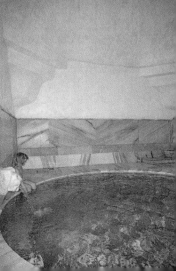

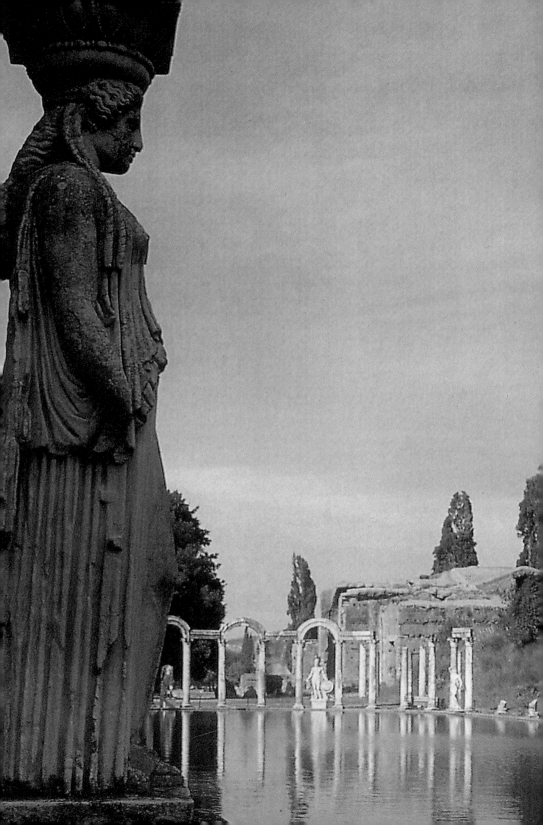

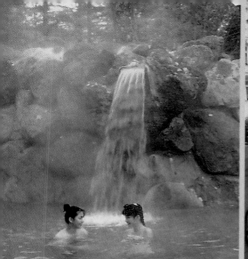

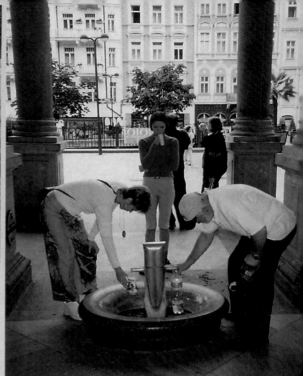

Opposite: Bagni di Tivoli, Italy

Above: Myoko Onsen, Japan

Right: Lower Castle Spring, Karlovy Vary,
     Czech Republic

Below: Oceanside hot spring, Ito Onsen,
     Japan

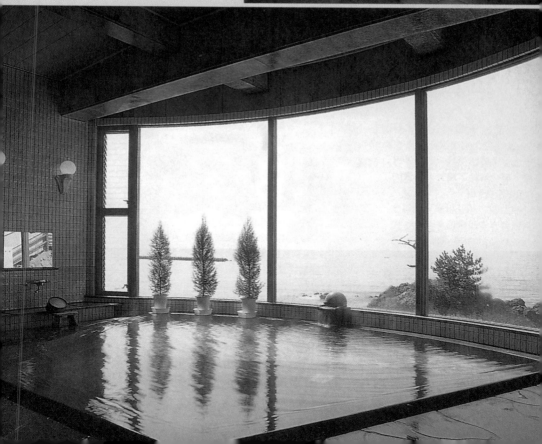

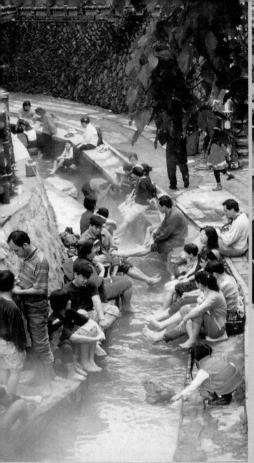

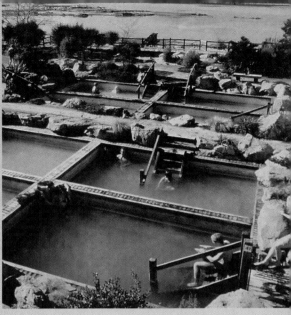

Above: Radium and Priest Hot Springs, Rotorua, New Zealand

Left : Hell Valley, Peitou, Taiwan

Below: Spencer Hot Springs, Nevada

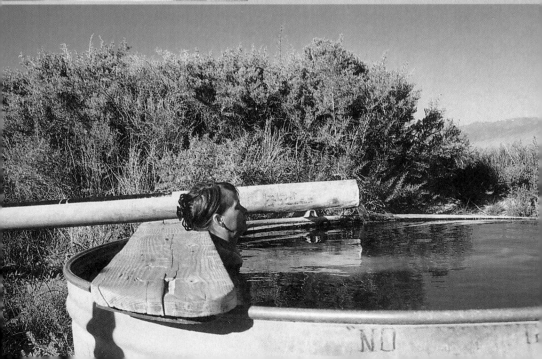

BAD ISCHL (UPPER AUSTRIA)

Waters: Sodium chloride, sodium, sulfur.

Facilities and services: Major resort offers balneology and hydrotherapy, including bathing, exercise, mud packs, drinking, inhalation.

Indications: Respiratory and vascular diseases; gynecological, rheumatic, and gastrointestinal problems; pediatric conditions.

BAD SCHALLERBACH (UPPER AUSTRIA)

Waters: Sodium bicarbonate, chloride, sulfate, sulfur.

Facilities and services: Full-service resort provides swimming, bathing, hydrotherapy, drinking, physical therapy.

Indications: Chronic rheumatic diseases, post-trauma recovery, polio.

BAD TATZMANNSDORF (BURGENLAND)

Waters: Sodium and calcium bicarbonate, carbon dioxide, iron; moor peat.

Facilities and services: Major resort offers bathing, hydrotherapy, drinking, mud and peat baths and packs, massage.

Indications: Gynecological diseases, cardiovascular diseases, rheumatic complaints, spinal disorders, rest, and convalescence.

SALZBURG (SALZBURG)

Waters: Brine water, saline; moor peat.

Facilities and services: Full-service spa offers balneotherapy and hydrotherapy, including moor packs, moor baths, brine baths, brine inhalations, steam and fog baths; research institutes.

Indications: Gynecological diseases, rheumatic diseases, diseases of the locomotor system, pediatric conditions, postoperative and post-trauma conditions.

WARMBAD-VILLACH (CARINTHIA)

Waters: Calcium bicarbonate; radon.

Facilities and services: Major spa with largest thermal pool in Europe; bathing, physiotherapy, massage.

Indications: Diseases of the nervous system, cardiovascular diseases, rheumatic disease, poliomyelitis.

For more information about Austrian spas, contact

Austrian National Tourist Office	Austrian National Tourist Office
P.O. Box 1142	2 Bloor Street East, #3330
New York, NY 10108	Toronto, Ontario M4W 1A8 Canada
(212) 944-6880	www.anto.com

Publishes *Endorsed by Body and Soul* and *Slim and Beautiful in Austria.*

BELGIUM

Belgium is the home of several spa towns, including the town where the name *spa* originated. Spa remains one of the most important hot springs resorts in the country, and ranks among the finest in Europe.

CHAUDFONTAINE (LIÈGE)
Waters: Bicarbonate, sodium, magnesium, sulfate.
Facilities and services: Thermal establishment provides balneotherapy, physiotherapy, drinking, pelotherapy.
Indications: Rheumatism, peripheral vascular disorders.

OOSTEND (WEST FLANDERS)
Waters: Alkaline chlorides, iodine, lithium, arsenic.
Facilities and services: Spa offers balneotherapy, including bathing, swimming, mud baths and packs.
Indications: Digestive problems, arthritis.

SPA (LIÈGE)
Waters: Sodium, magnesium, calcium, iron, bicarbonate.
Facilities and services: Major spa provides balneotherapy, including whirlpool baths, mud baths, peat applications, drinking, physiotherapy, inhalation, beauty program.
Indications: Stress, iron deficiency anemia, cardiovascular diseases, respiratory disorders, rheumatism, gynecological disorders.

For additional information about Belgian spas, contact

Belgian Tourist Office
780 Third Avenue
New York, NY 10017
(212) 758-8130

Office du Tourisme du Spa
Place Royale 41
4900 Spa, Belgium
www.colvert.be/spa

BOSNIA

There are numerous medicinal springs in Bosnia, including Guber, Ilidza, Vručica, Fojnica, Kiseljac Kod, Sarajeva, Koviljača, and Tuzla.

BULGARIA

Bulgaria, a small country with 230 spas and 570 sources of thermal waters, has a rich spa tradition that can be traced to pre-Roman times. Many spas have medical clinics with specialized medical services. Bulgaria is also rich in peloids, with mud therapy offered at many Black Sea resorts.

ALBENA (VARNA)

Waters: Sodium bicarbonate, chloride, sulfide.

Facilities and services: Major spa offers swimming, sea bathing, physical therapy.

Indications: Locomotor disturbances, peripheral nervous system disorders, cardiovascular problems, respiratory disease.

BANYA (SOFIA)

Waters: 2 springs; sodium, sulfate, bicarbonate, fluorine.

Facilities and services: Urban spa offers bathing, drinking.

Indications: Metabolic disorders, nervous system disorders, rheumatism.

BLAGOEVGRAD (DISTRICT TOWN)

Waters: 3 springs; sodium, sulfate bicarbonate.

Facilities and services: Bathing.

Indications: Peripheral nervous system disorders, locomotor disorders, gynecological disorders.

HISSARYA (PLOVDIV)

Waters: 24 springs; sodium bicarbonate, radon.

Facilities and services: Bathing, hydrotherapy, drinking; research centers.

Indications: Metabolic disorders, diseases of the liver, disorders of the urinary and gastrointestinal tracts.

KYUSTENDIL (SOFIA)

Waters: Sodium, sulfate, bicarbonate.

Facilities and services: Major spa offers bathing, massage, douches, physical therapy.

Indications: Skin diseases, diseases of the locomotor system, gynecological problems, heart and circulatory disorders, neurological disorders.

PAVEL BANYA (STARA ZAGORA)

Waters: 7 springs; bicarbonate, radon.

Facilities and services: Spa offers bathing, hydrotherapy, drinking.

Indications: Rheumatism, skin diseases, diseases of the locomotor system, genitourinary and gastrointestinal tract diseases.

SOPHIA (CAPITAL CITY)

Waters: 1 spring; sodium sulfate, sulfur, fluorine.

Facilities and services: Urban spa offers bathing, hydrotherapy, drinking.

Indications: Diseases of the locomotor system, diseases of the genitourinary and gastrointestinal systems.

VELINGRAD (PAZARDJIK)

Waters: 80 springs; sodium bicarbonate, sulfate, radon.

Facilities and services: Full-service spa offers bathing, hydrotherapy, drinking, physical therapy, massage.

Indications: Disorders of the gastrointestinal and genitourinary tracts, peripheral nerve disorders, respiratory tract disorders, diseases of the locomotor system.

CROATIA

LIPIK

Waters: Alkaline, chloride, iodine.

Facilities and services: Thermal establishment offers bathing, hydrotherapy, drinking.

Indications: Rheumatism.

IGALO

Waters: Sodium, radon.

Facilities and services: Small coastal resort offers swimming, bathing, hydrotherapy, drinking, pelotherapy.

Indications: Gastrointestinal complaints, rheumatism, gynecological diseases.

TOPUSCO

Waters: Lightly mineralized, radon.

Facilities and services: Bathing, hydrotherapy, mud baths, peat therapy, drinking.

Indications: Rheumatism, post-traumatic disorders, gynecological problems.

Other spas in Croatia include Stubičke Toplice, Sutinske Toplice, Tuheljske Toplice, and Varaždinske Toplice.

CZECH REPUBLIC

As part of the former Czechoslovakia, the Czech Republic has a rich bathing tradition: the medicalization of the Czech spas was initiated by Mladejovsky (1865–1935), professor of physical medicine and balneology at Charles University in Prague. Like their counterparts in neighboring Slovakia, Czech balneologists are among the best-trained in the world, and several spas are considered world class, particularly those at Karlovy Vary (Carlsbad) and Mariánské Lázně (Marienbad).

FRANTIŠKOVY LÁZNĚ [FRANZENBAD] (BOHEMIA)

Waters: 24 springs; sulfate, sodium, bicarbonate, chloride, calcium.

Facilities and services: Several fully-equipped thermal establishments offer bathing, hydrotherapy, physical therapy, mud baths and packs, dry carbon dioxide baths.

Indications: Cardiovascular disease, rheumatism, gynecological disorders.

JÁCHYMOV [JOACHIMSTHAL] (BOHEMIA)

Waters: Bicarbonate, sodium, radon.

Facilities and services: Full-service thermal center offers all forms of balneo-therapy and hydrotherapy, physical therapy, therapeutic exercise, drinking, inhalation.

Indications: Rheumatic diseases, gout, cardiovascular disorders.

KARLOVY VARY [CARLSBAD] (BOHEMIA)

Waters: 12 springs; bicarbonate, sulfate, sodium, chloride, calcium, magnesium.

Facilities and services: One of Europe's premier spa towns features several fully-equipped thermal establishments that offer bathing, hydrotherapy, physical therapy, mud packs, peat packs, oxygen therapy, drinking.

Indications: Digestive and hepatobiliary disorders, metabolic and endocrine disorders.

LÁZNĚ PODĚBRADY (BOHEMIA)

Waters: 18 wells; bicarbonate, sodium, calcium.

Facilities and services: Major spa offers carbon dioxide baths, inhalations, hydrotherapy, mud baths and packs, therapeutic exercise; research institute.

Indications: Cardiovascular disease, nervous disorders, convalescence.

MARIÁNSKÉ LÁZNĚ [MARIENBAD] (BOHEMIA)

Waters: 40 springs; carbon dioxide, sulfates, bicarbonate, sodium, calcium, magnesium, iron.

Facilities and services: An important spa town features several fully-equipped thermal establishments that offer all forms of bathing, hydrotherapy, physical therapy, mud packs, peat packs, drinking, oxygen therapy; research instutute.

Indications: Digestive disorders, urinary tract disorders, metabolic disorders (especially obesity), skin diseases, gout, allergy.

For more information about spas in the Czech Republic, contact

Czech Tourist Authority
1109 Madison Avenue
New York, NY 10111
(212) 288-0830

Kur-Info
Sprudel Collonnade
36001 Karlovy Vary
Czech Republic
(420) 17 322 4097, (420) 17 322 4667 (fax)

Provides information on spas and spa services, including accommodation assistance.

Medicinal Spa Mariánské Lázně Corporation
Masarykova 22, 35329 Mariánské Lázně, Czech Republic
(420) 165-655555, (420) 165-655500 (fax)
www.marienbad.cz

Provides information on spas and spa services, including accommodation assistance.

FINLAND

NAANTALI

Waters: Thermal.
Facilities and services: Largest spa resort in Scandinavia provides swimming, bathing, hydrotherapy, steam baths, sauna, mud baths, massage, beauty treatments, gym; treatments given under medical supervision.
Indications: Stress, rheumatic complaints, insomnia, obesity.

NOKIA

Waters: Thermal.
Facilities and services: Popular resort features swimming, bathing, saunas, sports.
Indications: Stress, rheumatology.

POORVOO

Waters: Thermal, bicarbonate.
Facilities and services: Major resort offers swimming, bathing, balneotherapy, physical therapy, beauty treatments, medical supervision.

TAMPERE

Waters: Thermal.
Facilities and services: Full-service resort offers bathing, hydrotherapy, fangotherapy, acupuncture, massage, beauty treatments, medical supervision.
Indications: Rheumatism, gout, arthritis, convalescence.

For more information about spas in Finland, contact

Scandinavian Tourist Board
655 Third Avenue, 18th Floor
New York, NY 10017
(212) 949-2333

FRANCE

Over 105 thermal centers are recognized by the French government. Although they vary in size and relative importance, all treatment facilities are operated under medical supervision and are regulated by the Ministry of Health. Some spas are affiliated with major university medical schools and other research institutions. In addition, most French spa towns offer a wide range of accommodations, as well as places to eat (after all, this is France), cultural attractions, and recreation opportunities. Some of the major French spas are listed below.

AIX-LES-BAINS (SAVOIE)
Waters: Calcium, bicarbonate, sulfur, radon.
Facilities and services: World-class spa offers bathing, hydrotherapy, pelotherapy, drinking, inhalations, physical therapy; several specialized hospitals and research centers, including one devoted to rheumatism.
Indications: Rheumatism, arthritis, post-trauma, gout.

AMÉLIE-LES-BAINS (PYRÉNÉES ORIENTALES)
Waters: 18 springs; sodium bicarbonate, hydrogen sulfide, radon.
Facilities and services: Several treatment centers provide swimming, bathing, hydrotherapy, physical therapy, massage, inhalations, drinking; research institute.
Indications: Respiratory tract diseases (especially emphysema and sinus problems), rheumatism, vertebral disk problems.

AX-LES-THERMES (ARIÈGE)
Waters: 80 springs; sodium bicarbonate, silica, radon.
Facilities and services: Major spa with 3 treatment centers provides bathing, hydrotherapy, inhalations, therapeutic showers, massage, physical therapy, drinking.
Indications: Rheumatology, respiratory tract disorders.

BAGNÈRES-DE-BIGORRE (HAUTES-PYRÉNÉES)
Waters: 60 springs; calcium and magnesium sulfate, iron, radon
Facilities and services: Three thermal treatment centers provide bathing, hydrotherapy, inhalations, physical therapy, pelotherapy.
Indications: Rheumatology, depression, stress-related disorders, chronic respiratory problems.

BALARUC-LES-BAINS (HERAULT)

Waters: 2 springs; sodium chloride, carbon dioxide.

Facilities and services: Thermal establishment offers bathing, hydrotherapy, steam, pelotherapy; university research center.

Indications: Rheumatology, nervous system disorders, gynecology, sequelae of phlebitis.

BARBOTAN-LES-THERMES (GERS)

Waters: 7 springs; sodium bicarbonate, carbon dioxide, iron, radon.

Facilities and services: Thermal establishment offers bathing, hydrotherapy, pelotherapy, massage, physical therapy, drinking.

Indications: Peripheral vascular problems, phlebitis, rheumatism.

BOURBON-LANCY (SAONE-ET-LOIRE)

Waters: 4 springs; sodium chloride, calcium bicarbonate, iron, radon.

Facilities and services: Three thermal establishments offer bathing, hydrotherapy, showers, mud packs, massage, drinking.

Indications: Rheumatology, cardiovascular diseases (especially hypertension and peripheral vascular disease), gynecological disorders.

BOURBON-L'ARCHAMBAULT (ALLIER)

Waters: 7 springs; sodium chloride, bicarbonate, calcium, magnesium, sulfate, iron.

Facilities and services: Three thermal establishments offer swimming, bathing, hydrotherapy, vaporarium (in a natural cave), irrigations, massage, mud packs.

Indications: Rheumatology, peripheral vascular disease, gynecological disorders.

LA BOURBOULLE (PUY-DE-DÔME)

Waters: 2 groups of springs; bicarbonate, carbon dioxide, sodium chloride, radon, arsenic.

Facilities and services: Important spa specializes in treating respiratory diseases, with two treatment centers that offer bathing, hydrotherapy, inhalations, irrigations, steam; centers for pulmonary research; special spa facilities for children.

Indications: Respiratory tract diseases (asthma, sinusitis, bronchial problems), allergy, skin diseases, burns.

CHÂTEL-GUYON (PUY-DE-DÔME)

Waters: 8 major springs; magnesium chloride, carbon dioxide, bicarbonate.

Facilities and services: Important spa for disorders of the digestive and urinary systems; four thermal treatment centers offer carbonated

bathing, hydrotherapy, pelotherapy, irrigations, massage, drinking.
Indications: Gastrointestinal problems (especially constipation), urinary
tract disorders, gynecology, obesity.

CONTREXÉVILLE (VOSGES)

Waters: Calcium sulfate.
Facilities and services: Small but famous spa known for its drinking cure;
bathing, hydrotherapy, massage, beauty treatments.
Indications: Urinary tract disorders, obesity, diabetes, gout.

DAX (LANDES)

Waters: 12 springs; sulfates, radon.
Facilities and services: 18 thermal establishments offer drinking cure, pelo-
therapy, bathing, hydrotherapy, irrigations, physical therapy, massage.
Indications: Rheumatology, phlebitis and post-phlebitis disorders, gynecology.

ENGHIEN-LES-BAINS (SEINE-ET-ORNE)

Waters: 10 springs; calcium sulfate, hydrogen sulfide.
Facilities and services: Spa 16 kilometers from Paris; treatment center offers
bathing, hydrotherapy (including nasal irrigation, filiform douches, and
inhalations), drinking cure, physical therapy.
Indications: Respiratory tract diseases, rheumatism, sequelae of fractures.

EUGÉNIE-LES-BAINS (LANDES)

Waters: 2 springs; sulfate, bicarbonate, calcium, magnesium.
Facilities and services: Thermal center offers bathing, showers, steam,
pelotherapy, drinking.
Indications: Rheumatology, urinary tract complaints, gastrointestinal
disorders, obesity.

EVIAN-LES-BAINS (HAUTE SAVOIE)

Waters: Bicarbonate, calcium, magnesium.
Facilities and services: Treatment center offers swimming, bathing, hydrotherapy, physical therapy, inhalations, pelotherapy.
Indications: Genitourinary tract complaints, digestive disorders, metabolic
disorders, rheumatology, sequelae of trauma to limbs and joints.

LUCHON (HAUTE-GARONNE)

Waters: 80 springs; chloride, sulfur, radon.
Facilities and services: Thermal establishment offers swimming, bathing,
hydrotherapy, vaporium, massage; university research laboratory.
Indications: Upper and lower respiratory tract disorders, chronic rheumatic
diseases.

LA ROCHE-POSAY (VIENNE)

Waters: 6 springs; calcium bicarbonate.

Facilities and services: Four thermal establishments offer bathing, hydrotherapy (including filiform douche and pulverizations), specialized
mouth treatments, massage, physical therapy, psychological counseling;
major dermatological research center.

Indications: Skin diseases (especially those that cause itching), hypertension, diseases of the mouth and gums.

ROYAT-CHAMALIÈRES (PUY-DE-DÔME)

Waters: 4 springs; bicarbonate, calcium, sodium chloride, carbon dioxide.

Facilities and services: Major center for treating heart diseases; four treatment centers offer bathing, therapeutic showers, subcutaneous gas
injections, physical therapy, pelotherapy, drinking, inhalation.

Indications: Peripheral vacular disease, including hypertension, cardiac
disease, arterial diseases.

SAINT HONORÉ (NIEVRE)

Waters: 3 major springs; bicarbonates, chlorides, carbon dioxide, arsenic.

Facilities and services: Six thermal establishments offers bathing, hydrotherapy, inhalations, insufflations, massage.

Indications: Diseases of the ear, nose, and throat; respiratory diseases;
rheumatology; special facilities for children and adolescents.

VICHY (ALLIER)

Waters: 6 cold and thermal springs; bicarbonates, carbon dioxide.

Facilities and services: Perhaps France's most important spa. Three thermal
establishments offer drinking cure, bathing, hydrotherapy (including
irrigations), pelotherapy, steam baths; major university research center.

Indications: Disorders of the digestive system, metabolic diseases (including diabetes, obesity), rheumatology, gallstones.

VITTEL (VOSGES)

Waters: 2 springs; calcium sulfate, carbon dioxide.

Facilities and services: Major spa offers all forms of balneotherapy, including
baths, showers, steam baths, fangotherapy, drinking cure; research center.

Indications: Digestive disorders, metabolic problems, rheumatology, sequelae
of trauma to joints and bones, kidney and urinary tract disorders.

For more detailed information about French spas, visit
www.thermae.fr

or contact

French Government Tourist Office
444 Madison Avenue

New York, NY 10022
(212) 838-7800
info@francetourism.com

GERMANY

Germany is one of the spa meccas of the world, boasting over 166 spas with mineral water or peat, as well as 52 health resorts specializing in Kneipp hydrotherapy treatment. Between 1973 and 1993, nearly 110 million people visited German spas as overnight guests, and nearly 10 million visitors enjoyed the waters at German spas for only the day. The vast majority of German spas are owned and operated either by local communities (78.2 percent) or by the German government (8.4 percent); many are under medical supervision. Those mentioned on the following list are full-service spas in towns that offer a wide range of accommodations.

BAD BERTRICH (RHINE-PFALZ)
Waters: Sodium, bicarbonate, sulfate.
Facilities and services: Spa resort offers bathing, hydrotherapy, steam, fangotherapy, solarium, fitness program, drinking.
Indications: Gastrointestinal problems, liver diseases, gallbladder disorders, metabolic disorders.

BAD EMS (HESSE)
Waters: 18 springs; bicarbonate, sodium, chloride, carbon dioxide.
Facilities and services: Several thermal establishments offer swimming, bathing, hydrotherapy, steam, massage, drinking.
Indications: Respiratory diseases (especially asthma), cardiovascular disorders.

BADEN-BADEN (BADEN-WÜRTTEMBURG)
Waters: Saline.
Facilities and services: Perhaps the world's most famous spa town, with two thermal establishments that offer swimming, bathing, hydrotherapy, mud packs, inhalation, drinking; research institutes; special facilities for children.
Indications: Rheumatism, gynecological problems, respiratory tract diseases, senility.

BAD GRIESBACH (BAVARIA)
Waters: 3 springs; bicarbonate, fluoride, sodium.
Facilities and services: Several thermal establishments offer swimming, bathing, hydrotherapy, inhalations, massage, sports medicine, mud packs, beauty treatment, oxygen therapy.
Indications: Rheumatism, sciatica, joint diseases, convalescence.

BAD HOMBURG (HESSE)

Waters: 9 springs; sodium chloride, bicarbonate, calcium, carbon dioxide.

Facilities and services: Major spa with two thermal establishments that offer bathing, hydrotherapy, inhalations, irrigations, fangotherapy, drinking; special facilities for children.

Indications: Gastrointestinal disorders, liver and gallbladder disease.

BAD KISSINGEN (BAVARIA)

Waters: Many springs; carbonated saline, carbon dioxide, sodium, chloride, calcium, iron.

Facilities and services: Full-service treatment center offers bathing, hydrotherapy, fangotherapy, inhalations, therapeutic exercise.

Indications: Gastrointestinal complaints, gallbladder disorders, metabolic disorders, rheumatism, gynecological diseases.

BAD KREUZNACH (RHINE-PFALZ)

Waters: Sodium, chloride, calcium, bicarbonate, radon.

Facilities and services: World-famous spa with several thermal centers that offer bathing, hydrotherapy, mud baths and packs, exercise, grape cure (autumn), inhalation, drinking; special services for children.

Indications: Rheumatism, gynecology, upper respiratory tract disorders, pediatric conditions.

BAD NAUHEIM (HESSE)

Waters: Bicarbonate, sodium, calcium.

Facilities and services: Major spa with several thermal establishments that provide carbonated baths, hydrotherapy, fangotherapy, peat baths, inhalations; research institutes.

Indications: Cardiovascular diseases, gynecological disorders, respiratory tract diseases, rheumatism.

BAD NENNDORF (HANNOVER)

Waters: 2 springs; bicarbonate, sulfate, calcium.

Facilities and services: Thermal establishment provides sulfur baths, hydrotherapy, mud baths, inhalation; special facilities for children.

Indications: Respiratory tract diseases, rheumatism, gynecological diseases, skin diseases, pediatric conditions.

BAD ORB (HESSEN)

Waters: Sodium chloride, carbon dioxide, iron.

Facilities and services: Public spa offers swimming, bathing, hydrotherapy, fitness center, pelotherapy, sauna, massage, drinking.

Indications: Cardiovascular diseases, rheumatism.

BAD PYRMONT (NIEDERSACHSEN)

Waters: Sodium chloride, carbon dioxide, iron.

Facilities and services: Thermal establishment offers bathing (including dry carbon dioxide baths), hydrotherapy, pelotherapy, massage, drinking.

Indications: Cardiovascular disease, gynecological problems, rheumatism, gastrointestinal diseases, anemia.

BAD REICHENHALL (BAVARIA)

Waters: 2 major springs; sodium chloride.

Facilities and services: Highly rated spa with several thermal establishments that offer bathing, hydrotherapy, inhalations, massages, beauty treatments, drinking.

Indications: Cardiovascular disease, respiratory diseases (especially asthma), gynecological disorders, rheumatism, pediatric conditions.

BAD SALZUFLEN (NORTH RHINE WESTPHALIA)

Waters: 4 major springs; sodium chloride, iron, carbon dioxide.

Facilities and services: Important spa known for treatment of respiratory diseases; thermal establishments offer bathing, hydrotherapy, fangotherapy, open-air inhalatorium (the largest in Germany), drinking; research institute.

Indications: Respiratory disease (especially asthma), cardiovascular diseases, gynecology, rheumatism.

BAD WILDBAD (BADEN-WÜRTTEMBURG)

Waters: Bicarbonate, chloride, sodium.

Facilities and services: Mountain spa with several thermal establishments that offer swimming, bathing, hydrotherapy, steam bath, sauna, inhalations, physical therapy, beauty treatments.

Indications: Rheumatism, senility, partial or complete paralysis.

BAD WILDUNGEN (HESSEN)

Waters: 2 springs; bicarbonate, sodium, chloride, carbon dioxide.

Facilities and services: Thermal establishment that provides bathing, hydrotherapy, fangotherapy, drinking.

Indications: Diseases of the genitourinary tract, cardiovascular diseases, metabolic disorders.

HINDELANG (BAVARIA)

Waters: Bicarbonate, sulfur, sulfate.

Facilities and services: Historic spa offers bathing, hydrotherapy, fangotherapy (including mud grotto), massage, inhalations, Kneipp therapy, beauty treatments, drinking.

Indications: Cardiovascular diseases, diseases of the digestive system, rheumatism, arthritis, convalescence, diseases of the bile system.

WIESBADEN (HESSEN)

Waters: 26 springs; chloride, sodium.

Facilities and services: World-famous 2,000-year-old spa town with thermal establishments that offer swimming, bathing (including carbon dioxide baths), hydrotheraoy, fangotherapy, drinking, inhalatorium, massage, sauna, solarium; research institute.

Indications: Rheumatology, locomotor conditons, respiratory diseases, metabolic disorders, sequelae of accidents.

WIESENBAD (SACHSEN)

Waters: 3 springs; thermal.

Facilities and services: Bathing, hydrotherapy, physical therapy, massage.

Indications: Rheumatism, arthritis, stress.

For German spa information, visit

www.kubis.de

or contact:

German National Tourist Office
122 East 42nd Street, 52nd Floor
New York, NY 10168
(212) 661-7200

175 Bloor Street East, North Tower, Suite 604
Toronto, Ontario M4W 3R8 Canada

P.O. Box 2695
London W1A 3TN, U.K.

Publishes *Our Spas and Health Resorts: Everything but Stress.*

GREAT BRITAIN

As in the United States, medical balneology is no longer recognized as a legitimate form of health care. Over the years, many British spas have closed to visitors. However, Bath will be able to offer spa treatment when it completes a contemporary health care facility in 2002, along with the restoration of five eighteenth-century spa buildings.

The following information is based on material appearing in *Medical Hydrology,* published in 1963. British medical authorities have since stopped using the spa waters for medicinal purposes. As the spas reopen, however, their water will have the same properties they have always had.

BATH (SOMERSETSHIRE)
Waters: 3 springs; calcium sulfate, radon.
Therapies used: Bathing, hydrotherapy, drinking.
Indications: Rheumatism, post-trauma, peripheral nerve lesions, orthopedic problems.

BUXTON (DERBYSHIRE)
Waters: 10 springs; carbon dioxide, radon, iron.
Therapies used: Swimming, hydrotherapy, pelotherapy.
Indications: Rheumatism, convalescence.

CHELTENHAM (GLOUCESTERSHIRE)
Waters: 3 major springs; magnesium sulfate, sodium, bicarbonate.
Therapies used: Drinking cure.
Indications: Gastritis.

DROITWICH (WORCESTERSHIRE)
Waters: Sodium (saline).
Therapies used: Hydrotherapy.
Indications: Rheumatism.

HARROGATE (YORKSHIRE)
Waters: 88 springs; sulfur, sulfide, iron.
Therapies used: Bathing, hydrotherapy, drinking, fangotherapy.
Indications: Rheumatism, obesity, convalescence.

LEAMINGTON SPA (WARWICKSHIRE)
Waters: Sodium, calcium sulfate.
Therapies used: Balneotherapy.
Indications: Rheumatism, locomotor disorders, gastrointestinal problems.

LLANDRINDOD WELLS (RADNORSHIRE)
Waters: 3 springs; hydrogen sulfide, sodium chloride.
Treatments used: Bathing, physical therapy, drinking.
Indications: Rheumatism, obesity.

WOODHALL (LINCOLNSHIRE)
Waters: Sodium chloride, iodide
Therapies used: Hydrotherapy, fangotherapy, inhalation.
Indications: Diseases of the respiratory tract, gynecological diseases.

GREECE

Some of the most ancient thermal spas in the world can be found in Greece. The major thermal centers include these:

AEDIPSOS (EUBOEA)

Waters: 60 major springs; sodium chloride, calcium chloride.
Facilities and services: Thermal center offers bathing, hydrotherapy, massage, drinking.
Indications: Rheumatism, joint diseases, gynecological complaints.

ICARIA (SAMOS)

Waters: 5 major springs; sodium chloride, radon.
Facilities and services: Island spa offers bathing.
Indications: Rheumatism, joint diseases (including arthritis), skin diseases.

LOUTRAKI (ATTICA)

Waters: 3 springs; sodium chloride, radon.
Facilities and services: Ancient spa town with a thermal establishment offers bathing, hydrotherapy, physical therapy, drinking.
Indications: Arthritis, gout, gallbladder and kidney stones, rheumatism, diabetes, skin conditions, gynecological problems.

THERMOPYLAE (THESSALY)

Waters: Sodium chloride, sulfur, radon.
Facilities and services: Ancient spa with a thermal establishment offers swimming, bathing, hydrotherapy, inhalation.
Indications: Rheumatism, arthritis, skin diseases, gynecological problems.

For more information about Greek hot springs and spas, contact

Greek National Tourist Office
645 Fifth Avenue
New York, NY 10022
(212) 421-5777

Hellenic Association of Municipalities and Communities of Curative Springs and Spas
Aristotelous Square
54623 Thessaloniki, Greece
(30) 31-230-933, (30) 31-285-962 fax

Provides information on spas and spa services, including accommodations.

HUNGARY

Authors of guidebooks have compared the hot springs of Hungary to oil in Texas: some 22 cities and 62 towns and villages have municipal baths that are officially recognized by the government, which can accommodate a total of 300,000 people at the same time. Budapest alone has 123 medicinal springs and 10 major thermal establishments. Hungary is also the home of ORFI National Institute for Rheumatism and Physiotherapy (Frankel Leo Utka 17-19, 1023 Budapest, [361] 212-4133 or 212-4627), a world-renowned research and treatment facility that uses the thermal waters of the Császár Baths.

BALATONFÜRED

Waters: 7 springs; bicarbonate of calcium, carbon dioxide.

Facilities and services: Known as the "cardiac mecca," thermal establishment offers bathing, hydrotherapy, drinking cure, physical therapy, diet therapy; State Cardiology Hospital.

Indications: Cardiovascular diseases, gynecological problems, gastrointestinal complaints, skin diseases.

BUDAPEST

Budapest may be the greatest spa city in the world, with 123 springs supplying 7 spas and 8 swimming pools. While the waters of each establishment vary as to temperature and proportion of medicinal elements, they mostly include calcium, bicarbonate, sulfur, sulfates, and chloride; some contain radon as well. The major spas include Gellért, Rudas, Rác, Király, Lukács, Császár, Széchenyi, the Danubius Thermal Hotel and Grand Hotel (Margaret Island), Hotel Aquincum Corinthia, and the Danubius Thermal Hotel Helia. All establishments offer hot spring bathing, and most provide swimming pools, complete balneotherapy treatments, hydrotherapy, steam rooms, pelotherapy, physical therapy, fitness centers, massage, and drinking cure (at Rudas, Lukács, Császár, and Margaret Island). Indications for the baths of Budapest include rheumatism and other locomotor diseases, gastrointestinal complaints, and respiratory diseases.

BÜKFÜRDO

Waters: Bicarbonate, iron, calcium, magnesium.

Facilities and services: Modern thermal establishment offers swimming, bathing, hydrotherapy, massage, fangotherapy, beauty treatments, drinking.

Indications: Rheumatism, arthritis, gastrointestinal diseases.

EGER

Waters: Bicarbonate, calcium, magnesium, radon.

Facilities and services: Thermal center offers bathing, hydrotherapy, massage.

Indications: Locomotor diseases, postoperative orthopedic rehabilitation.

HAJDÚSZOBOSZLÓ

Waters: Sodium chloride, bicarbonate, iodide.
Facilities and services: Treatment center offers swimming, bathing, hydrotherapy, massage, pelotherapy, drinking.
Indications: Locomotor diseases, gynecological complaints, skin diseases,
gastrointestinal problems.

HARKÁNY

Waters: Bicarbonate, sulfur, hydrogen sulfide.
Facilities and services: Thermal establishment offers swimming, bathing,
hydrotherapy, mud packs, physical therapy; rheumatic hospital and
research institute.
Indications: Locomotor diseases, gynecological disorders, skin diseases,
gastrointestinal complaints.

HÉVIZ

Waters: Unique 12-acre thermal lake fed by a hot spring; bicarbonate,
sulfate.
Facilities and services: Renowned spa town with several thermal establishments that offer swimming, bathing, hydrotherapy, mud baths, and mud
packs (the sulfur-rich radioactive mud here is legendary).
Indications: Locomotor disorders, sciatica, gout, post-trauma states, mouth
and gum diseases.

For more information about Hungarian spas, contact

Hungarian National Tourist Office
150 East 58th Street, 33rd Floor
New York, NY 10155
(212) 355-0240

46 Eaton Place
London SW1X 8AL, U.K.
(020) 7-823-1032
www.gotohungary.com

Publishes *Hungary: Land of Mineral Waters.*

ICELAND

Iceland is a country rich in hot springs, although there are only two thermal
establishments: a unique health facility set in a lagoon heated by thermal springs
(www.bluelagoon.is) and the NLFI Health and Rehabilitation Clinic, owned
by the Icelandic Nature Health Society (www.hnlfi.is).

THE BLUE LAGOON (GRINDAVIK)

Waters: Natural thermal salt-water lagoon located in a lava bed containing sodium, silica, calcium, potassium, and other minerals.

Facilities and services: A unique thermal establishment (recognized as an outpatient clinic by the Ministry of Health) that offers bathing, ultraviolet light therapy, steam cave, mud baths.

Indications: Psoriasis.

HVERAGERDI

Waters: Sodium chloride, hydrogen peroxide, carbon dioxide.

Facilities and services: Holistic resort and clinic offers swimming, hydrotherapy, physical therapy, mud baths, herbal baths, diet therapy, psychological counseling.

Indications: Rheumatic disease, stress-related problems, post-trauma care, convalescence.

IRELAND

Ireland is the home to one medicinal spa, Lisdoonvarna, in a picturesque town approximately 80 kilometers from Shannon Airport. There are plans to create a major health resort at this location.

LISDOONVARNA (COUNTY CLARE)

Waters: Several springs; sulfur, iron, iodine, magnesium.

Facilities and services: Spa contains bath house, sauna, pump room for drinking.

Indications: Arthritis, rheumatism, glandular and gastrointestinal diseases.

ITALY

Spa bathing in Italy dates back to pre-Roman times, and Roman baths—which were often large and luxurious bathing establishments containing separate sections for cold, tepid, and hot water—served as centers of entertainment, gymnastics, debating, and art throughout the Empire. Today, there are over 150 thermal spas in Italy, including some of the most famous in the world: Abano Terme, Montecatini, San Pellegrino, and Salsomaggiore. As in other European countries, Italian spas are operated under medical supervision, and many treatments are paid for by Social Security and private health insurance.

ABANO TERME (VENETO)

Waters: Lithium, bromide, iodide, radon.

Facilities and services: Major spa town offers bathing, hydrotherapy, fangotherapy, inhalations (in thermal caves), irrigations, massage, physical therapy.

Indications: Osteoarthritis, metabolic disorders, respiratory diseases, skin diseases, gynecological complaints.

ACQUI TERME (PIEDMONT)

Waters: Sulfur, bromide, iodide; radioactive mud.

Facilities and services: Full-service spa offers bathing, hydrotherapy, mud baths and packs, massage, physiotherapy, inhalation.

Indications: Rheumatism, arthritis, respiratory ailments, gynecological disorders, stomach disorders.

AGNANO TERME (CAMPANIA)

Waters: Bicarbonate, bromide, iodide.

Facilities and services: Major spa offers bathing, hydrotherapy, inhalation (thermal caves), mud baths and packs, massage, beauty treatments, drinking.

Indications: Rheumatism, arthritis, respiratory disorders, gynecological diseases, skin problems, metabolic disorders.

BAGNI DI LUCCA (TUSCANY)

Waters: Sulfate, radon.

Facilities and services: Several thermal establishments offer bathing, hydrotherapy, massage, mud baths and packs, thermal caves, inhalation, drinking.

Indications: Rheumatism, arthritis, digestive disorders, gynecological problems, respiratory illness, skin diseases, obesity.

CASTROCARO TERME (EMILIA-ROMAGNA)

Waters: Sulfur, bicarbonates, chloride, magnesium, sodium.

Facilities and services: Major thermal establishment offers bathing, hydrotherapy, mud baths and packs, massage, drinking, inhalation, beauty treatments.

Indications: Rheumatism, arthritis, disorders of the digestive system, liver complaints, vascular disorders.

CHIANCIANO TERME (TUSCANY)

Waters: Bicarbonate, sulfate, carbon dioxide, calcium.

Facilities and services: Major spa offers bathing, hydrotherapy, fangotherapy, drinking.

Indications: Disorders of the liver and digestive system, metabolic diseases, urinary tract disorders, circulatory diseases.

FIUGGI (LATIUM)

Waters: Lightly mineralized, radon.

Facilities and services: Several thermal establishments offer bathing, hydrotherapy, drinking.

Indications: Metabolic and bladder disorders, detoxification therapy.

ISCHIA TERME (CAMPANIA)

Waters: Bromide, chlorides, iodide, sulfate, radon.

Facilities and services: Thermal establishment offers bathing, hydrotherapy, mud baths and packs, massage, inhalation, physiotherapy, drinking.

Indications: Rheumatism, arthritis, metabolic disorders, gynecological problems, respiratory illness, vascular problems.

LURISIA TERME (PIEDMONT)

Waters: Lightly mineralized, radon.

Facilities and services: Thermal establishment offers bathing, hydrotherapy, mud baths and packs, massage, inhalation, physiotherapy, drinking.

Indications: Respiratory ailments, digestive and bladder disorders, liver problems, gynecological disorders, skin problems.

MONTECATINI TERME (TUSCANY)

Waters: Many springs; sulfates, bicarbonates.

Facilities and services: Italy's most famous spa, with several thermal establishments that offer bathing, hydrotherapy, mud baths and packs, massage, physical therapy, inhalation, drinking; research institutes.

Indications: Digestive disorders, liver and urinary tract complaints, gynecological problems, convalescence.

MONTEGROTTO TERME (VENETO)

Waters: Bromide, iodide.

Facilities and services: Many thermal establishments offer bathing, hydrotherapy, thermal caves, inhalation, physical therapy, beauty treatments.

Indications: Rheumatism, arthritis, metabolic disorders, cardiovascular diseases, gynecological problems, respiratory illnesses.

SALSOMAGGIORE TERME (EMILIA-ROMAGNA)

Waters: Sodium, iodide, bromide.

Facilities and services: World-famous spa with numerous thermal establishments that offer bathing, hydrotherapy, mud baths and packs, inhalations, massage, physiotherapy, beauty treatments; special facilities for children.

Indications: Rheumatism, arthritis, gynecological problems, vascular disorders, metabolic disorders, diseases of the mouth and gums, pediatric conditions.

SAN PELLEGRINO TERME (LOMBARDY)

Waters: Sulfate.

Facilities and services: A spa town best known for its bottled waters; several thermal establishments offer bathing, hydrotherapy, massage, physical therapy, drinking.

Indications: Digestive and liver disorders, urinary tract diseases, metabolic disorders.

SIRMIONE TERME (LOMBARDY)

Waters: Sulfur, bromide, iodide.

Facilities and services: Thermal establishment offers bathing, hydrotherapy, mud baths and packs, massage, inhalation, physical therapy, drinking.

Indications: Skin diseases, gynecological disorders, rheumatism, arthritis, respiratory problems.

For more information about Italian spas, contact

Italian Government Travel Office
630 Fifth Avenue, #1565
New York, NY 10111
(212) 245-4822

1 Place Ville Marie
Montreal, Quebec, Canada
(514) 866-7667

1 Princess Street
London W1R 8AY, U.K.
(020) 7-408-1254

Publishes *Thermal Regions Italia* and *Atlas of Italian Spas.*

LUXEMBOURG

The only thermal spa in Luxembourg can be found just across the border from France. Located in a beautiful park setting, it was extensively renovated and enlarged in 1988.

MONDORF-LES-BAINS

Waters: 2 springs; sodium, calcium chloride, calcium sulfate.

Facilities and services: Large, full-service thermal establishment offers swimming, bathing, hydrotherapy, fangotherapy, massage, physiotherapy, inhalations, steam and sauna, fitness center, diet therapy, drinking.

Indications: Digestive disorders, rheumatism, circulatory problems, respiratory disorders, diabetes.

For more information, contact

Mondorf Les Thermes
B.P. 52
5601 Mondorf-les-Bains
Luxembourg
(352) 66 12 12

NETHERLANDS

Holland has one thermal spa, Nieueschans, located near the city of Groningen.

NIEUESCHANS
Waters: Thermal, containing sulfate, iron, iodine, calcium.
Facilities and services: Modern facility under medical supervision offers
swimming, bathing, balneotherapy, thalassotherapy, massage. solarium,
ultraviolet light therapy, beauty treatments.
Indications: Skin diseases (especially psoriasis).

POLAND

There are over 40 spas in Poland, many of them located in beautiful natural
surroundings. Spas are under medical supervision, and many collaborate with
medical schools for research.

BUSKO-ZDRÓJ (KIELCE)
Waters: 13 springs; chloride, sulfide, sodium, iodide, selenium.
Facilities and services: Highly rated spa offers bathing, hydrotherapy,
physical therapy, fangotherapy, drinking; special facilities for children;
university research center.
Indications: Cardiovascular problems, rheumatism and arthritis, skin
diseases, cerebral palsy in children.

CIECHOCINEK (BYDGOSZCZ)
Waters: 5 springs; sodium, sulfate, bromide, iodide.
Facilities and services: Major spa offers saline swimming and bathing,
hydrotherapy, inhalations; several scientific medical centers.
Indications: Cardiovascular diseases, respiratory problems, rheumatism,
arthritis.

CIEPLICE ŚLĄSKIE-ZDRÓJ (WROCLAW)
Waters: 6 springs; silica, fluoride, sodium, bicarbonate, sulfate.
Facilities and services: Large thermal establishment offers swimming,

bathing, hydrotherapy, massage, orthopedic rehabilitation; special facilities for children.

Indications: Rheumatism, urinary tract disorders, eye diseases, pediatric conditions (especially cardiovascular diseases, arthritis).

KOLOBRZEG (KOSZALIN)

Waters: 45 springs; saline, iodide, bromide.

Facilities and services: Seaside resort offers bathing in saline water, hydrotherapy, physiotherapy, inhalations, fangotherapy; special therapeutic program for children.

Indications: Cardiovascular, respiratory and locomotor diseases, diabetes, obesity, pediatric conditions (skin allergies, obesity).

KRYNICA (KRAKOW)

Waters: 10 springs; low mineralization, bicarbonate, iron, iodide, bromide.

Facilities and services: Known as the "Pearl of Polish Spas," treatment center offers swimming, bathing, hydrotherapy, fangotherapy, physical therapy, drinking; affiliated with medical school.

Indications: Cardiovascular disease, diseases of the urinary and digestive systems, endocrine gland disorders, diabetes, gynecological problems.

KUDOWA-ZDRÓJ (WROCLAW)

Waters: 5 springs; bicarbonate, calcium, magnesium, arsenic, radioactive iron.

Facilities and services: Six health resort hospitals and sanitoria offer bathing, hydrotherapy, physical therapy, inhalatorium, drinking; special treatment program for children.

Indications: Cardiovascular problems, metabolic diseases, disorders of the endocrine glands, diseases of the digestive system (children).

POLANICA-ZDRÓJ (WROCLAW)

Waters: Carbon dioxide, bicarbonate, calcium.

Facilities and services: Known for its bottled water, Polanica is a major health spa that offers bathing, hydrotherapy, physical therapy, drinking.

Indications: Cardiovascular diseases, disorders of the digestive system, inflammatory diseases of the gallbladder and pancreas.

POTCZYN-ZDRÓJ (KOSZALIN)

Waters: Lightly mineralized, iron.

Facilities and services: Thermal establishment offers bathing, hydrotherapy, pelotherapy, physical therapy, massage.

Indications: Diseases of the locomotor system, rheumatism, gynecological problems.

For more information about spas in Poland, contact

Polish National Tourist Office
275 Madison Avenue
New York, NY 10016
(212) 338-9412

310-312 Regent Street
London W1R 5AJ, U.K.
(020) 7-580-8811
www.polandtour.org

Publishes *Health Spas in Poland.*

Polish Resorts Chamber of Commerce
(Izba Gospodarcza "Uzdrowiska Polskie")
ul. Rolna 179/181
02-729 Warsaw, Poland
(48) 22-433460, (48) 22-432171 (fax)

Provides information on spas and spa services, including free reservation assistance.

PORTUGAL

Though a small country, Portugal has an abundance of hot springs within its borders: a total of 55 thermal spas can be found in continental Portugal as well as on the islands of Madeira and the Azores. Many of the Portuguese spas are in beautiful natural surroundings. Spas are under the supervision of the General Direction (Ministry) of Health. The Portuguese Tourist Board publishes an informative 135-page directory of thermal spas.

CALDAS DA RAINHA (LEIRIA)
Waters: 5 springs; sulfur, chlorides, sulfates, sodium, calcium, magnesium.
Facilities and services: Historic spa town with two treatment centers (one is the Spa Hospital) that offer bathing, hydrotherapy, drinking, inhalations, irrigations.
Indications: Rheumatism, musculoskeletal problems, disorders of the respiratory tract and gastrointestinal system.

CALDAS DO GERES (BRAGA)
Waters: Bicarbonate, sodium, fluoride, sulfates, radon.
Facilities and services: Two thermal centers offer bathing, hydrotherapy (including irrigations), gargles.
Indications: Digestive tract disorders, obesity, circulatory problems (especially hypertension).

TERMAS DAS FURNAS (SÃO MIGUEL, AZORES)

Waters: Bicarbonate, sodium, fluorides.
Facilities and services: Thermal establishment offers swimming, bathing, hydrotherapy.
Indications: Rheumatism, musculoskeletal problems, respiratory diseases.

TERMAS DA CURIA (AVEIRO)

Waters: 2 springs; sulfates, calcium, magnesium, carbon dioxide, radon.
Facilities and services: Beautiful thermal establishment offers bathing, hydrotherapy, physical therapy, drinking.
Indications: Diseases of the urinary tract (especially kidney stones), hypertension, rheumatism and musculoskeletal complaints, skin diseases.

TERMAS DOS CUCOS (LISBOA)

Waters: 2 springs; chlorides, sodium, fluorides.
Facilities and services: Thermal establishment offers bathing, hydrotherapy, drinking, mud baths and packs.
Indications: Metabolic disorders, rheumatism, musculoskeletal complaints.

TERMAS DE LUSO (AVEIRO)

Waters: Lightly mineralized, saline, silica, radon.
Facilities and services: Major spa with several thermal establishments that offer swimming, bathing (including radioactive baths), hydrotherapy, massage, inhalation, drinking.
Indications: Circulatory problems, rheumatism, diseases of the kidneys and urinary tract, musculoskeletal complaints.

TERMAS DE MONTE REAL (LEIRIA)

Waters: Several springs; sulfur, sulfates, calcium.
Facilities and services: Thermal center offers bathing, hydrotherapy, physical therapy.
Indications: Digestive disorders, rheumatism, liver and gallbladder diseases, musculoskeletal complaints.

TERMAS DE SÃO PEDRO DO SUL (VISEU)

Waters: Several springs; sulfur, bicarbonate, sodium, fluorides.
Facilities and services: Modern spa offers bathing, hydrotherapy (including irrigations), massage, inhalations.
Indications: Rheumatism, musculoskeletal complaints, respiratory disorders, disorders of the endocrine glands.

TERMAS DE VIDAGO (CHAVES)

Waters: 3 springs; carbon dioxide, bicarbonate, sodium, iron, fluorides.
Facilities and services: Large thermal establishment offers bathing, hydrotherapy, drinking.
Indications: Stomach, liver, and bile duct disorders; respiratory problems; skin diseases; nervous system disorders.

For more information about hot springs in Portugal, contact

Portuguese National Tourist Office
590 Fifth Avenue, 4th floor
New York, NY 10036
(212) 354-4403

60 Bloor Street West, Suite 1005
Toronto M4W 3B8, Ontario, Canada
(416) 921-7376

22-25A Sackville Street, 4th Floor
London W1 X1DE, U.K.
(020) 7-494-1441

Publishes *Estancias Termais* (a directory in four languages).

ROMANIA

Romania has an ancient spa tradition dating back to Roman times. There are approximately 600 mineral and thermal springs (a third of the natural springs existing in Europe) and 150 health resorts, many of them quite large. All spas are under the supervision of the Ministry of Health, and treatments are directed by a qualified medical doctor.

BĂILE FELIX

Waters: Bicarbonate, sulfur, calcium, sodium.
Facilities and services: Romania's largest resort; modern thermal establishment offers swimming, bathing, hydrotherapy, massage, fangotherapy, Aslan therapy, fitness center.
Indications: Rheumatism, neurological conditions, metabolic disease, gynecological disorders.

BĂILE HERCULANE

Waters: 17 springs; lightly mineralized, sulfur, sulfate, bicarbonate.
Facilities and services: Large, historic spa and resort offers swimming, bathing, hydrotherapy, pelotherapy, inhalation, drinking, Aslan therapy.
Indications: Rheumatism, peripheral nervous system disorders, post-trauma effects, cardiovascular disorders, gynecological problems, digestive complaints.

BĂILE OLĂNEŞTI

Waters: 30 springs; sodium, chloride, sulfur.

Facilities and services: Modern thermal establishments offer swimming, bathing, hydrotherapy, physical therapy, heliotherapy, therapeutic exercise, drinking, injections.

Indications: Diseases of the urinary tract, digestive, hepatobiliary and respiratory problems, metabolic problems (including obesity), gynecological disorders, allergy, rheumatism.

CĂLIMĂNEŞTI

Waters: 12 springs; sulfur, bicarbonate, iodine, magnesium, calcium.

Facilities and services: Major spa offers swimming, bathing, hydrotherapy, drinking; Aslan therapy.

Indications: Digestive, urinary tract, renal, and liver disorders; rheumatism, arthritis; gynecological problems; skin diseases.

GEOAGIU BAI

Waters: Bicarbonate, calcium, magnesium; peat mud.

Facilities and services: Large, historic thermal resort offers swimming, bathing, hydrotherapy, therapeutic exercise, pelotherapy, drinking.

Indications: Rheumatism, gynecological problems, skin diseases, metabolic disorders.

SOVATA

Waters: Sodium, bicarbonates, sulfur; mud.

Facilities and services: Major mountain resort offers swimming, bathing, hydrotherapy, physiotherapy, mud baths, mud packs, heliotherapy, Aslan therapy.

Indications: Gynecological disorders, arthritis, cardiovascular disorders, stress-related problems.

For more information about Romanian spas, contact

Romanian Tourist Information Bureau
342 Madison Avenue, Suite 210
New York, NY 10173
(212) 545-8484

83A Marylebone High Street
London W1M 3DE, U.K.
www.rezq.com/ronto

Publishes *Spa Cures in Romania.*

RUSSIA (INCLUDING FORMER SOVIET REPUBLICS)

The development of spas in the former Soviet Union began in 1919, shortly after the Russian Revolution. Several hundred thermal spas were developed for both the prevention and treatment of disease, and have been operated as both resorts and sanitoria. Many of these spas have served as medical research centers; a large volume of research has been published in Russian medical journals on many aspects of balneotherapy. At present, many spas are becoming privatized, and some are undergoing renovation. Few efforts have been made to attract foreign visitors, but this should change in the future. The most popular spa region in Russia is Kavkazskie Mineralnye Vody (Caucasian Mineral Waters), and its best-known spa towns include Kislovodsk, Pyatigorsk, Zheleznovodsk, and Essentuki.

ESSENTUKI (STAVROPOL)
Waters: Several springs; bicarbonate, chloride; mud.
Facilities and services: Russia's largest thermal resort features bathing, balneotherapy, drinking, fangotherapy.
Indications: Digestive disorders, liver problems, metabolic disease.

KISLOVODSK (STAVROPOL)
Waters: Bicarbonate, carbon dioxide, calcium sulfate, magnesium.
Facilities and services: Established in 1802, thermal establishment offers bathing, hydrotherapy, mud baths, inhalation rooms, fitness center, physical therapy, beauty treatments, drinking.
Indications: Cardiovascular disease, metabolic and endocrine disorders, respiratory diseases.

PYATIGORSK (STAVROPOL)
Waters: Carbon dioxide, bicarbonate, radon; mud.
Facilities and services: Several thermal establishments offers bathing, hydrotherapy, mud baths, inhalations, massage, fitness center.
Indications: Locomotor disorders, digestive and metabolic disorders, gynecological problems, skin diseases, cardiovascular and nervous syetsm diseases.

REPINO (ST. PETERSBURG)
Waters: Bicarbonate.
Facilities and services: Resort offers thermal bathing, hydrotherapy, inhalation, massage, beauty treatments.
Indications: Cardiovascular disorders, rheumatism and arthritis, nontubercular respiratory diseases.

SOCHI (KRASNODAR)

Waters: Many springs; sodium chloride.

Facilities and services: Major Black Sea resort with many thermal establishments offers salt water swimming and bathing, hydrotherapy, heliotherapy, massage, injections, poultices.

Indications: Cardiovascular disease, rheumatism, arthritis, gynecological disorders, skin diseases.

ZHELEZNOVODSK (STAVROPOL)

Waters: Several springs; bicarbonate, sulfates, carbon dioxide; mud.

Facilities and services: Major spa features several sanitoria that offer swimming, bathing, hydrotherapy, physical therapy, fangotherapy, inhalations, drinking.

Indications: Gastrointestinal diseases, liver and gallbladder problems, urological diseases.

Other spas featuring medicinal waters in the former Soviet Union include the following:

Armenia: Arzni, Dzhermuk

Azerbaijan: Badamly, Itsi-Su, Naftalan, Shikhov

Belarus: Bobruisk, Minsk

Estonia: Pyarnu

Georgia: Borzhomi, Mendzhi, Sairmye, Tbilisi, Tsaishi, Tzkhaltubo

Kazakhstan: Alma-Arasan, Arasan-Kopal

Latvia: Baldone, Kemeri, Valmiera

Lithuania: Birshtonas, Druskininkai, Likennai

Moldavia: Ungenyi

Russia: Anapa (Krasnodar), Byelokurikha (Altai), Darasun (Chita), Dorokhovo (Moscow), Evpatoria (Crimea), Gagre (Abkhasia), Goryachy Kluch (Krasnodar), Issyk-ata (Kirghizstan), Karachi (Novosibirsk), Kislovodosk (Stavropol), Krainka (Tula), Kuldur (Khabarovsk), Moscow (Moskow), Nalchik (Kabardino-Balkaria), Sadgorod (Vladivostok), Saki (Crimea), Sergievskye (Kuibyshev), Sestroretzk (St. Petersburg), Shira (Krasnoyarsk), Shmakovka (Vladivostok), Staraya Russa (Novgorod), Talatya (Magadan), Usolye (Irtutsk), Ust-Kachka (Perm), Yangan-Tau (Bashkiria), and Zvenigorod (Moscow)

Tadzhikistan: Garm-Chashma, Khodzha-Obi-Garm

Ukraine: Beriosovskie, Cherche, Chernovsky, Gornaya Tissa, Khmelnik, Kuyalnitzky, Lugansk, Lyuben-Vyeliki, Mirgorod, Mironovka, Nemirov, Polyana, Shayan, Sinyak, Soimy, Slavyansk, Starobyelsk, Truskavetz

Uzbekistan: Chartak, Tashkent

SERBIA

Serbia is a land of many medicinal springs. Major thermal spas include Bukovička Banja, Koviljača, Mataruška Banja, Mladenovačka Banja, Niška Banja, Rusanda, and Soko Banja.

SLOVAKIA

As part of the former Czechoslovakia, Slovakia has a rich bathing tradition. Its balneologists are among the best-trained in the world, and many of its spas are highly regarded for their healing waters and therapeutic treatments.

BARDEJOV

Waters: Saline, iron.
Facilities and services: Bathing, hydrotherapy, mud baths.
Indications: Disease of the alimentary tract, obesity, occupational diseases, diabetes.

BOJNICE

Waters: Simple thermal.
Facilities and services: Bathing, hydrotherapy, swimming, mud baths.
Indications: Rheumatism, nervous diseases.

ČIZ

Waters: Chlorides, bicarbonates, iodide, sodium.
Facilities and services: Bathing, drinking.
Indications: Arteriosclerosis, joint disorders.

PIEŠTANY

Waters: Sulfate, calcium, hydrogen sulfide; mud.
Facilities and services: Slovokia's premiere spa offers bathing, hydrotherapy, physical therapy, massage, mud baths and packs, oxygen therapy; rehabilitation institute for children; sanitoria specializing in rheumatology, traumatology, and neurology. Its therapeutic muds are world renowned.
Indications: Rheumatism, osteoporosis, diseases of the nervous system.

SLIAČ

Waters: Sulfate, bicarbonate, calcium, radon.
Facilities and services: Full-service spa offers bathing, hydrotherapy, carbonic dry baths, mud packs, therapeutic exercise, drinking.
Indications: Cardiovascular problems (special treatment centers for children and adolescents).

TRENČIANSKÉ TEPLICE

Waters: 4 springs; sulfate, calcium, sulfur, radon.

Facilities and services: Bathing, hydrotherapy, mud baths, drinking; rehabilitation institutes.

Indications: Diseases of the locomotor system, disorders of the nervous system.

SLOVENIA

Slovenia has an ancient spa tradition that is constantly being modernized and improved. There are over 100 spas and resorts, all under medical supervision, with the major establishments providing a holistic approach to disease prevention and healing. In addition to balneotherapy and related therapies, spas offer programs geared to beauty and fitness, as well as a wide range of recreational and cultural activities. The Slovenian Tourist Board is actively promoting health resort holidays to foreigners and provides attractive, informative brochures in English.

ČATEŽ

Waters: Thermal, lightly mineralized.

Facilities and services: Large modern spa complex offers swimming (including wave pool), bathing, hydrotherapy, fangotherapy, physiotherapy, acupuncture, massage; spondylitis clinic.

Indications: Rheumatism, post-trauma conditions, postoperative treatment for cancer, nervous system disorders, stress.

DOBRNA

Waters: Thermal, lightly mineralized.

Facilities and services: Discovered in the twelfth century, this historic spa offers swimming, bathing, hydrotherapy, mud and peat packs, acupuncture, massage, hyperbaric oxygen therapy, Kneipp treatments, laser therapy.

Indications: Rheumatic and orthopedic problems, gynecology (including infertility), psychosomatic diseases, post-traumatic and postoperative conditons, microcirculatory disorders.

MORAVSKE TOPLICE

Waters: 4 springs; bicarbonate.

Facilities and services: Major resort offers swimming, bathing, hydrotherapy, fangotherapy, massage, nutrition, physical therapy; sports park.

Indications: Rheumatism, post-traumatic and postoperative joint conditions, chronic obstructive lung disease, skin diseases.

RADENCI

Waters: Sodium chloride, bicarbonate.

Facilities and services: Major resort offers 10 swimming pools, balneo-therapy, massage, Kneipp treatments, physiotherapy, fangotherapy with sulfur-rich mud, drinking.

Indications: Heart and circulatory diseases, kidney and urinary tract disorders, rheumatism, metabolic disorders.

ROGAŠKA

Waters: Sodium bicarbonate, carbon dioxide, magnesium.

Facilities and services: Known for its famous "Donat Mg" bottled waters, this major spa has several thermal establishments that offer bathing, hydrotherapy, inhalations, fitness center, beauty center, drinking; staffed by a broad range of medical specialists.

Indications: Liver, gallbladder, and biliary disorders; digestive problems; metabolic disorders; stress-related diseases; diabetes; prevention of kidney stones.

ŠMARJEŠKE TOPLICE

Waters: Carbon dioxide, magnesium, calcium, potassium.

Facilities and services: Major spa offers swimming, bathing, hydrotherapy, massage, beauty treatments, fitness studio, diet therapy; specialist clinics in cardiology, orthopedics, pain management, neurology, psychology.

Indications: Cardiovascular diseases, rheumatism and arthritis, diseases of the central and peripheral nervous system, psychosomatic diseases, sports injuries.

For more information about spas in Slovenia, contact

Slovenian Tourist Office
345 East 12 Street
New York, NY 10003
(212) 358-9686

49 Conduit Street
London W1R 9FB, U.K.
(020) 7-287-7133
www.tourist-board.si

Publishes *Slovenia's Health Resorts.*

Slovenian Spas Community
(Skupnost Slovenskih Zdravilisc)
Ljubljanska 14, p.p. 269
3000 Celje, Slovenia
(386) 63 442 111, (386) 63 442 918 (fax)

SPAIN

A country rich in thermal and medicinal springs, Spain includes over 80 established spas. Many are smaller than those in the famous spa towns of France, Germany, Italy, or the Czech Republic and are located in picturesque towns far from noisy urban centers. Balneology is part of the medical mainstream in Spain, and research is constantly being undertaken in conjunction with major medical schools and universities. Spas are under medical supervision. When a spa contains more than one thermal establishment, not all the services mentioned are necessarily offered at each spa. The Tourist Board of Spain publishes an excellent 174-page *Guide to Health Spas.*

ALHAMA DE ARAGÓN (ZARAGOZA)

Waters: Many springs: light mineralization, bicarbonate, magnesium, calcium.

Facilities and services: Ancient spa used by the Celts and Romans; three thermal establishments offer bathing, hydrotherapy, inhalations, electrotherapy, massage, acupuncture, mud, drinking.

Indications: Rheumatism, arthritis, diseases of the respiratory tract, disorders of the nervous system.

ARCHENA (MURCIA)

Waters: Sodium chloride, sulfur; mud.

Facilities and services: Thermal center offers bathing, hydrotherapy, mud and peat therapy, inhalations, gargling, physiotherapy, fitness center.

Indications: Rheumatism, arthritis, respiratory disorders, skin diseases.

ARTEIJO (LA CORUÑA)

Waters: Sodium chloride, iron, iodide.

Facilities and services: Small spa offers bathing, hydrotherapy, drinking, inhalations.

Indications: Skin diseases, rheumatism, respiratory disorders, nervous system diseases.

CALDES DE MONTBUI (BARCELONA)

Waters: Sodium chloride.

Facilities and services: Historic 200-year-old spa town, visited in the early twentieth century by King Alfonso XIII. Five thermal establishments offer bathing, hydrotherapy, inhalations, physiotherapy, fangotherapy, massage, fitness centers, beauty treatments.

Indications: Rheumatism, post-traumaic conditions, neurological diseases, gynecology, respiratory disorders, stress.

CALDES DE MALAVELLA (GERONA)

Waters: 3 major springs; bicarbonate, sodium chloride.

Facilities and services: Vichy Catalan spa at Caldes de Malavella offers bathing, hydrotherapy, mud baths, sauna, steam, physical therapy, ultraviolet light treatments, beauty treatments.

Indications: Rheumatism, arthritis, obesity, stress, disorders of the respiratory and digestive systems.

FITERO (NAVARRA)

Waters: Sodium, chloride, radon.

Facilities and services: Spa offers bathing, hydrotherapy, inhalations, drinking, mud baths, massage.

Indications: Rheumatism, arthritis, osteoporosis, post-traumatic conditions, respiratory disorders, peripheral arterial disease, obesity.

JARABA (ZARAGOZA)

Waters: Many springs; bicarbonate, calcium, radon.

Facilities and services: Three thermal establishments offer bathing, hydrotherapy, massage, inhalations, drinking, mud therapy, ultraviolet light therapy.

Indications: Rheumatism, arthritis, kidney problems, cardiovascular diseases.

LEDESMA (SALAMANCA)

Waters: Low mineralization, carbon dioxide, sulfate, radon.

Facilities and services: Large thermal establishment and hotel offers bathing, hydrotherapy, inhalations, mud baths, UV therapy, massage.

Indications: Rheumatism, nervous system disorders, gynecological disorders, respiratory diseases, skin diseases (especially eczema and psoriasis).

For more information about hot springs in Spain, contact

The Tourist Office of Spain
666 Fifth Avenue
New York, NY 10036

102 Bloor Street West, 14th Floor
Toronto, Ontario M5S 1M8, Canada
(416) 961-3131

57-58 St. James Street
London SW1A 1LD, U.K.
(020) 7-499-1169

Publishes *Guide to Health Spas.*

SWITZERLAND

Although there are over 250 mineral springs in Switzerland, only a small percentage qualify as health resorts according to government regulations. In addition to satisfying strict government hygienic regulations and medical requirements, a spa must receive scientific verification of the waters' therapeutic value. Thermal establishments are all under medical supervision. Although many believe that all Swiss spas are located in exclusive health resorts that are beyond the means of all but the rich, many can be enjoyed for day use. The major thermal establishments include the following:

BAD RAGAZ (ST. GALLEN)

Waters: Calcium, magnesium, sodium, chloride, bicarbonate.

Facilities and services: Famous resort with several thermal establishments offers swimming, bathing, hydrotherapy, sauna, massage, solarium, fitness center, beauty treatments, stress-reduction programs, special medical departments.

Indications: Rheumatism, circulatory problems, post-trauma injuries, paralysis.

BAD SCHINZNACH (AARGAU)

Waters: Sulfur, fluoride.

Facilities and services: Thermal establishment offers bathing, hydrotherapy, inhalations, sauna, massage, physiotherapy, beauty treatments.

Indications: Rheumatism, stress, postoperative disorders, diabetes.

BAD SCOUL-TARASP-VULPERA (GRAUBÜNDEN)

Waters: 20 springs; carbon dioxide, sodium sulfate, sodium chloride, calcium, magnesium, iron.

Facilities and services: Public thermal establishment offers bathing, hydrotheraoy, fangotherapy, physiotherapy, therapeutic exercise, massage, drinking.

Indications: Diseases of the liver, gallbladder, pancreas, gastrointestinal and urinary tracts; cardiovascular disorders; metabolic diseases.

BADEN (AARGAU)

Waters: 18 springs; sodium chloride, calcium chloride, sulfate.

Facilities and services: Switzerland's oldest spa offers swimming, bathing, hydrotherapy, fangotherapy, electrotherapy, massage, therapeutic exercise.

Indications: Rheumatism, gout, osteoporosis, neurological problems, metabolic disorders, convalescence after surgery or accident.

LEUKERBAD (VALAIS)

Waters: Calcium, magnesium, sulfate, fluoride.

Facilities and services: Several thermal establishments offer bathing, hydrotherapy, inhalation, massage, physiotherapy.

Indications: Rheumatism, gout, paralysis, circulatory problems, stress.

RHEINFELDEN (BASEL)

Waters: 3 major types; sodium (brine); calcium, magnesium sulfate, carbon dioxide, iron.

Facilities and services: Thermal establishments and several hotels offer brine bathing and swimming, hydrotherapy (including brine packs), inhalations, physiotherapy, drinking, fitness centers, beauty treatments, therapeutic exercise.

Indications: Rheumatism; convalescence after illness, surgery or accident; circulatory diseases; gynecological disorders; geriatric conditions; diseases of the eye, ears, and throat; respiratory diseases; stress.

YVERDON-LES-BAINS (VAUD)

Waters: Chlorides, calcium, magnesium.

Facilities and services: Old Roman bath with a modern thermal establishment offers swimming, bathing, hydrotherapy, sports massage, steam, sauna, solarium.

Indications: Rheumatism, neurological disorders, effects of orthopedic surgery, respiratory diseases.

For more information about spas in Switzerland, contact

Swiss National Tourist Office
608 Fifth Avenue
New York, NY 10020
(212) 757-5944
www.switzerlandtourism.com

Publishes *Wellness Vacation.*

24

HEALING SPRINGS OF ASIA, OCEANIA, AFRICA, AND THE MIDDLE EAST

AUSTRALIA

The vast majority of Australia's hot and mineral springs are located in "Spa Country," an area in the Victorian Central Highlands about 120 kilometers northeast of Melbourne. The most famous are Daylesford and nearby Hepburn Springs, which provide the country's most extensive range of spa services and facilities.

DAYLESFORD (VICTORIA)

Waters: Carbon dioxide, calcium, magnesium, sodium bicarbonate.
Facilities and services: Bathing, drinking.
Indications: Rheumatism, stress.

HEPBURN SPRINGS (VICTORIA)

Waters: Carbon dioxide, calcium, magnesium, sodium bicarbonate, sulfate.
Facilities and services: Bathing, drinking.
Indications: Rheumatism, stress.

MOREE (NEW SOUTH WALES)

Waters: Sodium bicarbonate.
Facilities: Bathing.
Indications: Rheumatism.

PEOPLE'S REPUBLIC OF CHINA

Several public hot springs are found in the People's Republic of China. At Chinese spas, the government provides complex therapy for several chronic diseases, including balneotherapy combined with acupuncture and other physical therapies.

HUANQING (XIAN)
Waters: 4 springs; thermal, radon.
Facilities and services: Sanitarium.
Indications: Rheumatic disease, mild hypertension, skin diseases, digestive disorders, stress.

LONGMEN (LUOYANG)
Waters: Simple thermal.
Facilities and services: Bathing, sanitarium.
Indications: Stress.

Other springs include Lu Chan, considered a simple thermal spring, and Chung Hwa, which contains radioactive waters. Here, as with other Chinese spas, balneotherapy is often combined with physical therapy and traditional acupuncture treatments.

REPUBLIC OF CHINA (TAIWAN)

Taiwan is an island known for its volcanic activity and is thus the home of literally hundreds of hot springs, many convenient to the capital, Taipei. Hot springs were developed by the Japanese during their occupation of Taiwan between 1895 and 1945. Although many springs experienced a decline in visitors after the end of World War II, several important hot springs areas are being redeveloped for both Taiwanese and foreign visitors. The ROC Tourism Bureau declared 1999 "The Year of Hot Spring Tourism."

PEITOU (TAIPEI)
Waters: Sulfur, sulfate.
Facilities and services: Famous spa town with several luxury spa hotels and smaller thermal establishments; traditional Japanese-style bathing is popular here.
Indications: Rheumatism, arthritis, stress.

CHIHPEN (TAITUNG)

Waters: Bicarbonate, sulfate.

Facilities and services: Popular resort features luxury spa hotels that offer bathing, hydrotherapy, and massage, and simple thermal establishments that provide hot pools for bathing.

Indications: Rheumatism, arthritis, skin diseases, digestive complaints.

WULAI (TAIPEI)

Waters: Bicarbonate, sulfate.

Facilities and services: A popular tourist resort; many hotels offer thermal pools for bathing; natural bathing pools by the river are free.

Indications: Rheumatism, arthritis, skin diseases, digestive complaints.

YANGMINGSHAN (TAIPEI)

Waters: Sulfur, sulfate.

Facilities and services: Several major resorts in Yangmingshan National Park offer bathing, balneotherapy, and massage; dozens of smaller private hot springs offer bathing facilities.

Indications: Rheumatism, arthritis, stress.

For more information about hot springs in Taiwan, contact

Taiwan Visitors Association
1 World Trade Center, Suite 7953
New York, NY 10048
(212) 466-0691 • (312) 346-1037 (Chicago) • (415) 989-8677 (San Francisco)

Suite 1904, Level 19
MLC Center, Martin Place
Sydney 2000, NSW, Australia
(02) 9231-6942
www.tbroc.gov.tw

ETHIOPIA

The African country of Ethiopia is rich in hot springs, although current information about their facilities is difficult to come by.

BATE (WOLLO)

Several thermal springs.

FILWOHA (ADDIS ABABA)

Over 100 springs, some containing sodium bicarbonate. Bathing.

HAGERE HIWOT (AMBO)

Resort features weakly mineralized waters containing some sodium bicarbonate and carbon dioxide. Bathing and swimming.

INDIA

People have been bathing in Indian hot springs for over 2,500 years; the therapeutic uses of the springs were known under the name of *jalachikitsa,* similar to what balneotherapy is today. Current information about Indian hot springs and spas is difficult to come by, but natural medicinal springs can be found in the following locations:

Aravali (Maharasthra)

Bakreswar (West Bengal)

Barbmasia (Bihar)

Bariapur (Bihar)

Bhimbandi (Bihar)

Chormara (Bihar)

Darjeeling (West Bengal)

Jarom (Bihar)

Jharipani (Bihar)

Kajra (Bihar)

Kalobathan (Bihar)

Kanki (Bihar)

Khed (Maharashtra)

Kodarma (Bihar)

Kopili (Assam)

Monghyr (Bihar)

Mussoori (Uttar Pradesh)

Nambor (Assam)

Nowada (Bihar)

Pali (Maharashtra)

Patalsur (Bihar)

Rajgir (Bihar)

Rajwadi (Maharashtra)

Rampur (Bihar)

Sangameshwar (Maharasthra)

Sohna (Punjab)

Sov (Maharashtra)

Suarj Kund (Bihar)

Tanteswari (Bihar)

Tantloi (Bihar)

Tapoban (Bihar)

Tural (Maharashtra)

Unhara (Maharasthra)

Vajreswari (Maharashtra)

Varanasi (Uttar Pradesh)

ISRAEL

Israel is the home of several ancient hot springs, and the spas of the Dead Sea have made the region a healing mecca, especially for people with rheumatism, arthritis, and skin diseases. The clinical procedures at several Dead Sea spas have been subject to extensive medical research over the last 20 years; treatments are under medical supervision.

EIN BOKEK (NEGEV)

Waters: Sulfur, sodium.

Facilities and services: Famous Dead Sea resort with thermal establishment offers bathing, hydrotherapy, massage, mud packs, ultraviolet light therapy, beauty treatments.

Indications: Skin diseases (especially psoriasis), respiratory problems (especially asthma).

EIN GEDI (MASADA)

Waters: Sulfur, sulfate, sodium.

Facilities and services: Dead Sea resort offers bathing, hydrotherpy, massage, mud packs, ultraviolet light therapy, beauty treatments.

Indications: Skin diseases (especially psoriasis), respiratory problems (especially asthma).

HAMME ZOHAR (NEGEV)

Waters: Sodium, magnesium, calcium, chloride, sulfate.

Facilities and services: Dead Sea resort features swimming, bathing, hydrotherapy, mud packs, massage.

Indications: Skin diseases (especially psoriasis and neurodermatitis), rheumatism.

TIBERIAS (GALILEE)

Waters: 18 springs; sulfur, sodium, calcium, sulfate, chloride, radon.

Facilities and services: Ancient spa with modern thermal establishments offers bathing, hydrotherapy, physiotherapy; fitness and recreation center.

Indications: Rheumatism, arthritis, gynecological diseases, respiratory disorders.

For more information about spas in Israel, contact

Israeli Government Tourist Office
800 Second Avenue
New York, NY 10017
(888) 774-7732, (212) 499-5650

180 Bloor Street West
Toronto, Ontario M5S 2V6, Canada
(800) 669-2369, (416) 964-3784

180 Oxford Street
London W1N 9DJ, U.K.
(020) 7-299-1113
www.infotour.co.il

JAPAN

Japan is blessed with over 10,000 hot springs located in 1,133 thermal areas. They range from simple hot pools in the remote countryside to major luxury resorts and are visited more than 100 million times a year. Some spa towns such as Beppu, Hakone, and Noboribetsu have a variety of waters and attract people with a wide range of health problems. However, most of Japan's hot springs are enjoyed for pleasure and relaxation. Visiting a traditional hot spring in Japan is a special experience for Westerners because it offers unique insights into authentic Japanese life and culture.

ARIMA ONSEN (HYOGO PREFECTURE)

Waters: 2 major springs; sodium chloride, iron, radon.
Facilities and services: A 1,300-year-old spa town with one municipal
   onsen and hot springs in many hotels; bathing, hydrotherapy, drinking.
Indications: Cardiovascular disease, anemia, nervous system disorders.

ATAMI (SHIZUOKA)

Waters: Sulfate, chloride, sodium.
Facilities and services: Vacation resort features bathing, hydrotherapy,
   drinking.
Indications: Rheumatism, gastrointestinal disorders, liver and gallbladder
   problems.

BEPPU (OITA)

Waters: 8 different groups of thermal springs feature sodium, chloride,
   sulfur, iron, hydrogen sulfide, aluminum.
Facilities and services: One of the most thermally active places on earth,
   with over 70 thermal establishments that offer bathing, hydrotherapy,
   sand baths, steam baths, cascade baths, mud baths, massage; balneological institute connected to Kyushu University; many bubbling "hell
   pools."
Indications: Rheumatism and orthopedic disorders, gastrointestinal
   problems, skin diseases, genitourinary disorders, gynecological problems, stress.

DOGO (EHIME)

Waters: Simple thermal.
Facilities and services: Historic resort offers numerous bathing facilities.
Indications: Digestive complaints, rheumatism, stress.

HAKONE (KANAGAWA)

Waters: Many springs that contain sodium chloride, calcium, sulfate,
   hydrogen sulfide, bicarbonate.
Facilities and services: A popular resort with many bathhouses and swimming pools.
Indications: Rheumatism, stress, orthopedics.

IBUSUKI (KAGOSHIMA)

Waters: Calcium, chloride, sodium, radon.

Facilities and services: Resort facing Kinko Bay offers 12 public hot spring baths; natural hot sand baths.

Indications: Rheumatism, stress, convalescence.

ITO (SHIZUOKA)

Waters: Sodium chloride.

Facilities and services: Springs for bathing, hydrotherapy, physical therapy, rehabilitation.

Indications: Rheumatism, orthopedic problems.

KATSUURA (WAKAYAMA)

Waters: 6 springs; sulfur, sulfate.

Facilities and services: Several indoor and outdoor thermal establishments offer bathing, hydrotherapy, drinking; unique cave bath.

Indications: Joint problems, stress-related complaints, skin diseases, gastrointestinal disorders.

KUSATSU (GUMMA)

Waters: Many springs containing sulfate, chloride, hydrogen sulfide, aluminum, iron.

Facilities and services: Numerous indoor and outdoor bathhouses for bathing, hydrotherapy, physical therapy; famous "time bath"; balneological research institute and hospital connected to Gumma University.

Indications: Rheumatism, skin diseases.

NARUGO (MIYAGI)

Waters: 4 springs; sodium chloride, sodium bicarbonate, sulfate, carbon dioxide.

Facilities and services: Several bathhouses offer bathing, cascade bath, hydrotherapy; research institute connected to Tohoko University.

Indications: Rheumatism, skin diseases, gastrointestinal disorders, orthopedics.

NIKKO YUMOTO (TOCHIGI)

Waters: Many springs containing bicarbonate, sulfate, calcium, hydrogen sulfide, carbon dioxide.

Facilities and services: Historic spa town with many indoor and outdoor bathing facilities.

Indications: Rheumatism, skin diseases, diabetes, respiratory diseases.

NOBORIBETSU (HOKKAIDO)

Waters: 3 major springs; sodium sulfate, iron, sodium chloride, bicarbonate.

Facilities and services: Major thermal resort offers facilities for bathing, swimming, hydrotherapy, inhalations, drinking, physical therapy; balneological hospital connected to Hokkaido University.

Indications: Gynecological, respiratory, gastrointestinal and skin diseases, rheumatism, orthopedic conditions, anemia.

SHIOBARA (TOCHIGI)

Waters: 4 major springs; oligomineral, sulfide, sulfate, bicarbonate, chloride, potassium.

Facilities and services: Historic spa town with six main bathing areas offers indoor and outdoor bathing, hydrotherapy.

Indications: Gynecological complains, gastrointestinal disorders (especially constipation), rheumatism.

SHIRAHAMA (WAKAYAMA)

Waters: Sodium bicarbonate, chloride, carbon dioxide.

Facilities and services: Ancient spa town offers bathing facilities, hydrotherapy.

Indications: Rheumatism, gynecological problems, skin diseases, gastrointestinal problems, orthopedics.

TAMAGAWA (IWATE)

Waters: 2 springs; sulfur, sodium chloride, sulfate, calcium, iron, radon.

Facilities and services: Bathing, hydrotherapy, steam baths, mud baths, drinking.

Indications: Rheumatism, asthma, gastrointestinal complaints, skin diseases, hemorrhoids.

UNZEN (NAGASAKI)

Waters: 3 springs; sulfur, carbon dioxide, hydrogen sulfide. Many bubbling "hell pools."

Facilities and services: Several public baths, and thermal bathing in nearly every hotel.

Indications: Skin diseases, rheumatism.

YUFUIN (OITA)

Waters: Simple thermal.

Facilities and services: Quaint, historic spa at the foot of Mt. Yufu; many thermal establishments that offer indoor and outdoor bathing, including rock bath.

Indications: Stress.

YUGAWARA (KANAGAWA)

Waters: Bicarbonate, sodium sulfate.

Facilities and services: Several bathing establishments; orthopedic hospital offers balneotherapy, hydrotherapy, and physical therapy.

Indications: Orthopedic problems.

ZAO (YAMAGATA)

Waters: Thermal, acidic.

Facilities and services: Popular ski resort with three public bathing establishments.

Indications: Skin diseases, high blood pressure, stress.

For more information about Japanese hot springs and related accommodations, contact

Japan National Tourist Organization
1 Rockefeller Plaza, Suite 1250
New York, NY 10020
(212) 757-5640

165 University Avenue
Toronto, Ontario M5H 3B8, Canada
(416) 366-7140

20 Savile Row
London, W1X 1AE, U.K.
(020) 7-734-9638

2 Chiefly Square, Level 33
Sydney 2000, NSW, Australia
(02) 9232-4522
www.jnto.go.jp

Publishes *Japanese Hot Springs.*

KOREA (SOUTH)

There are more than 20 thermal establishments in South Korea, some of them dating back more than 500 years. The Oonyang Spa, for example, dates from 1458, when King Sejong of the Lee Dynasty bathed in its waters to cure his chronic skin disease.

Unlike the Japanese hot springs, the waters in Korea are not volcanically related and tend to be cooler with low mineral content; some exceptions are Bugok (sometimes translated as Pugok), Tongnae, and Onyang. Many are characterized as carbonate mineral springs with free carbon dioxide, similar to the waters of Saratoga Springs in New York or Vichy in France, which are popular for relieving circulation problems, skin diseases, and arthritis.

Specific information about spa facilities and services is difficult to come by, with the best source being country guidebooks to Korea. Some are large resorts such as Bugok and Onyang (both known for treating skin disorders) and Tongnae (favored by arthritis sufferers), with complete spa services, lodging, and entertainment. Others, such as Suanbo, have smaller bathing facilities.

If you visit Korea, you may want to explore some of the following medicinal thermal springs:

Osaek (Kangwan-do)	Tokgu (Kyongsangbuk-do)
Ich'on (Kyonggi-do)	Raekam (Kyongsangbuk-do)
Onyang (Kyongsangnam-do)	Tongnae (Pusan)
Suanbo (Ch'ungju)	Haendae (Pusan)
Bugoc (Yongman Alps)	

There are also several cold mineral springs that are noted for their therapeutic value, including Myongam, Chojong, and Pugang (all in Ch'ungch'ongbuk-do) and Talgi (Kyongsangbuk-do).

NEPAL

Although they are rarely known outside the country, there are several natural hot water springs in the Kingdom of Nepal. These thermal springs are locally known as *tatopani*, meaning "hot water." The thermal waters are used to treat a variety of health complaints, including paralysis and diseases relating to the stomach and skin. Local residents often celebrate festivals during which they take a bath in the hope of remaining healthy.

The most famous is Tatopani Hot Spring, which is located near the Friendship Bridge by the border between Nepal and China. Other hot springs include

Hotiyana (Sankhuwasabha, Koshi zone, eastern Nepal)
Syabrubesi and Chilime (Rasuwa, north of Kathmandu)
Bhurung, Do Khola, Singha, Chhumrung and Dhadkharka (Myagdi district)
Jomsom and Dhima (Mustang)
Chame and La Ta (Manang district)
Bhulbhule Khar (Tanahu district)
Tapoban (Bajhang district)
Dhanachauri (Luma)
Srikaar, Sina and Chamlaiya (Darchula)
Riar, Saghu Khola, and Sarai Khola (in what is known as the middle
    development region of Nepal)

NEW ZEALAND

New Zealand is a country rich in thermal resources, with many geothermal facilities for heating, agriculture, recreation, and the generation of electric power. The city of Rotorua is known as "geyserland" because of its many geysers and bubbling mud.

HAMNER SPRINGS (SOUTH ISLAND)

Waters: Sulfate, sodium chloride, bicarbonate.
Facilities and services: Day spa offers bathing, swimming, hydrotherapy, massage.
Indications: Rheumatism, stress.

MIRANDA HOT SPRINGS (NORTH ISLAND)

Waters: Chlorides, silica, borax.
Facilities and services: Bathing, swimming, "sauna pool."
Indications: Rheumatism, stress.

ROTORUA (NORTH ISLAND)

Waters: Sulfate.
Facilities and services: Spa provides 35 hot mineral outdoor pools for bathing, swimming, massage.
Indications: Rheumatism, arthritis, muscle aches, stress.

TAUPO HOT SPRINGS (NORTH ISLAND)

Waters: Carbonates, sulfate, silica.
Facilities and services: Day spa offers soaking pools, water slide, massage, acupressure, reflexology.
Indications: Skin problems, stress, arthritis.

SOUTH AFRICA

There are many thermal medicinal springs in South Africa, but current information about facilities and services is difficult to come by. Current information can be found in any annual tourist guidebook to South Africa. The most important medicinal springs in the country include these:

Aliwal North (Eastern Cape Province)
Badplaas (Mpumalanga)
Cradock (Eastern Cape)
Malmesbury (Western Cape)
Montagu (Western Cape)
Tugela (Kwazulu-Natal)
Warmbad (Northern Transvaal)

TURKEY

Asiatic Turkey (Anatolia) has more than 500 mineral springs, some of which have been used therapeutically since ancient times. Some of Turkey's major spas are these:

BURSA

Waters: Bicarbonate, calcium, magnesium sulfate.

Facilities and services: Historic spa with several thermal establishments offers bathing, hydrotherapy, Turkish bath, massage, electrotherapy, physical therapy.

Indications: Rheumatism, liver and gallbladder disorders, gynecological diseases, metabolic disorders, postoperative problems.

IZMIR-BALCOVA

Waters: Sodium chloride, calcium bicarbonate.

Facilities and services: Located at the site of the ancient baths of Agamemnon, large, modern thermal center offers swimming, bathing, sauna, steam baths, massage, hydrotherapy, physical therapy, therapeutic exercise.

Indications: Rheumatism, skin diseases, stress.

IZMIR-ÇESME

Waters: Chloride, sulfate, bicarbonate; mud.

Facilities and services: Swimming, bathing, hydrotherapy, massage, physical therapy, electrotherapy, mud treatments.

Indications: Rheumatism, skin diseases, gynecological disorders, stress.

PAMUKKALE

Waters: Sulfates, bicarbonate, radon.

Facilities and services: Several thermal establishments offer swimming, bathing, hydrotherapy, drinking.

Indications: Rheumatism, skin disease, gynecological disorders, stress, digestive and nutritional disorders.

YALOVA

Waters: Sodium chloride, calcium sulfate, radon.

Facilities and services: Large thermal complex offers swimming, bathing, massage, drinking.

Indications: Rheumatism, gastrointestinal disorders, metabolic problems, urological complaints.

For more information about spas in Turkey, contact

Turkish Tourism and Information Bureau
821 United Nations Plaza
New York, NY 10017
(212) 687-2194

360 Albert Street, Suite 801
Ottawa, ON K1R 7X7, Canada
(613) 230-8654
www.turkey.org

Publishes *Hot Springs & Spas.*

GLOSSARY

Acupressure A form of Oriental finger massage that is designed to both relieve tension and stimulate the energy centers of the body. It is often used as part of shiatsu and traditional Chinese massage.

Aslan therapy A type of anti-aging therapy developed by Ana Aslan, a Romanian physician. It involves the use of Gerovital H_3 and Aslavital cures, which are applied as tablets and injections. Aslan therapy is offered at numerous Eastern European spas, especially in Romania.

Aromatherapy The use of scented oils made from the essence of different flowers, often in massage. It is based on the ancient art of using perfumes for healing; certain smells are believed to promote relaxation, relieve anxiety, and relieve depression.

Balneology The study of the medicinal uses of mineral water and thermal water that involves bathing.

Balneotherapy The use of hot spring water, gases, mud, and climactic factors (such as heat) as therapeutic elements for healing.

Cavitosonic ionization The use of aerosol inhalation devices with the benefit of internal cleansing and energy building.

Climatotherapy A type of treatment that uses environmental features, such as the atmosphere, temperature, humidity, and light, for healing.

Colonic irrigation A specialized type of enema that cleanses high into the colon. Some holistic spas utilize thermal spring water for this cleansing treatment.

Crenotherapy A general term to describe healing with mineral and thermal waters.

Fangotherapy The use of a mud pack or coating parts of the body with mud; also known as pelotherapy. It is believed that mud helps remove toxins from the body, helps relieve arthritic and muscle pain, and helps heal the skin. In some spas, such as those in Calistoga and Palm Springs, California, fangotherapy involves being totally immersed in a tub of warm mud made with water from the mineral springs.

Fasting   The use of a supervised diet of water, juice, and possibly fruit to improve health and lose weight.

Filiform douche   A shower involving a fine jet of water.

Grottotherapy   A type of treatment using mineral springs that evaporate quickly; such springs are often found in caves.

Heliotherapy   A form of treatment using exposure to sunlight.

Herbal wraps   Wrapping the body in warm sheets and blankets infused with herbal essences, which penetrate the skin, promoting cleansing, healing, and relaxation. These wraps are a popular adjunct to bathing.

Hydrotherapy   Several types of water therapies, including underwater massage with jets of water (hydromassage), alternating hot and cold showers or baths, hot and/or cold compresses, steam baths, colonic irrigations, or applying jets of water under pressure to various parts of the body; often an essential part of balneotherapy.

Hydrotherapy tub   A special bathtub designed for a single person that uses air jets, water jets, and a jet hose for underwater massage.

Hypotonic   Characterizing water with a low osmotic pressure, meaning that it is easily absorbed by the intestine.

Ionization   An aspect of thalassotherapy involving the use of marine spray using negative ions. Seawater particles ionized with negative electrons are believed to be beneficial, especially for the upper respiratory tract.

Kneipp kur   A specialized program of hydrotherapy that also includes a natural foods diet, exercise, and herbs. Developed by German cleric Sebastian Kneipp during the mid-1800s, it is still widely used in European spas today.

Massage   Manipulation, methodical pressure, friction, and kneading of different parts of the body. It is designed to relax the muscles, reduce stress, and improve body flexibility. Massage is a popular adjunct to different forms of balneotherapy.

Mineral salt bathing   Soaking in a tub filled with bath salts (especially sodium chloride and sodium sulfate) that have been extracted from places such as the Dead Sea, Great Salt Lake, Saratoga Springs, or Karlovy Vary. Although many (including this author) have testified to the therapeutic value of bathing in mineral salts, balneologists believe that they are not nearly as useful as bathing at the original source from which they came: considerations need to be given to the water's pH as well as its temperature and total chemical composition, which is rarely, if ever, duplicated in one's own bathtub.

Mineral water A type of spring or well water that contains significant amounts of inorganic matter such as iron, sulfates, or chlorides. In order to be classified as a mineral water, it must contain between 0.2 and 1 gram of minerals per liter of water. "True" mineral water contains more than 1 gram of minerals per liter of water.

Oligomineral waters Lightly mineralized waters, usually containing less than 0.2 grams of minerals per liter of water.

Oxygen therapy The therapeutic use of supplemental oxygen, medical-grade hydrogen peroxide, or ozone therapy to improve oxygenation and oxidation.

Ozone therapy The use of mixing a small amount of therapeutic ozone and oxygen with the patient's blood, which is then reinfused into the patient; it may also be given by rectal insufflation or administered by means of allowing ozone and oxygen to flow into a steam cabinet. It has been used to treat a wide variety of diseases, including cancer, high blood pressure, HIV-related problems, circulatory disorders, and diabetes.

Pelotherapy Health or beauty treatment using mud packs or mud baths.

pH A measure of how acidic or basic a type of water is. The range goes from 0 to 14, with 7 being neutral. A pH of less than 7 indicates acidity; a pH of greater than 7 indicates a base. The pH is a measure of the relative amount of free hydrogen and hydroxyl ions in the water. Water that has more free hydrogen ions is acidic, whereas water that has more free hydroxyl ions is basic. Chemicals in the water can affect pH. The pH is reported in logarithmic units, with each number representing a ten-fold change in the acidity/basicness of the water: water with a pH of 5 is ten times more acidic than water having a pH of 6.

Scotch hose Projection of water through a jet hose to stimulate the client from 10 to 12 feet away. Therapists are trained to massage the client in specific patterns.

Sitz bath A type of bath involving immersing the lower part of the body in a warm bath followed by cold water. It is intended to stimulate the immune system.

Spa   A resort or health facility that uses mineral water or seawater for facilitating health and healing.

Spa cuisine   A general term used to describe healthy natural foods with an emphasis on fresh fruits and vegetables, low-fat animal products, and a minimum of salt, artificial flavorings, and colorings.

Swiss shower   A type of shower in which the client stands inside a circular or triangular shower that has many shower nozzles from three or more directions.

Thalassotherapy   A type of therapy using seawater, seaweed wraps, and breathing sea air.

Vaporium   A steam bath.

Vichy shower   A type of shower that uses several shower nozzles (five or more) in a horizontal pattern over the client to create a gentle or vigorous rain shower. Usually used with body treatments such as seaweed wraps, body exfoliation, and wet massage therapy.

Watsu   A unique type of body massage conducted in a thermal pool, using gentle, fluid movements and deep breathing.

RESOURCES

GUIDES TO HOT SPRINGS
AND MINERAL SPRINGS

Fodor's Healthy Escapes (1997) **by Bernard Burt (Fodor's Travel Publications, Inc., New York).**
A comprehensive and highly rated guide to 244 spas, fitness resorts, and cruises in the United States, Canada, and Mexico, including many retreats, resorts, and spas that have thermal and mineral springs.

Great Hot Springs of the West (1994) **by Bill Kaysing (Capra Press, P.O. Box 2068, Santa Barbara, CA 93120).**
First published in 1984, this comprehensive guide offers detailed information about more than 200 hot springs in Arizona, California, Colorado, Montana, Idaho, Nevada, New Mexico, Oregon, Utah, Washington, and Wyoming.

Hot Springs and Hot Pools of the Southwest (1998) **and** *Hot Springs and Hot Pools of the Northwest* (1999) **by Marjorie Gersh-Young (Aqua Thermal Access, 55 Azalia Lane, Santa Cruz, CA 95060).**
These invaluable guides list both noncommercial and commercial hot springs throughout the United States, Canada, and Baja California in Mexico. Includes detailed maps.

Hiking Hot Springs of the Pacific Northwest (1998) **by Evie Litton (Falcon Publishing, Helena, MT).**
Offers detailed descriptions of 118 primitive, noncommerical hot springs in Idaho, Oregon, Washington, and British Columbia that can be reached via hiking trails.

Enchanted Waters: A Guide to New Mexico's Hot Springs (1998) **by Craig Martin (Pruett Publishing Co., Boulder, CO).**
A guide to both commercial and noncommercial springs in New Mexico.

Colorado's Hot Springs (1996) by Deborah Frazier (Pruett Publishing Co., Boulder, CO).

A guide to both commercial and noncommercial springs in Colorado.

Touring California and Nevada Hot Springs (1997) by Matt C. Bishcoff (Falcon Publishing, Helena, MT).

A guide to both commercial and noncommercial springs in California and Nevada.

Touring Montana and Wyoming Hot Springs (1999) by Jeff Birkby (Falcon Publishing, Helena, MT).

A guide to both commercial and noncommercial springs in Montana and Wyoming.

The Spa Guide (1988) by Ed and Judy Colbert (Globe Pequot Press, 138 West Main Street, Chester, CT 06412)

A well-researched guide to spas, fitness resorts, and cruises in the United States, Canada, and Mexico, including those that offer thermal and mineral springs.

Spas & Hot Springs of Mexico (1998) by "Mexico" Mike Nelson (Roads Scholar Press, 2022 Amy Street, Mission, TX 78572)

An entertaining and useful guide to the diverse variety of spas and mineral springs of Mexico, including many that are off the beaten track.

Spas: The International Spa Guide (B.D.I.T. Inc., P.O. Box 1405, Port Washington, NY 11050).

Published every two years, this guide offers detailed information on spas and hot springs resorts in many parts of the world, with primary emphasis on Europe, the United States, and Israel.

Hot Springs of Western Canada by Glenn Woodsworth (Gordon Soules Book Publishers Ltd., 1354-B Marine Drive, West Vancouver, B.C. V7T 1B5; or 1916 Pike Place, Suite 620, Seattle, WA 98101).

A comprehensive guide to both commercial and noncommercial hot springs in British Columbia, Alberta, the Yukon, and Northwest Territories in Canada, along with some entries from Washington and Alaska in the United States. Includes detailed maps.

A Guide to Japanese Hot Springs (1986) by Anne Hotta with Yoko Ishiguro (Kodansha International, Tokyo and New York).

A comprehensive and highly readable guide to the major hot springs throughout Japan, including information about transportation and lodging.

Japan's Hidden Hot Springs (1995) by Robert Neff (Charles E. Tuttle Company, Rutland, VT, and Tokyo).

A fascinating guide to Japan's lesser-known hot springs, many of which are off the beaten path. Includes useful information about transportation and lodging.

Guide du Thermalisme edited by Brigitte Martin (Groupe Impact Medecin, 1, rue Paul Cézanne, 75375 Paris Cedex 08, France).

Published annually, this lavishly illustrated guide contains detailed information about each of France's 105 thermal spas, including a description of the waters, types of therapies offered, contact numbers, and accommodations. In French.

Karlovy Vary: A World Famous Spa (Promenada Publishing, T.G. Masaryka 12, 36001 Karlovy Vary, Czech Republic; fax [420] 17-322-2175).

Publishes excellent and inexpensive full-color guides (including spa listings and descriptions) to the spa towns of Karlovy Vary, Mariánské Lázně, and Františkovy Lázně in a variety of languages, including English.

OTHER BOOKS ABOUT WATER AND HEALING SPRINGS

The Complete Book of Water Therapy (1994) by Dian Dincin Buchman (Keats Publishing, Inc., New Canaan, CT).

Written by an expert in the field of natural health and medicine, this well-written and comprehensive book explores how baths, showers, and the use of steam, wet packs, drinking, and other natural methods can cure hundreds of common ailments.

Healing Waters (1998) by Linda Troeller (Aperture, NY).

A beautiful book of photographs taken at hot springs and spas around the world.

Taking the Waters (1992) by Alev Lytle Croutier (Abbeville Press, NY).
A well-researched, informative, and beautifully illustrated book about bathing, hot springs, and mineral waters. Presently out of print, but may be available in libraries.

The Drinking Water Book: A Complete Guide to Safe Drinking Water (1991) by Colin Ingram (Ten Speed Press, Berkeley, CA).
The author addresses the dangers of tap water and offers information about cancer-causing chemicals in public water supplies, home water purifiers, and the need for better state and federal water standards. He also tells us how to test our tap water, rates various brands of water filters, and compares different types of bottled water.

The Good Water Guide (1996) by Timothy and Maureen Green (Seven Hills Books, Cincinnati, OH).
This guide contains many color pictures of bottled water labels, with detailed profiles of bottlers, both international and domestic.

Harbin Hot Springs: Healing Waters Sacred Land (1993) by Ellen Klages (Harbin Springs Publishing, Middletown, CA).
A well-written and entertaining book that traces the colorful history of Harbin Hot Springs from its earliest days as a meeting place for Native Americans through its successive uses as a Victorian resort, a boxer's training camp, and a hippie commune to a unique healing and spiritual community.

The Healing Energies of Water (2000) by Charlies Ryrie (Journey Editions, Boston, MA).
This intelligent and insightful book explores our relationship to water from both the scientific and the spiritual viewpoints. The author also discusses healing with water through drinking and bathing.

Saratoga: Queen of Spas (1998) by Grace Maguire Swanner, M.D. (North Country Books, Utica, NY).
A comprehensive and highly detailed book about Saratoga Spa and its history by a physician who served as medical consultant there.

Your Body's Many Cries for Water (1995) by F. Batmanghelidj, M.D. (Global Health Solutions, Falls Church, VA).
A controversial book based on a physician's 12 years of clinical research. The author maintains that chronic dehydration is a major cause of illness and that drinking lots of pure water can both prevent and cure disease.

MAGAZINES AND JOURNALS

Spa Finder Magazine
Spa Finders
(800) ALL-SPAS; (212) 924-6800
www.spafinders.com

> A magazine providing information about more than 200 spas around the world, including some featuring natural mineral waters. Publishes annual *Spa Finder Directory.*

Geo-Heat Center Quarterly Bulletin
Geo-Heat Center
Oregon Institute of Technology
Klamath Falls, OR 97601-8801

> Published at a respected university, this is primarily a journal dealing with the direct uses of geothermal resources. It often contains well-researched and highly readable articles about various hot springs around the world.

Hot Springs Gazette
2188 Chapman Ranch Road
Henderson, NV 89012
www.hotspringsgazette.com

> A folksy magazine focusing on often overlooked, smaller, and off-the-road hot springs.

INTERNET RESOURCES

Healingsprings.com
www.healingsprings.com

> The author's home page with the latest information about balneology and online links to hot springs in the United States and abroad.

Spa Reporter
www.primenet.com/spareporter/index.html

> An interesting website featuring travel writer Steve Bergsman's informal (and sometimes irreverent) reviews of spas in the United States and abroad.

Spamagazine.com
www.spamagazine.com

> An online world spa directory.

International Society for Medical Hydrology and Climatology (I.S.M.H.)
www.med.uni-muenchen.de/ismh

The home page of the I.S.M.H., an international organization of health professionals dedicated to research of spa therapy and health resort medicine for prevention, treatment, and rehabilitation.

International Spa Association (I.S.P.A.)
www.experienceispa.com

The I.S.P.A. is the professional association of the spa industry, representing hot spring resorts and other health and wellness establishments. It maintains the Global Spa Guide.

Bottledwaterweb.com
www.bottledwaterweb.com

Providing both consumers and researchers with the most current and accurate information about bottled water.

NOTES

INTRODUCTION

1. *Spas in Japan* (Tokyo: Japan Spa Association, 1983), 4.

2. Derek Freedman and Michael A Waugh, "The Spa and Sexually Transmitted Diseases," *Clinics in Dermatology* 14 (1996): 577–82.

3. I. Ghersetich and T. Lotti, "Immunology of Mineral Water Spas," *Clinics in Dermatology* 14 (1996): 563–66.

4. M. F. Rogers et al., "Lack of transmission of human immunodeficiency virus from infected children to their household contacts," *Pediatrics* 85, No. 2 (February 1990): 210–14.

5. T. M. Courville et al., "Lack of evidence of transmission of HIV-1 to family contacts of HIV-1 infected children," *Clinical Pediatrics* 37, No. 3 (March 1998): 175–78.

6. R. M. Gershon et al., "HIV infection risk to non-healthcare workers," *American Industrial Hygiene Association Journal* 51, No. 12 (December 1990): A807–9.

7. Oskar Baudisch, *The Magic and Science of Natural Healing Waters,* No. 10 (Saratoga Springs, N.Y.: Saratoga Springs Authority, 1940).

CHAPTER 1

1. Leonard M. Rosenfeld, "Physiology of Water," *Clinics in Dermatology* 14 (1996): 555–61.

2. Hirak Bihari Routh et al., "Balneology, Mineral Water and Spas in Historical Perspective," *Clinics in Dermatology* 14 (1996): 550–56.

3. M. Lamarche, *Hydrologie et climatologie médicale* (Paris: Edition Marketing, 1977), 28.

4. *Spas in Japan* (Tokyo: Japan Spa Association, 1983), 3.

5. Yuko Agishi, "Effects of Thermal Stimuli by Total Body Water Immersion and Balneotherapy on Endocrine and Autonomic Nervous Functions," *Journal of the Japanese Association of Physical Medicine, Balneology and Climatology* (in Japanese) 42, Nos. 1, 2 (1978): 30.

6. Jinichi Suzuki and Yuichi Yamauchi, "Endocrinological Changes in Psychosomatic Patients after Balneotherapy in a Hot Sulfate Spring," *Journal of the Japanese Association of Physical Medicine, Balneology and Climatology* (in Japanese) 42, Nos. 1, 2 (1978): 33.

7. Yuko Agishi and Yoshinori Ohtsuka, *Recent Progress in Medical Balneology and Climatology* (Sapporo: Hokkaido University School of Medicine, 1995), 8.

8. Yuko Agishi, "Hot Springs and the Physiological Functions of Humans," *Asian Medical Journal* 38, No. 3 (March 1995): 115–24.

9. Sidney Licht, ed., *Medical Hydrology* (New Haven, Conn.: Elizabeth Licht, 1963), 111.

10. Agishi and Ohtsuka, *Medical Balneology,* 8.

11. Ibid.

12. Glenn Woodsworth, *Hot Springs of Western Canada* (W. Vancouver and Seattle: Gordon Soules Book Publishers Ltd., 1997), 27–28.

13. V. Digiesi, "Dietetic Prevention and Therapy with Mineral Waters," in *Proceedings: 33rd World Congress of the International Society of Medical Hydrology and Climatology* (Prague: Lubomar Houdek and Nakadatelstvi Galen, 1998), 176.

14. Yasumitsu Uzumasa, *Chemical Investigations of Hot Springs in Japan* (Tokyo: T. Skokan, 1965), 148.

15. Bohuslav Kocab, *Spa Treatment in Czechoslovakia* (Prague: Balnea, 1972), 27–28.

16. Ibid., 30

17. Ian Bartholomew, "Beitou—Center of Taiwan's Hot Springs Culture," *Travel in Taiwan* 14, No. 10 (May 1998): 4–6.

18. Akira Okada, "Viewpoint of Preventive Medicine," in Y. Agishi and Y. Ohtsuka, eds., *New Frontiers in Health Resort Medicine* (Sapporo: Hokkaido University Medical School, 1996), 49–56.

CHAPTER 2

1. John W. Lund, "Spas and Balneology in the United States," *Geo-Heat Center Quarterly Bulletin* 14, No. 4 (March 1993): 1–3.

2. A. V. Benedetto and L. E. Millikan, "World Survey of Mineral Waters and Spas," *Clinics in Dermatology* 14 (1996): 586–89.

3. John W. Lund, "Hot Springs, Arkansas," *Geo-Heat Center Quarterly Bulletin* 14, No. 4 (March 1993): 12–15.

4. J. J. Moorman, *Mineral Springs of North America* (Philadelphia: J. B. Lippincott & Co., 1873), 214.

5. Benedetto and Millikan, "Mineral Waters and Spas," 586.

6. Alev Lytle Croutier, *Taking the Waters* (New York: Abbeville Press, 1992), 150.

7. Ellen Klages, *Harbin Hot Springs: Healing Waters Sacred Land* (Middletown, Calif.: Harbin Springs Publishing, 1993), 4.

8. Yuko Agishi and Yoshinori Ohtsuka, "Present Factors of Balneology in Japan," *Global Environmental Resources* 2 (1998).

CHAPTER 3

1. Roy Porter, ed., *The Medical History of Waters and Spas* (London: Wellcome Institute for the History of Medicine, 1990), 1–13.

2. Andreas Rubovszky, *Hotel Gellért* (Budapest: Artunion/Szechenyi Publishing House, 1988), 12–13.

3. Goichi Fujinami, *Hot Springs in Japan* (Tokyo: Japan Government Railways, 1936), 17–25.

4. Yoshio Oshima, *Thermalism in Japan* (Tokyo: The Forum on Thermalism in Japan, 1988), 6.

5. Laurette Sejourné, *Thought and Religion in Ancient Mexico* (in Spanish) (Mexico: Fondo de Cultura Económica, 1957), 15.

6. John W. Lund, "Hot Springs, Arkansas," *Geo-Heat Center Quarterly Bulletin* 14, No. 4 (March 1993): 12–15.

7. Klages, *Harbin Hot Springs,* 55.

8. Agishi, "Hot Springs," 122.

9. John W. Lund, "White Sulphur Springs, West Virginia" and "Hot Springs, Virginia," *Geo-Heat Center Quarterly Bulletin,* 17, No. 2 (May 1996): 11–20.

10. Henry E. Sigerist, "American Spas in Historical Perspective," in *Bulletin of the History of Medicine,* Vol. IX (Baltimore: Johns Hopkins University Press, 1942), 133–47.

11. Edwina Walls, "Hot Springs Waters and the Treatment of Venereal Diseases: The U.S. Public Health Service Clinic and Camp Garraday," *Journal of the Arkansas Medical Society,* 91, No. 9 (February 1995): 430–37.

12. John W. Lund, "Thermopolis, Wyoming," *Geo-Heat Center Quarterly Bulletin* 14, No. 4 (March 1993), 19–21.

13. Herman L. Kamenetz, "History of American Spas and Hydrotherapy," in Licht, ed., *Medical Hydrology* (New Haven, Conn.: Elizabeth Licht, 1963), 160–85.

14. *Hand-Book of Calistoga Springs* (San Francisco: Alta California Book and Job Printing House, 1871), 11–12.

15. Kamenetz, "History of American Spas," 182.

16. Sigerist, "American Spas," 133–47.

17. Grace Maguire Swanner, *Saratoga: Queen of Spas* (Utica, N.Y.: North Country Books, 1988), 239–50.

18. George Kersley, "The History of Spas," *Journal of the Royal Society of Health,* 109, No. 1 (February 1989): 3.

19. Sigerist, "American Spas," 146–47.

CHAPTER 4

1. M. Armijo and J. San Martín, *La salud por las aguas termales* (Madrid: Ediciones EDAF, 1984), 40–47.

2. Michel Boulangé, *Les vertus des cures thermales* (Montpellier: Editions Espaces 34, 1998), 24–25.

3. M. Lamarche, *Hydrologie et climatologie médicale* (Paris: Edition Marketing, 1977), 32.

4. Gerard Katz and Alain Maurin, *Santé et thermalisme* (St. Jean-de-Braye: Editions Dangles, 1988), 17.

5. Sigmund Forster, "The Prescription of Spa Therapy" in Licht, ed., *Medical Hydrology* (New Haven, Conn.: Elizabeth Licht, 1963), 403.

CHAPTER 5

1. M. Armijo and J. San Martín, *La salud por las aguas termales* (Madrid: Ediciones EDAF, 1984), 37–39, 48–50.

2. Michel Boulangé, *Les vertus des cures thermales* (Montpellier: Editions Espaces 34, 1998), 21–22.

3. M. Lamarche, *Hydrologie et climatologie médicale* (Paris: Edition Marketing, 1977), 31.

4. Gerard Katz and Alain Maurin, *Santé et thermalisme* (St. Jean-de-Braye: Editions Dangles, 1988), 17–18.

CHAPTER 6

1. Roberta Larson Duyff, *The American Dietetic Association's Complete Food and Nutrition Guide* (Minneapolis: Chronimed Publishing, 1976), 97.

2. Sigmund Forster, "The Prescription of Spa Therapy" in Licht, ed., *Medical Hydrology* (New Haven, Conn.: Elizabeth Licht, 1963), 403.

3. J. J. Moorman, *Mineral Springs of North America* (Philadelphia: J. B. Lippincott & Co., 1873), 283.

4. M. Armijo and J. San Martín, *La salud por las aguas termales* (Madrid: Ediciones EDAF, 1984), 31–34.

5. Michel Boulangé, *Les vertus des cures thermales* (Montpellier: Editions Espaces 34, 1998), 22.

6. M. Lamarche, *Hydrologie et climatologie médicale* (Paris: Edition Marketing, 1977), 31.

7. Gerard Katz and Alain Maurin, *Santé et thermalisme* (St. Jean-de-Braye: Editions Dangles, 1988), 18.

CHAPTER 7

1. Michel Boulangé, *Les vertus des cures thermales* (Montpellier: Editions Espaces 34, 1998), 24.

2. Ibid., 24–25.

3. Yvonne Boucomont, "The Treatment of Arteriopathies with the Royat Cure" (in French), *Presse Thermal et Climatique* 108, No. 4 (1971): 257.

4. Grace Maguire Swanner, *Saratoga: Queen of Spas* (Utica, N.Y.: North Country Books, 1988), 249.

5. *Saratoga Mineral Springs and Baths* (Albany: State of New York Conservation Department, n.d.) 15.

6. G. Bernatzky et al., "Analgesic Effect After Therapy at Radon Spa," in *Proceedings: Internationales Symposium fur Spelaeotherapie,* October 1992.

7. A. Falkenbach et al., "Radon Exposure for Treatment of Rheumatoid Arthritis," *Scandinavian Journal of Rheumatology* Supplement 106 (1996): 27.

8. Sidney Licht, ed., *Medical Hydrology* (New Haven, Conn.: Elizabeth Licht, 1963), 460.

9. Sigmund Forster, "The Prescription of Spa Therapy" in Licht, ed., *Medical Hydrology* (New Haven, Conn.: Elizabeth Licht, 1963), 404.

CHAPTER 8

1. Françoise Davrainville, *Pelotherapy and a Study of Cutaneous Exchanges* (in French), Doctoral Thesis, Department of Pharmaceutical and Biological Sciences, University of Nancy, France, 1989, 52–54.

2. Bohuslav Kocab, *Spa Treatment in Czechoslovakia* (Prague: Balnea, 1972), 12–13.

3. *The Treatments* (Abano and Montegrotto: Abano Terme and Montegrotto Terme, n.d.), 4.

4. J. Gyarmati, "Peat Balneology in Hungary," in *Proceedings: 33rd World Congress of the International Society of Medical Hydrology and Climatology* (Prague: Lubomar Houdek and Nakadatelstvi Galen, 1998), 40.

5. Sigmund Forster, "The Prescription of Spa Therapy" in Licht, ed., *Medical Hydrology* (New Haven, Conn.: Elizabeth Licht, 1963), 404.

CHAPTER 9

1. M. Armijo and J. San Martín, *La salud por las aguas termales* (Madrid: Ediciones EDAF, 1984), 59–60.

2. Michel Boulangé, *Les vertus des cures thermales* (Montpellier: Editions Espaces 34, 1998), 23.

3. Roberta Larson Duyff, *The American Dietetic Association's Complete Food and Nutrition Guide* (Minneapolis: Chronimed Publishing, 1976), 168–72.

4. F. Batmanghelidj, *Your Body's Many Cries for Water* (Falls Church, Va.: Global Health Solutions, Inc., 1992), 27.

5. Robert Garrison Jr., and Elizabeth Somer, *The Nutrition Desk Reference,* 3rd ed. (New Canaan, Conn.: Keats Publishing, Inc., 1995), 197–205.

6. Duyff, *Complete Food and Nutrition Guide,* 93.

7. Ibid., 96–97.

8. Ibid., 97.

9. Ibid., 98.

10. *Mosby's Medical, Nursing and Allied Health Dictionary* (St. Louis: C. V. Mosby Company, 1998), 5084.

11. John Harte et al., *Toxics A to Z* (Berkeley: University of California Press, 1991), 217.

12. Klages, *Harbin Hot Springs,* 109–10.

13. Garrison and Somer, *Nutrition Desk Reference,* 226–27.

CHAPTER 11

1. Joel E. Bernstein, "Dermatological Aspects of Mineral Water," *Clinics in Dermatology* 14 (1996): 567–69.

2. Paula Karam, "Mineral Water and Spas in France," *Clinics in Dermatology* 14 (1996): 607.

3. Hilaria Ghersetich and Torello M. Lotti, "Immunological Aspects: Immunology of Mineral Water Spas," *Clinics in Dermatology* 14 (1996): 565.

4. Ibid., 563–64.

5. Kazuo Kabota et al., "Treatment of 100 Cases of Adult-type Atopic Dermatitis with Kusatsu Balneotherapy," *Journal of the Japanese Association of Physical Medicine, Balneology and Climatology* (in Japanese) 62, No. 2 (February 1999): 71–79.

6. Kazuo Kabota et al., "Treatment of Refractory Cases of Atopic dermatitis with Acidic Hot-Spring Bathing," *Acta Dermato-Venerealogica* 77 (1997): 452–54.

7. Kazuo Kubota et al., "Case Report: Dependence on Very Hot Hot-Spring Bathing in a Refractory Case of Atopic Dermatitis," *Journal of Medicine* 25, No. 5 (1994): 333–38.

8. N. K. Tsankov and J. A. Kamarashev, "Spa Therapy in Bulgaria," *Clinics in Dermatology* 14 (1996): 677.

9. Anastazy Omulecki et al., "Spa Therapy in Poland," *Clinics in Dermatology* 14 (1996): 682.

10. J. B. Ubugui, "Experience in Copahué (Argentina) Volcanic Muds and Mineral Waters," in *Proceedings: 2nd Symposium, Sulfur in Health Resort Medicine* (Geretsried, Germany: I.S.M.H. Verlag, 1994), 171.

11. N. K. Tsankov and J. A. Kamarashev, "Spa Therapy in Bulgaria," *Clinics in Dermatology* 14 (1996): 676.

12. David J. Abels et al., "Treatment of Psoriasis at a Dead Sea Dermatology Clinic," *International Journal of Dermatology* 33 (1995): 134–37.

13. O. Y. Oumeish, "Climatotherapy at the Dead Sea in Jordan," *Clinics in Dermatology* 14 (1996): 662–64.

14. Jon Hjaltalin Olaffson, "The Blue Lagoon in Iceland and Psoriasis," *Clinics in Dermatology* 14 (1996): 647–51.

15. V. Streit and W. Wiedow, "Effect of Brine Bathing in Psoriasis," in *Proceedings: 32nd World Congress of the International Society of Medical Hydrology and Climatology* (Geretsried, Germany: I.S.M.H. Verlag, 1994), 442–43.

16. N. Storojenko et al., "Treatment of Patients Affected by Burns with Hydro-sulphur Mineral Water Irrigation at Health Resorts of Sochi (Russia)," in *Proceedings: 2nd Symposium, Sulfur in Health Resort Medicine* (Geretsried, Germany: I.S.M.H. Verlag, 1994), 163–64.

17. Alberto López Rocha, "Hydrological Techniques in the Treatment of Hydrolipidistrophy" (in Spanish), *Boletín de la Sociedad Española de Hidrología Médica* 9, No. 2 (May 1994): 75–78.

CHAPTER 12

1. D. Hours and P. Brillat, "Indications of Crenotherapy in Arthrosis" (in French), *Presse thermale et climatique* 134, No. 1 (1997) 46–49.

2. Florence Constant et al., "Measurement Methods on Drug Consumption as a Secondary Judgement Criterion for Clinical Trials in Chronic Rheumatic Diseases," *American Journal of Epidemiology* 145, No. 9 (1997): 826–33.

3. Florence Constant et al., "Effectiveness of Spa Therapy in Chronic Low Back Pain: A Randomozed Clinical Trial," *The Journal of Rheumatology* 22, No. 7 (1995): 1315–20.

4. B. Graver-Duvernay et al., "Evaluation of the Efficacy of the Thermal Cure at Aix-les-Bains for the Treatment of Chronic Low Back Pain in Adults" (in French), *Presse thermale et climatique* 134, No. 3 (1997): 170–77.

5. Bernard Allery and Michel Picard, "Interest in Crenotherapy to Treat Lower Back Pain after Surgery for Herniated Disc" (in French), *Presse thermal et climatique* 125, No. 5 (1988): 275–77.

6. Grace Maguire Swanner, *Saratoga: Queen of Spas* (Utica, N.Y.: North Country Books, 1988), 237.

7. Laszlo Szucs et al., "Double-Blind Trial on the Effectiveness of the Puspokladay Thermal Water on Arthritis of the Knee Joints," *Journal of the Royal Society of Health* 1 (1989): 7–9.

8. D. Fabiani et al., "Rheumatolgical Aspects of Mineral Water," *Clinics in Dermatology* 14 (1996): 573.

9. M. Kanaan, "Comparative Study of the Effect of the Dead Sea Salt Aqueous Solution Heat Compresses at Different Concentrations on Patients with Knee-Joint Osteoarthritis," in *Proceedings: 2nd Symposium, Sulfur in Health Resort Medicine* (Geretsried, Germany: I.S.M.H. Verlag, 1994), 203–5.

10. R. Meijide Failde et al, "Evaluation of the Thermal Cure at Caldas de Lugo (Spain) on Rheumatoid Pathology" (in Spanish), in *Proceedings: 2nd Symposium, Sulfur in Health Resort Medicine* (Geretsried, Germany: I.S.M.H. Verlag, 1994), 221.

11. Masasashi Nobunaga et al., "Balneotherapy for Patients with Rheumatoid Arthritis, Especially the Effects of Cold Water Bathing," in Y. Agishi and Y. Ohtsuka, *New Frontiers in Health Resort Medicine* (Sapporo: Hokkaido University Medical School, 1996), 109–14.

12. R. Akbashev et al., "Natural Stream Thermal Bath in the Process of the Complex Treatment of Patients with Rheumatoid Arthritis," in *Proceedings: 2nd Symposium, Sulfur in Health Resort Medicine* (Geretsried, Germany: I.S.M.H. Verlag, 1994), 219–20.

13. M. Harari and J. Horowitz, "Climatotherapy of Psoriasis Arthritis at the Dead Sea" in *Proceedings: 2nd Symposium, Sulfur in Health Resort Medicine* (Geretsried, Germany: I.S.M.H. Verlag, 1994), 461.

14. Bokusha Kobal, *Spa Treatment in Czechoslovakia* (Prague: Balnea, 1972), 47–49.

15. Joanna Trevelyan, "Taking the Waters," *Nursing Times* 86, No. 40 (October 3, 1990): 38–39.

CHAPTER 13

1. Karl Luhr, "Spa Therapy of Gastrointestinal Disorders" in Licht, ed., *Medical Hydrology* (New Haven, Conn.: Elizabeth Licht, 1963), 374–79.

2. Yuko Agishi, "Hot Springs and Their Physiological Functions of Humans," *Asian Medical Journal* 38, No. 3 (March, 1995): 121–22.

3. Christophe Gutenbrunner, "Present Features of Drinking Cure," in Y. Agishi and Y. Ohtsuka, *Recent Progress in Medical Balneology and Climatology* (Sapporo: Hokkaido University School of Medicine, 1995), 135–48.

4. Constantin Stoicescu and Laviniu Munteahu, *Natural Curative Factors of the Main Balneoclimatic Resorts in Romania* (Bucharest: Editura Sport-Turism, 1977), 121.

5. Bohuslav Kocab, *Spa Treatment in Czechoslovakia* (Prague: Balnea, 1972), 41.

6. Mario Gonçalves, "Mineral Spring Therapy for the Treatment of Diseases of the Digestive System" (in Spanish), in *Thermalism in Galicia in the Decade of the Eighties* (Santiago de Compostela: Consellería de Sanidade, 1988), 225–33.

7. Seraphin Pérez Pombo, "Thermalism in Gastrointestinal Processes" (in Spanish), in *Thermalism in Galicia in the Decade of the Eighties* (in Spanish) (Santiago de Compostela: Consellería de Sanidade, 1988), 237–39.

8. Sannosuke Tarusawa et al., *Text Book of Cures at Tamagawa Hot Springs in Towada-Hachimantai National Park* (Kazuno City: Tamagawa Hot Springs Research Center, 1998), 48–54, 64.

9. Ibid.

10. G. N. Ponomarenko et al., "Mineral Water Ekateringofskaya in the Gastritic and Ulcer Disease Treatment," in *Proceedings: 33rd World Congress of the International Society of Medical Hydrology and Climatology* (Prague: Lubomar Houdek and Nakadatelstvi Galen, 1998), 109.

11. J. B. Chareyras et al., "Survey on the Quality of Life of Patients Suffering from Colon Problems" (in French), *Press thermale et climatique* 135, No. 3 (1998): 151–54.

12. *Spas in Japan* (Tokyo: Japan Spa Association, 1983), 11–12.

CHAPTER 14

1. Constantin Stoicescu and Laviniu Munteanu, in Pratzel, *Health Resort Medicine* (Geretsried: I.S.M.H. Verlag, 1994), 124–25.

2. Z. Z. Faizullin, "Rehabilitation of Patients with Chronic Persistent Hepatitis by Means of Sulphide-Chloride-Sodium Baths at the Sanitorium Stage," in *Sulfur in Health Resort Medicine* (Geretsried: I.S.M.H. Verlag, 1995), 129–30.

3. Christoph Gutenbrunner, "Present Features of the Drinking Cure," in Y. Agishi and Y. Ohtsuka, *Recent Progress in Medical Balneology and Climatology* (Sapporo: Hokkaido University School of Medicine, 1995), 144.

4. V. Edreva, "Advances in Contemporary Aspects of the Drinking Cure in Bulgaria" (in French), in *Proceedings: 2nd Symposium, Sulfur in Health Resort Medicine* (Geretsried, Germany: I.S.M.H. Verlag, 1994), 269–70.

5. Joseph Mates, "Spa Therapy of Urologic Disorders" in Licht, ed., *Medical Hydrology* (New Haven, Conn.: Elizabeth Licht, 1963), 383–89.

6. Nicole Poset et. al., "Is Kidney Function Affected by the Composition of Ingested Water?" (in French), *Presse thermal et climatique,* 131, No. 1 (1994): 5–9.

7. Mates, "Spa Therapy," 383–89.

8. Ibid.

9. Bohuslav Kocab, *Spa Treatment in Czechoslovakia* (Prague: Balnea, 1972), 51.

CHAPTER 15

1. J. P. O'Hare et al., "Observations on the Effects of immersion in Bath Spa Water," *British Medical Journal* 291 (December 21–28, 1985): 1747.

2. B. Bhambhra et al., "Thermal Environment and Evolution of Factors of Cardiovascular Risk Concerning 223 Patients After a Three-Week Stay at the Paul Ribeyre Specialized Hospital at Vals-les-Bains" (in French), *Presse thermale et climatique* 132, No. 3 (1995): 176–77.

3. Yoshimasa Yabe, "Studies on the Effects of Hot-Spring Bathing on the Functions of the Circulatory System," [*Journal of the Japanese Association of Physical Medicine, Balneology and Climatology* 33], No. 47 (1970).

4. C. Ambrosi et al., "Functional Readaptation of Patients with Intermittent Claudication Treated at Royat" (in French), in Herisson, [*Crenotheraopy and Readaptation*] (Paris: Masson, S.A., 1989), 176–82.

5. S. Zhukovsky, "Sulphur Spa Treatment for the Rehabilitation of Patients after Acute Infarction of the Myocardium," in *Proceedings: 2nd Symposium, Sulfur in Health Resort Medicine* (Geretsried, Germany: I.S.M.H. Verlag, 1994), 70.

6. E. L. Sedenco et al., "The Treatment with Sulphurous Waters in the Hemo-dynamical Improvement of the Diabetical Arteriopathies," in *Proceedings: 2nd Symposium, Sulfur in Health Resort Medicine* (Geretsried, Germany: I.S.M.H. Verlag, 1994), 69.

7. Bernard Graber-Duverndy, ed., *Le Thermalisme, Face aux Défis de l'Evaluation* (Paris: Fédération Thermale et Climatique Française, 1996), 9.

8. K. Tanmura et al., "Effects of Hyperthermal Stress on the Fibrinolytic System," *International Journal of Hyperthermia* 12, No. 1 (1996): 31–36.

9. Kazuo Kabota et al., "Effects of Hot Spring Bathing on Blood Pressure, Heart Rate, Plasma Cortisol and Hematocrit at Kusatsu," *Journal of the Japanese Association of Physical Medicine, Balneology and Climatology* (in Japanese) 60, No. 2 (1998): 61–68.

10. Kazuo Kubota et al., "Acute Myocardial Infarction and Cerebral Infarction at Kusatsu-Spa," *Japanese Journal of Geriatrics* 34 (1997): 23–29.

11. Kazuo Kubota et al., "A Transient Rise in Plasma Beta Endorphin After a Traditional 47°C. Hot-Spring Bath in Kusatsu-Spa, Japan," *Life Sciences* 51 (1992): 1877–80.

12. Yvonne Boucomont, "The Treatment of Arterial Problems with the Royat Cure" (in French), *Presse thermal et climatique* 108, No. 4 (1971): 257–58.

13. Brigitte Martin, ed., *Guide du Thermalisme* (Paris: Edinter, 1998), 156.

14. Victor R. Ott, "Spa Therapy in Cardiovascular Disorders," in Licht, ed., *Medical Hydrology* (New Haven, Conn.: Elizabeth Licht, 1963), 363–66.

15. Kurt Franke, "Kneipp Treatment," in Licht, ed., *Medical Hydrology* (New Haven, Conn.: Elizabeth Licht, 1963), 321–31.

16. Ibid., 330.

17. Bernd Hartmann, "The Role of Thermalism in Cardiovascular Diseases" (in French), *Cinesiologie* 34, No. 159 (January–February 1995), 18.

18. E. Rubenowitz et al., "Magnesium in Drinking Water and Death from Acute Myocardial Infarction," in *American Journal of Epidemiology* 143 (1996): 456–62.

19. Bohuslav Kocab, *Spa Treatment in Czechoslovakia* (Prague: Balnea, 1972), 37–39.

20. Martin, *Guide du Thermalisme,* 168.

21. Ott, "Spa Therapy," 357–67.

CHAPTER 16

1. R. Capudoro and C. Althofer-Starke, "Present-Day Status of the French Thermal Cure for Gynecology" (in French), in *Proceedings: 2nd Symposium, Sulfur in Health Resort Medicine* (Geretsried, Germany: I.S.M.H. Verlag, 1994), 307–9.

2. M. Armijo and J. San Martín, *La salud por las aguas termales* (Madrid: Ediciones EDAF, 1984), 107–8.

3. Ibid.

CHAPTER 17

1. Tsukasa Asoh, "Cold Spring Therapy in Kan-no-Jigoku" in Y. Agishi and Y. Ohtsuka, eds., *New Frontiers in Health Resort Medicine* (Sapporo: Hokkaido University Medical School, 1996), 117–25.

2. Hajime Ide et al., "Balneotherapy in Diabetes," in Y. Oshima, *Thermalism in Japan* (Tokyo: The Forum on Thermalism in Japan, 1988), 26.

3. E. L. Sidenco et al., "The Biochemical Evolution of the Patients with Diabetes Mellitus Treated by Sulphurous Waters" in *Proceedings: 2nd Symposium, Sulfur in Health Resort Medicine* (Geretsried, Germany: I.S.M.H. Verlag, 1994), 67.

4. I. Baican et al., "Health Resort Treatment with Sulphurous Bath in Complicated Diabetes Mellitus" in *Proceedings: 2nd Symposium, Sulfur in Health Resort Medicine* (Geretsried, Germany: I.S.M.H. Verlag, 1994), 65–66.

5. Yuko Agishi et al., "Chronobiological Studies on Balneotherapy in Patients with Non-Insulin-Dependent Diabetes Mellitus" in Y. Agishi and Y. Ohtsuka, *New Frontiers in Health Resort Medicine* (Sapporo: Hokkaido University Medical School, 1996), 13–25.

6. Y. Miyazaki and Y. Motohashi, "Forest Environment and Physiological Response," in Y. Agishi and Y. Ohtsuka, *New Frontiers in Health Resort Medicine* (Sapporo: Hokkaido University Medical School, 1996), 67–77.

7. Yoshinori Ohtsuka et al., "Significance of Shinrinyoku (Forest-Air Bathing and Walking) as an Exercise Therapy for Elderly Patients with Diabetes Mellitus," *Journal of the Japanese Association of Physical Medicine, Balneology and Climatology* (in Japanese) 61, No. 2 (1998): 101–5.

8. P. Jeanjean and J. M. Benoit, "Results of la Preste Spa Therapy in Prostatitis" (in French), *Presse thermal et climatique* 135, No. 1 (1998): 14–18.

9. D. Fabiani et al., "Rheumatologic Aspects of Mineral Water," *Clinics in Dermatology* 14 (1996): 573.

10. George D. Kersley, "Spa Therapy for Rheumatologic Diseases" in Licht, ed., *Medical Hydrology* (New Haven, Conn.: Elizabeth Licht, 1963), 371.

11. I. M. Kasianova, "Hydrotherapy in the Treatment of Obesity," in *Proceedings: 2nd Symposium, Sulfur in Health Resort Medicine* (Geretsried, Germany: I.S.M.H. Verlag, 1994), 131–33.

CHAPTER 18

1. Armijo Valenzuela, "Crenotherapy for Respiratory Afflictions" (in Spanish), in *Thermalism in Galicia in the Decade of the Eighties* (Santiago de Compostela: Consellería de Sanidade, 1988), 257–63.

2. Ibid.

3. Nathaniel Altman, *What You Can Do About Asthma* (New York: Dell Medical Library, 1991), 67–116.

4. Y. Petrovska, "The Results from Climatic and Balneological Therapy of Bronchial Asthma Patients Depending on Season and Form of Disease," in *Proceedings: 2nd Symposium, Sulfur in Health Resort Medicine* (Geretsried, Germany: I.S.M.H. Verlag, 1994), 361–63.

5. Yoshiro Tanizaki et al., "Intractable Asthma and Swimming Training in a Hot Spring Pool," *Journal of the Japanese Association of Physical Medicine, Balneology and Climatology* (in Japanese) 47, No. 3–4 (1984): 115–22.

6. Yoshiro Tanizaki et al., "Changes of Ventilatory Function in Patients with Bronchial Asthma During Swimming Training in a Hot Spring Pool," *Journal of the Japanese Association of Physical Medicine, Balneology and Climatology* (in Japanese) 47, No. 2 (1984): 99–103.

7. Yoshiro Tanizaki, "Improvement of Ventilatory Function by Spa Therapy in Patients with Intractable Asthma," *Acta Medica Okayama* 40, No. 1 (1986): 55–59.

8. R. Jean et al., "Essai d'evaluation de la qualité de vie des dilates bronchiques en cure thermal à allevard les bains," in *Proceedings: 2nd Symposium, Sulfur in Health Resort Medicine* (Geretsried, Germany: I.S.M.H. Verlag, 1994), 373–77.

9. Constantin Stoicescu and Laviniu Munteahu, *Natural Curative Factors of the Main Balneoclimatic Resorts in Romania* (Bucharest: Editura Sport-Turism, 1977), 74–75.

10. Ibid.

11. R. Jean et al., "Spa treatment in pediatric pneumoallergologic and ENT diseases" (in French), *Annales de Pédiatrie* 39, No. 5 (1992): 293–99.

12. P. Shiller and G. Bardelay, *The Thermal Cure: How to Evaluate and Prescribe* (in French) (Paris: Editions Frison-Roche, 1990), 173–77.

13. Centre d'étude sur la therapeutique, le thermalisme et l'enfant, *Mieux connaître les cures thermales chez l'enfant* (Paris: Expansion Scientifique Française, 1991), 70.

CHAPTER 19

1. Helmut G. Pratzel, "Advantages and Disadvantages of Crenotherapy Treatment for Patients Suffering from Neoplasm" (in Spanish), *Bulletin of the Spanish Society of Medical Hydrology* 12, No. 1 (1997): 49–50.

2. E. Tomb et al., "How We Treat Migraines at Vittel" (in French), in *Proceedings: 2nd Symposium, Sulfur in Health Resort Medicine* (Geretsried, Germany: I.S.M.H. Verlag, 1994), 289–92.

3. C. Loisy et al., "Rehabilitation of Patients Suffering from Migraine in Spas" (in French), in Herisson, *Crenotherapy and Readaptation* (in French) (Paris: Masson, S.A., 1989), 198–203.

4. C. Loissy and S. Beorchia, "Migraines Among Children and Their Treatment with the Thermal Cure" (in French), *Presse thermal et climatique* 125 (1988), 17–19.

5. J. Constant et al., "Study on the Efficacy of the Thermal Cure at Divonne-les-Bains on Depression" (in French), *Presse thermal et climatique* 134, No. 3 (1997): 181–85.

6. Josefina San Martín Baciacoa, "Considerations regarding Psychalgias and Bathing Cures" (in Spanish), *Bulletin of the Spanish Society of Medical Hydrology* (in Spanish) 9, No. 1 (1966), 9.

7. Bohuslav Kocab, *Spa Treatment in Czechoslovakia* (Prague: Balnea, 1972), 47.

8. José Antonio Frias Fernández et al., "Parkinson's Disease: Present Status and Treatment at the Fitero Spa (Navarra)" (in Spanish), *Bulletin of the Spanish Society of Medical Hydrology* (in Spanish) 9, No. 3 (1996): 127–34.

9. Philippe Schilliger and Gilles Bardelay, *Know How to Evaluate and Prescribe a Thermal Cure* (in French) (Paris: Editions Frison-Roche, 1990), 215–17.

10. G. Nappi et al., "Thermal Treatment of Chronic Otitis by Insufflation" (in Spanish), *Bulletin of the Spanish Society of Medical Hydrology* (in Spanish) 10, No. 2 (1995): 75–78.

11. Sidney Licht, ed., *Medical Hydrology* (New Haven, Conn.: Elizabeth Licht, 1963), 111.

12. V. Edreva, "Advances in Contemporary Aspects of the Drinking Cure in Bulgaria" (in French), in *Proceedings: 2nd Symposium, Sulfur in Health Resort Medicine* (Geretsreid, Germany: ISMH Verlag, 1994), 269–70.

CHAPTER 20

1. Yuko Agishi, "Hot Springs and the Physiological Functions of Humans," *Asian Medical Journal* 38, No. 3 (March 1995): 115–24.

2. Nathaniel Altman, *Oxygen Healing Therapies* (Rochester, Vt.: Healing Arts Press, 1995), 11.

3. Jinichi Suzuki and Yuichi Yamauchi, "Endocrinological Changes in Psychosomatic Patients after Balneotherapy in a Hot Sulfate Spring," *Journal of the Japanese Association of Physical Medicine, Balneology and Climatology* (in Japanese) 42, Nos. 1, 2 (1978): 33.

4. Yuko Agishi, "Effects of Thermal Stimuli by Total Body Water Immersion and Balneotherapy on Endocrine and Autonomic Nervous Functions," *Journal of the Japanese Association of Physical Medicine, Balneology and Climatology* (in Japanese) 42, Nos. 1, 2 (1978): 30.

5. Ibid.

6. Yuko Agishi and Yoshinori Ohtsuka, *Recent Progress in Medical Balneology and Climatology* (Sapporo: Hokkaido University School of Medicine, 1995), 8.

7. "Negative ions and positive vibes," *Technology Review* 86, No. 1 (January 1983): 74.

8. Sidney Licht, ed., *Medical Hydrology* (New Haven, Conn.: Elizabeth Licht, 1963), 111.

INDEX

Abano Terme, Italy, 74–75, 78, 116, 124, 148, 160, 227–28
accident, sequelae of, 73
Acqua Panna water, 88
acupressure, 26, 259
acupuncture, 26
aerobic exercise, 21
aerosol, 25, 157–58
Agishi, Yuko, 19, 170
Agua Hedionda, Mexico, 40, 72, 125, 160, 162, 204
Aix-en-Province, France, 147
Aix-les-Bains, France, 32, 38, 58, 62, 72, 119, 165, 215
Alaska, springs in, 186
Alberta, springs in, 184
Alhambra water, 88
Allevard Spa, France, 158
angina, 141
Anne of Austria, 43
Apollinaris water, 55
Aquincum, 39
Argentina, springs in, 198–99
Arima Onsen, Japan, 72, 81, 145, 170, 251
Arizona, springs in, 186–87
Arkansas, springs in, 176–77
aromatherapy, 26, 259
Arrowhead Spring water, 3, 79, 88
arsenic, 85–86
  spas containing, 86
Artemis Thermia, 38
arthritis, 71, 73, 120–23
  osteoarthritis, 120–21
  psoriatic, 122–23
  rheumatoid, 121–22
Asclepiades, 38
Aslan therapy, 259
asthma, 156–57
Atami Onsen, Japan, 40, 62, 125, 131, 251
Aulus-les-Bains, France, 139
Australia, springs in, 246
Austria, springs in, 207–9

back pain, 119–20
bacteria in hot springs, 20
Bad Ems, Germany, 55, 58, 65, 160, 219

Baden-Baden, Germany, 7, 32, 44, 64, 65, 72, 78, 124, 148, 219
Bad Gastein, Austria, 7, 62, 70–71, 124, 208
Badgastein-Bockstein-Thermalstollen, Austria, 58, 70–71
Bad Griesbach, Germany, 7, 219
Bad Ischl, Austria, 64, 65, 78, 130, 145, 148, 209
Bad Kissingen, Germany, 58, 65, 130, 133, 148, 154, 161, 220
Bad Nauheim, Germany, 69, 72, 148, 160, 220
Bad Wildbad, Germany, 17, 58, 65, 80, 124, 221
Badoit water, 55, 87, 89
Bagnères-de-Bigorre, France, 62, 72, 78, 81, 124, 215
Bagnoles de l'Orne, France, 144, 147
Băile Olăneşti. *See* Olăneşti
Balaruc-les-Bains, France, 65, 69, 78, 124, 147, 216
balneology, 2, 8–9, 259
balneotherapy, 3, 18–26, 171, 259
  contraindications to, 20
  drinking, 22–24
  indications for, 19
Balneotherapy Institute, Japan, 43
Banff, Alberta, 3, 47, 58, 62, 124, 184
Baruch, Simon, 49, 68
Baruch Institute, New York, 49–50
Bath, England, 42, 50, 62, 69, 124, 137, 223
bathing, 21, 57
  adjuncts to, 21
  Christian aversion to, 41
  decline of, 49–50
  in Japan, 39–40
  Native Americans and, 40–41
  safety advice when, 20
Batmanghelidj, F., 79–80
Baudisch, Oskar, 9
Beethoven, Ludwig von, 44
Belgium, springs in, 210
Bell, John, 47
Beppu, Japan, 35–37, 43, 77–78, 81, 116, 122, 125, 131, 136, 149, 251
Berkeley Springs, WV, 45, 62, 125, 148, 182